INTRODUCTION TO
HEALTH PROMOTION

INTRODUCTION TO HEALTH PROMOTION

Anastasia Snelling, Editor

JB JOSSEY-BASS™

A Wiley Brand

Published by Jossey-Bass
A Wiley Brand
One Montgomery Street, Suite 1200, San Francisco, CA 94104-4594—www.josseybass.com

Limit of Liability/Disclaimer of Warranty: While the publisher and author have used their best efforts in preparing this book, they make no representations or warranties with respect to the accuracy or completeness of the contents of this book and specifically disclaim any implied warranties of merchantability or fitness for a particular purpose. No warranty may be created or extended by sales representatives or written sales materials. The advice and strategies contained herein may not be suitable for your situation. You should consult with a professional where appropriate. Neither the publisher nor author shall be liable for any loss of profit or any other commercial damages, including but not limited to special, incidental, consequential, or other damages. Readers should be aware that Internet Web sites offered as citations and/or sources for further information may have changed or disappeared between the time this was written and when it is read.

Jossey-Bass books and products are available through most bookstores. To contact Jossey-Bass directly call our Customer Care Department within the U.S. at 800-956-7739, outside the U.S. at 317-572-3986, or fax 317-572-4002.

Wiley publishes in a variety of print and electronic formats and by print-on-demand. Some material included with standard print versions of this book may not be included in e-books or in print-on-demand. If this book refers to media such as a CD or DVD that is not included in the version you purchased, you may download this material at http://booksupport.wiley.com. For more information about Wiley products, visit www.wiley.com.

Library of Congress Cataloging-in-Publication Data
Introduction to health promotion/Anastasia Snelling, editor.
    p.; cm.
Includes bibliographical references and index.
    ISBN 978-1-118-45529-6 (paperback) – ISBN 978-1-118-45528-9 (pdf) – ISBN 978-1-118-45530-2 (epub)
    I. Snelling, Anastasia, 1957- editor.
    [DNLM: 1. Health Promotion–methods–United States. 2. Health Behavior–United States. 3. Health Planning–methods–United States. 4. Health Promotion–trends–United States. 5. Preventive Health Services– methods–United States. WA 590]
    RA427.8
    362.1–dc23
                                                        2014010406

CONTENTS

Chapter 11 Health Promotion–Related Organizations, Associations, and Certifications **299**

Anastasia Snelling and Michelle Kalicki

Chapter 12 Trends in Health Promotion **321**

David Hunnicutt

TABLES AND FIGURES

Tables

Figures

This introductory text will be a perfect fit for many of the rapidly emerging professional degree programs in health promotion and allied professions that regard health promotion as a core responsibility. The convergence of focus on health promotion in recent years has been spurred by the inescapable reality that behavior is the primary pathway through which society can have a positive influence on the prevailing health problems of today's world. Professor Snelling and her collaborating authors have represented that reality in the first part of the book with a chapter on each of the leading behavioral determinants of chronic health conditions. Then they have shown how state-of-the-art theories, models, and experience-based strategies for health promotion can be applied in systematic ways to address those problems.

One feature that makes this book stand out among many others is the selection of a balanced roster of authors from academia and practice. The role of practicing health professionals who lead important organizations and programs in health promotion should help bring the theories and research evidence of academics to life for students. Indeed, it has been my lament that too many evidence-based guidelines for practice in health promotion have been produced by academic research without sufficient attention to the context in which the evidence would be applied. My argument to those who sponsor health promotion research and those who fund health promotion programs is that if we want more evidence-based practice, we need more practice-based evidence. This book will help point the way and inspire some students to plan, implement, and evaluate theory-based and evidence-based health promotion interventions and programs that will, in turn, produce the complementary practice-based evidence we desperately need in this field.

Lawrence W. Green, DrPh, Scd (Hon.)
Professor, Department of Epidemiology and Biostatistics
School of Medicine
University of California at San Francisco

The health promotion field emerged during the second half of the twentieth century as medicine and science became successful treating infectious diseases with antibiotics, advancing maternal and child health, and improving sanitation practices. These gains significantly improved the quality and quantity of life for all. Yet, now we face the next medical crisis: chronic disease. Medicine and science research have continued to manage disease conditions through a number of procedures, surgeries, and pharmaceuticals. All of these approaches come with a very high cost to the individual through reduced quality of life and economic cost to organizations and the federal government responsible for providing health insurance. At this time, health care costs account for 17.6% of the gross domestic product. This means that the United States spends almost seventeen cents of every dollar on providing health care to Americans. Controlling these health care costs is a continuing priority for the nation. Consider that over 70% of all health care costs are related to chronic disease and that many risk factors for chronic disease are considered modifiable, such as tobacco use, physical inactivity, food choices, and managing stress. These modifiable risk factors are the core behaviors that the field of health promotion focuses on to improve the quality of people's lives and to manage rising health care costs.

Changing individual and societal health behavior is a very complex process. Since the 1980s, more research has shown that for individuals to successfully adopt healthy behaviors, social, behavioral, and environmental factors also must be part of the process of change. The healthy choice must be the easy choice in our homes, schools, work sites, and communities. The vision is to live in a country where a culture of health is seen, practiced, and supported throughout the life span.

The unique contribution of this book is to introduce students to the individual and societal forces that have transformed the factors that influence one's health, including social and physical environments, medical advances, personal lifestyle choices, and legislation. The book identifies and discusses the innovative health campaigns, strategies, and policies that are being implemented and enacted to improve health behaviors and practices that ultimately improve the quality of life.

It is my sincere desire that the writings in this book inspire you to either embark on a career in health promotion or, at the very least, provide you with an understanding of the ways in which many disciplines intersect with health promotion, so that whatever discipline you study, you will better understand how your work interacts with the promotion of health. Almost every discipline intersects with the field of health promotion. Further, health promotion professionals do not work in isolation. The nature of health promotion is to work across multiple disciplines to design and develop strategies that use the best knowledge we know and apply it to health behaviors. Table P.1 lists diverse areas of study and identifies the related work of health promotion, whether you study exercise or nutrition science to understand how to advise consumers on health behaviors to improve their health status or if you study communication or marketing to design health campaigns that inform the general public about health risks associated with smoking or drinking and driving or public policy to understand or evaluate how public health policy decreases health disparities by providing consumers with healthful foods or access to affordable health care.

This introductory textbook for health promotion students is designed and written to be distinctly different from other textbooks. It provides readers with an in-depth examination of the forces that have changed our

Table P.1 Disciplines and the Relationship with Health Fields

Discipline	Contribution	Example
Communication and marketing	Social marketing campaigns	Campaigns to reduce smoking or promote physical activity
Public policy	Local, state, and national policy promoting health	Affordable Care Act
Human resources	Health benefits offered through employers	Work site health
Biology	Understanding the changes in the body from food and exercise	Healthy behavior identification
Psychology	Understanding why people make the choices they do and how to facilitate behavior change	Health promotion models
Sociology	Understanding how human society functions and influences behavior	Health promotion models
Medicine and allied health	Monitoring health, identifying risk factors, and restoring health	Annual physicals; clinical preventive services
Economics	Behavioral economics	Encouraging healthy food choices

lifestyles and environments over the past century, which in turn have resulted in changes in individual health behaviors that affect the onset of chronic conditions. During this same time frame, there were also considerable medical advances, improving early detection of disease and developing progressive treatments for chronic conditions. These changes are ones that health promoters must understand and address. Ultimately, the framework for the development of social and physical environments that support healthy lifestyle choices will guide the transformation of communities where people are empowered to make healthy choices, so they can live longer lives free of preventable disease, disability, and premature death.

The book is divided into three parts. Part 1, "The Foundation of Health Promotion," introduces the framework of health promotion and provides the student to a number of key terms, models, and trends related to the field. Chapter 2 introduces health behavior change theories that offer constructs on how individuals approach personal behavior change, that is, the essence of health promotion—engaging individuals to actively promote their own health through daily actions such as being physically active or selecting healthy foods to eat. Program planning models (chapter 3) are essential tools to successfully reaching large groups of people through social marketing campaigns to interventions to enacting policies to create environments in which people can practice healthy behaviors.

Part 2, "Health Behaviors," describes those actions that promote health and prevent disease. These chapters introduce the short history of how tobacco use, eating, physical activity, and emotional health have evolved as a result of the changes in our social and physical environments. These chapters provide a comprehensive discussion of the health behaviors that influence the onset of chronic disease in our country and how and why these behaviors have changed over time. Chapter 8 highlights the important role clinical preventive services also have on promoting health by monitoring chronic disease development and overall health status. Health promotion professionals are promoting healthful living, hence, the inclusion of preventive services (immunizations and age-appropriate screenings) available through the medical community need to be understood and promoted.

These health behavior chapters examine how changes in our environment and society over the past several decades have affected behaviors and how those changed behaviors affect health and disease. By understanding the historical perspective of each of these behaviors, health promotion professionals will possess a richer context for their work, understanding that multiple forces have shaped, and continue to affect, the health of individuals and our society. Health behavior change is complex; in order to advance innovative solutions, it is critical that health promoters fully understand the history of these behaviors. Within each chapter, examples of policies and programs that exemplify health promotion in action are provided.

Part 3, "Health Promotion in Action," presents how state and federal governments engage in promoting healthful living for their consumers, what associations and certifications support the health promotion profession, where health promotion is taking place and the job opportunities available for this profession, and closing out with future trends in health promotion as we move through the twenty-first century. There are a plethora of national activities that promote health and prevent disease. The federal agencies monitor health status, provide broad guidelines, conduct research, and fund programs to promote health. Collectively, there are thousands of federal employees who work across disciplines to study or implement new approaches to improve the health of our society.

Chapter 10 discusses the setting where health promotion takes place, which further exemplifies that health promotion is beginning to be seen everywhere such as in day care centers, schools, colleges, work sites, food stores, retirement homes, and communities. Again, thousands of professionals believe in the vision of a country in which people are practicing healthy behaviors every day because the healthy choice is the easy choice. Staying current within the discipline will be important after you graduate. Chapter 11 discusses associations, journals, and certifications that provide important information for your life beyond the borders of an academic institution. In time, reading a textbook or listening to a professor's lecture will be in the past. But as a professional, you will need to stay current and this chapter is full of associations and journals that will facilitate your continued professional development. The final chapter is a look into the future predicting some trends that will help to create a culture of health to ensure that the Healthy People 2020 goals to "attain high-quality, longer lives free of preventable disease, to improve the health of all groups, to create social and physical environments that promote good health for all, and to promote healthy behaviors across all life stages" will be achieved.

At the end of each chapter, the student will find a brief summary and list of key terms of the information presented in the chapter. After the summary and key terms are a list of student questions and activities. Both the questions and activities are written to extend the learning and understanding of the material presented in the chapter. By completing the questions and activities, students will gain a deeper understanding of the breadth and depth of the health promotion field. All references used in each chapter are at the end and students are encouraged to seek out these articles, book chapters, and books for additional information.

My goal for this textbook is to enhance the academic preparation of students who are pursuing degrees in health promotion, public health, health education, and other degrees that address or affect the health status of individuals, communities, and societies nationally as well as around the world. Although this textbook focuses on behaviors, trends, and resources in the United States to promote health, many of them are applicable to cultures and settings around the world. There is a universal desire to live a healthful life, and this desire can be found in people of every age, gender, race, and ethnicity.

The book provides a foundation of knowledge for the health promotion professional. Many students are excited to learn such a field exists and ask where they can begin. My response is always with themselves! Being a role model and learning to practice what health promotion professionals teach is a great starting point. I do not expect that you will set a perfect example of health every day, but by practicing health-promoting behaviors you will personally experience the process and the benefits and become healthy as a result.

An instructor's supplement is available at www.josseybass.com/go /snelling. Additional materials such as videos, podcasts, and readings can be found at www.josseybasspublichealth.com. Comments about this book are invited and can be sent to publichealth@wiley.com.

Acknowledgments

I would like to first thank all of the contributing authors of this book whose expertise in their respective areas has enhanced the content in this book. Many of the contributing authors have spent time at American University, and the health promotion programs have been enriched as a result of their work. Also, I would like to thank all the faculty, staff, and students in the School of Education, Teaching, and Health at American University for their encouragement and support along this journey. A special recognition to my team of graduate assistants, especially Michelle Kalicki and Stephanie Sunderlin, who are always willing to work with me on this and the many projects I accept. Last, I want to thank Laura Aden Caldwell, whose editorial and organizational work has enhanced this book.

I would also like to thank Jossey-Bass for producing this book with me. The entire team has been valuable in making this a reality, and I would like to acknowledge especially Andy Pasternack, Seth Schwartz, Susan Geraghty, and Justin Frahm.

Reviewers Lori Francis, Christina R. Johnson, and Steve McClaran provided thoughtful and constructive comments on the complete draft manuscript.

Finally, this book is dedicated to my family who inspire me to make a difference in people's lives through my work. My husband, Roger; my children, Trevor, Anastasia, and Amelia; my parents, John and Amelia Mustone; my siblings, John, Lisa, Paul, Mary Ellen, and Jessica; and my extended Mustone and Snelling family members. May we all live a life full of love, happiness, and good health.

"To laugh often and much; to win the respect of intelligent people and the affection of children; to earn the appreciation of honest critics and endure the betrayal of false friends; to appreciate beauty; to find the best in others; to leave the world a bit better, whether by a healthy child, a garden patch or a redeemed social condition; to know even one life has breathed easier because you have lived. This is to have succeeded."

Ralph Waldo Emerson

Dr. Anastasia Snelling is a professor and the Associate Dean in the School of Education, Teaching, and Health at American University. She has been a member of the Academy of Nutrition and Dietetics as a registered dietitian for over thirty years and a fellow in the American College of Nutrition. Dr. Snelling teaches courses including nutrition, health promotion, and health communication at both the undergraduate and graduate level.

Her research focuses on methods of behavior change in nutrition education to manage risk factors related to chronic disease. Specifically, her research focuses on using the school environment to improve the health status of children. Grounded in the Social Ecological Model, her work in school health examines different levels of influence that can improve the health and food environment, leading to improved health and weight status. By addressing the needs of the child within the social, economic, and cultural contexts where they live, the research aligns health *and* education to enable students to reach their full potential. Reliable evidence indicates that healthy students are better learners, and, consequently, good health is fundamental to ensuring an effective education.

Dr. Snelling regularly presents her research at national and international conferences. Her research is published in many highly-regarded journals focusing on nutrition, health promotion, and school health. She has appeared on *C-Span* to discuss food labeling regulation and her opinions and expertise have appeared in such media outlets as *Education Week*, the *Washington Post, US World and News Report*, and *Fox Business News.*

Jennifer Childress is the owner of Patina Esprit Wellness, LLC, where she provides health coaching, personal training, and consulting services to her clients. In addition to her training and coaching practice, Jen also serves as an independent consultant to the Alliance to Make US Healthiest, where she works on implementing and advancing the HealthLead Workplace Accreditation Program. Jen has a master's degree in health promotion management (American University, Washington, DC) and holds certificates in personal fitness training (Aerobics and Fitness Association of America [AFAA]), coaching (Coach Training Alliance), and health education (National Commission for Health Education Credentialing [NCHEC]).

She has been an author on articles published in the *American Journal of Public Health,* the *North Carolina Medical Journal,* and the Wellness Councils of America (WELCOA) Absolute Advantage. Jen has taught as an adjunct professor in the Department of Health and Physical Education at Grand View University in Des Moines, Iowa. She is involved within the business community and has served on the National Board of the American Business Women's Association (ABWA).

Laurie DiRosa is a faculty member of the Department of Health and Exercise Science at Rowan University, teaching undergraduate and graduate health promotion courses. She also serves as the research and nutrition consultant for a grant-funded program titled GetFIT, which is a fitness and nutrition program that serves individuals with disabilities and their caregivers. For this program, Dr. DiRosa trains community members and undergraduate students in the counseling techniques of motivational interviewing using the training program she developed specifically for this population. Dr. DiRosa holds an EdD from Wilmington University, an MS in health promotion management from American University, and a BS in exercise and sport science from Ursinus College.

Jill Dombrowski is a clinical assistant professor at The Catholic University of America in the School of Nursing. Dr. Dombrowski holds a BSN from Georgetown University and an MSN and PhD from The Catholic University of America, as well as an MS from American University in health and fitness management. She teaches undergraduate- and graduate-level health promotion courses and coordinates interprofessional wellness committees in the university and DC communities. Dr. Dombrowski's research interests include work site health promotion interventions, physical activity in working mothers, self-efficacy, and time management.

David Hunnicutt has been the president of the Wellness Council of America (WELCOA), one of the largest and most respected work site wellness organizations in the United States since 1995. With more than five thousand corporate members, WELCOA is the industry leader when it comes to keeping the nation's employers up-to-date on issues related to improving health, enhancing productivity, and containing health care costs.

A gifted teacher and writer, David travels extensively and has keynoted many of the most important business and health events in the country. With more than five hundred national keynote addresses since 2000, David has presented to such audiences as the National Chamber of Commerce, the United Nations, the National Institutes of Health, the Centers for Disease Control and Prevention, the US Department of Defense, as well as many of the major Fortune 500 companies.

Dr. Hunnicutt has written, edited, and produced more than a dozen books, including a best-selling medical self-care book that has sold more than six hundred thousand copies. Dr. Hunnicutt's opinions, expertise, and work have appeared in such media as the *Wall Street Journal,* MSN, CBS News, CBS MarketWatch, *Business Week, CIO Magazine, Business and Health, American Medical News, Workforce Magazine,* and numerous local and national newspapers.

Michelle Kalicki received her BS in sport management from the University of Florida and her MS in health promotion management from American University. Thanks to funding from the USDA's Economic Research Service, she has been part of a research team focused on childhood obesity and, in particular, vegetable consumption in low-income elementary schools. Her areas of interest in health promotion include physical activity, nutrition education, and health policy.

Casey Korba is director of prevention and population health at America's Health Insurance Plans (AHIP). Casey works with AHIP member health plans and health care stakeholder partners to support and advance health insurance plans' initiatives and partnerships in the areas of clinical and community preventive services, wellness, and disease management activities and programs. Casey's key areas of interest include promoting physical activity and healthy eating initiatives, tobacco cessation, and work site and community health programs. Casey received a BA in English literature from Dickinson College and an MS in health promotion management at American University.

Marty Loy is professor of health promotion and dean of the College of Professional Studies at the University of Wisconsin–Stevens Point. Prior to becoming dean, Marty served as the associate dean of the School of Health Promotion and Human Development. His teaching and research are in the areas of stress management, including mindfulness meditation, grief, and loss. He has published extensively in these areas, authoring two books: *Childhood Stress: A Handbook for Parents, Teachers and Therapists* (Whole Person Associates, 2010) and with Amy Boelk, *Losing a Parent to Suicide: Using Lived Experiences to Inform Bereavement Counseling* (Routledge, 2013).

Marty won the University Excellence in Teaching Award in 2001. He is past president and currently serves on the board of directors for the National Wellness Institute. He and his wife, Becky, are cofounders of Camp Hope, a camp for grieving children that has served as a model for similar camps around the country.

Maya Maroto is the academic director of the nutrition program at the Maryland University of Integrative Health. Maya's instructional focus includes nutrition education, holistic nutrition, public health nutrition, and health policy. Her research areas include food insecurity, school nutrition policies, and school-based food pantries. Maya holds a BS in nutrition and food science from Auburn University, an MPH in nutrition from the University of North Carolina at Chapel Hill, an EdD in community college leadership from Morgan State University, and is also a registered dietitian nutritionist (RDN).

David Stevenson serves as the president and CEO of the Central Connecticut Coast YMCA, one of the largest Ys in the United States. As part of a worldwide movement, each Y serves unique community needs with a special focus on youth development, healthy living, and social responsibility. In 2013, 2,400 Central Connecticut Coast Y volunteers and staff served 87,000 children and families through twelve branches and fifty program sites. Dr. Stevenson began his Y career in Ohio and has also served at Ys in Washington, DC; Baltimore, Maryland; Pittsburgh, Pennsylvania; and most recently in Connecticut. Dr. Stevenson holds a BS in recreation management from Ithaca College, an MS in health and fitness management from American University, and a PhD in educational administration from American University.

Maura Stevenson is currently an associate professor of biological sciences at Quinnipiac University in Hamden, Connecticut, where she teaches and serves as academic coordinator for anatomy and physiology. She has a BS degree from Ithaca College, an MS degree from the University of Wisconsin–LaCrosse, and her PhD was earned at American University. She was previously involved in work site health promotion research at American University. She is a coauthor of "Using Theories and Models to Support Program Planning" in *ACSM's Worksite Health Promotion Manual: A Guide to Building and Sustaining Healthy Worksites* and "The Weight Management Triad: Dietary Intervention, Behavior Change, and Daily Activity" in *Journal of the American Association of Physician Assistants.* She has presented "Past and Future Trends of Health Promotion" at the Association for Worksite Health Promotion Conference and "Trends in School-based Health Promotion" at the Keystone Health Promotion Conference. Dr. Stevenson had previous academic appointments at Community College of Allegheny County and Robert Morris University in Pittsburgh, Pennsylvania, and at McDaniel College in Westminster, Maryland.

INTRODUCTION TO HEALTH PROMOTION

PART ONE

THE FOUNDATION OF HEALTH PROMOTION

Health promotion is a relatively new field and works in conjunction with the fields of health education and public health to improve the health and well-being of individuals, communities, and society. Collectively, professionals in these fields take a leadership role in collaborating with public health departments, communities, work sites, health care organizations, schools, and other entities to deliver programs and create healthful environments that lead to an improved health status of individuals. The chapters in this part provide an overview of the changes in our environment that have prompted more attention to the prevention of disease and the promotion of health. To accomplish this, key terminology and, most important, select theories and models used to promote behavior change and how to design, implement, and evaluate programs are discussed. In many academic programs, you may have additional course work to study behavior change theories and models as well as a program planning class.

Chapter 1 is a broad overview of select environmental changes occurring after World War II that significantly changed the way people lived, moved, worked, and obtained food. These changes in our society were aligned with shifts in the causes of death and disability in the United States. As medical treatment for infectious diseases were being discovered, personal health choices emerged as an important part to support healthful living. You will find an introduction to many key terms and concepts that are part of the language of health promotion and other related fields. The chapter ends with how the Patient Protection and Affordable Care Act is galvanizing the field of health promotion because the act prioritizes prevention of disease and promotion of healthful lifestyles.

Chapter 2 introduces health behavior change theories and models that offer constructs on how individuals approach personal behavior change, that is, the essence of health promotion—engaging individuals to actively promote their own health through daily actions such as being physically active or selecting healthy foods to eat. These models and theories will assist you in understanding the motivation that drives individuals to engage in behavior change. Tapping into key behavior change theories enables you to deliver theory-based programs to a target audience that will result in people successfully making the changes they set out to make.

Chapter 3 introduces you to program planning models, which incorporate behavior change theories within the intervention. Again, as a health promotion professional, the use of program planning models will set you apart from other practitioners. These models are essential tools to successfully reaching large groups of people through social marketing campaigns to creating effective interventions to enacting policies to create environments where people can practice healthy behaviors.

Collectively, these three chapters introduce you to the foundation of the field of health promotion, and you will study and use this information many times both in your academic work and in your professional life.

CHAPTER 1

HEALTH PROMOTION

An Emerging Field

Anastasia Snelling

The field of health promotion has a relatively short history compared to public health or medicine. However, it is clear that promoting health is an important component of public health and the medical field. Over the past century, US society has changed dramatically in the ways we work, live, and study. In recent decades, these societal changes have affected individual health choices and disease patterns, and as a result the field of health promotion has emerged as a distinct discipline to work in synergy with the fields of public health and health education. The purpose of this textbook is to familiarize students with the history of health patterns, with an emphasis on personal health behaviors, and to identify the social and environmental forces that can create a culture of health to promote a citizenry with longer, healthier lives that are free of disability and disease.

Brief Overview of Health in the Twentieth Century

A critical examination of the history of health issues related to death and disability in the United States provides us with an appreciation of how social and environmental factors influence disease patterns (see US Department of Health and Human Services, National Center for Health Statistics, 2010). This section briefly examines US health in the first

LEARNING OBJECTIVES

After reading this chapter, the student will be able to:

* **Identify health trends related to chronic disease during the second half of the twentieth century.**

* **Explain primary, secondary, and tertiary care.**

* **Explain modifiable and nonmodifiable risk factors.**

* **Identify the leading causes of death in the United States.**

* **Describe how the Affordable Care Act is working to improve healthy lifestyles.**

* **Explain the determinants of health.**

half of the twentieth century and provides a more in-depth investigation of US health in the second half of the twentieth century.

1900–1950s

During the first half of the twentieth century (1900–1950s), the topic of health in the nation focused on developing the medical profession and establishing hospitals to treat patients. Public health departments focused on sanitation, disease control, and health education. During this time, public health functions included child immunization programs, community health services, substance abuse programs, and sexually transmitted disease control.

Life Expectancy

By examining the life expectancy of men and women in the United States over time (see table 1.1), one can understand how medical and health advances have affected the health of a population. **Life expectancy** is a measure of the health status of a given population and is defined as "the average number of years a person from a specific cohort is projected to live from a given point of time" (McKenzie, Pinger, & Kotecki, 1999). At the beginning of the twentieth century, the life expectancies of men and women were 46.3 and 48.3 years, respectively. Infectious diseases such as influenza, pneumonia, tuberculosis, and gastrointestinal infections were the leading causes of death in the United States. The discovery of antibiotics and

Life expectancy
the average number of years that a person from a specific group is projected to live

Table 1.1   Life Expectancy at Birth, at Sixty-Five Years of Age, and at Seventy-Five Years of Age

	At Birth			At Sixty-Five Years			At Seventy-Five Years		
Year	Both sexes	Male	Female	Both sexes	Male	Female	Both Sexes	Male	Female
1900	47.3	46.3	48.3	11.9	11.5	12.2	*	*	*
1950	68.2	65.6	71.1	13.9	12.8	15.0	*	*	*
1960	69.7	66.6	73.1	14.3	12.8	15.8	*	*	*
1970	70.8	67.1	74.7	15.2	13.1	17.0	*	*	*
1980	73.7	70.7	77.4	16.4	14.1	18.4	10.4	8.8	11.5
1990	75.4	71.8	78.8	17.2	15.1	18.9	10.9	9.4	12.0
1995	75.8	72.5	78.9	17.4	15.6	18.9	11.0	9.7	11.9
2000	77.0	74.3	79.7	18.0	16.2	19.3	11.4	10.1	12.3

Source: US Department of Health and Human Services, National Center for Health Statistics (2010).

improved sanitation practices significantly contributed to increasing life expectancies by the 1950s, reaching sixty-five and seventy-one years for men and women, respectively.

Chronic Disease

As a result of the advances of immunizations, antibiotics, maternal and child health, and improved sanitation practices, life expectancy increased. Extending years of life was a positive advancement. However, one result of a longer life expectancy is the more significant impact that personal health choices and environmental factors have on the development of chronic conditions, sometimes referred to as **noncommunicable diseases**, which are not infectious or transferable from one person to another. **Chronic disease** is defined as a health condition or disease that lasts for a long period of time, usually for longer than three months. Chronic diseases also tend to take a long period to develop. Chronic conditions such as high cholesterol have developed over years of consuming high saturated fat and cholesterol foods, which leads to high blood cholesterol levels and is a risk factor for cardiovascular disease. These chronic conditions are usually managed with lifestyle changes, medication, or surgical approaches, depending on the disease.

One of the first studies conducted to measure the impact of personal health choices on cardiovascular disease was the Seven Countries Studies conducted by Ancel Keys in the 1950s (Keys et al., 1986). Keys recruited researchers in seven countries to launch the first cross-cultural comparison of heart attack risk in populations of men engaged in traditional occupations, comparing their diet and fat intake. The Seven Countries Study indicated that the risk and rates of heart attack and cardiovascular risk at the population and individual levels were directly and independently related to the level of total serum cholesterol. It demonstrated that the association between blood cholesterol level and coronary heart disease risk in the five- to forty-year follow-up was found consistently across different cultures. Cholesterol and overweight or obesity was also associated with increased mortality from cancer. The Seven Countries Study, along with other important large studies such as the Framingham Heart Study, the Nurses' Health Study, and the Women's Health Initiative, confirmed not only the importance of healthy diet but also identified weight status and regular physical activity as important factors for maintaining good general health. These studies were conducted in the mid-1950s and begin to establish the influence of personal health choices on disease patterns. Since that time, hundreds of studies have been done and are now being conducted to

noncommunicable diseases
not passed from one person to another, also known as chronic diseases

chronic disease
a health condition or disease that lasts for a long period of time, usually for longer than three months

improve our understandings of the influence of lifestyle behaviors on chronic disease.

1960s–2000s

During the second half of the twentieth century, a number of social and environmental changes occurred that influenced consumer health choices and behaviors. Changes in the way we live are inevitable; however, health promotion professionals must examine how these changes influence health status and respond to these changes to maintain and improve health for individuals and society.

Employment

Americans were prosperous after World War II; the end of the war generated enormous advances in technology, medicine, and communications that led to new job opportunities for returning soldiers and for all citizens. Starting in the 1950s, for the first time in American history, a majority of US workers were white-collar rather than blue-collar workers (McColloch, 1983). White-collar workers tended to be involved in positions that required less physical activity than workers in blue-collar positions. People working in white-collar positions are typically sedentary for most of their day; there is a need to build physical activity back into their daily routines.

A blue-collar worker is someone who performs manual labor. Blue-collar work may involve skilled or unskilled labor, such as mining, mechanical, construction, or manufacturing jobs. A white-collar worker is someone who performs professional, managerial, or administrative work; examples include teachers, managers, and secretaries.

Suburbs and Cars

The housing industry boomed and shifted families into new suburban neighborhoods; the explosion of the automobile industry accompanied this shift. As people moved from urban to suburban areas, cars became more popular and necessary. Between 1945 and 1947, car production increased from 70,000 to 3.5 million (Weiner, 1992). As people moved out of the city and started owning cars, the reliance on transportation negatively influenced their daily physical activity.

Supermarkets, Food Choices, and Eating Patterns

As suburban neighborhoods were built, supermarkets and the food industry began to develop and shift to meet this new demand. In 1958, there were approximately fifteen thousand supermarkets; this number roughly doubled by the 1980s (Ellickson, 2011). In the 1960s, women began to enter the workforce, which shifted their role of preparing daily meals for the family. Then, frozen foods became more readily available at the retail level and the fast food industry was born. In 1968, McDonalds operated approximately one thousand restaurants; by 2012 there were thirty thousand McDonalds around the world. Along with the emergence of fast food restaurants, the microwave was introduced into the family kitchen. The shift from eating what one grew during the growing season to being able to purchase large quantities of foods at any time promoted increased calorie consumption. The food environment, from the prevalence and size of supermarkets to the growth of the fast food industry, underwent significant changes during this period.

Entertainment and Leisure Time

A shift in the physical activity patterns of adults and children also occurred. Advancing technology brought televisions into American living rooms. In 1950, less than 1% of homes had televisions. In 2012, over 83% of homes had at least one television. Between 1975 and 1985, video games such as Atari and Nintendo became available and IBM introduced the first personal computer. People of all ages are entertained with televisions, computers, and video games, again decreasing our daily physical activity time.

Tobacco Use

Although Americans had been smoking throughout the entire twentieth century, by 1950 more women were smoking than ever before and approximately 42% of all Americans smoked. Smoking was permitted everywhere, in office buildings, schools, restaurants, and airplanes. However, research started to suggest dangers associated with smoking. In 1964, the first surgeon general's report was written that clearly documented the effects of smoking on health. Early into the 1970s, concerns regarding secondhand smoke were validated and the negative effects of smoking became clear. As a result, clean indoor air legislation and higher cigarette taxes were put into effect in an attempt to reduce the prevalence of smoking. As a nation, we continue to limit where people can smoke and require higher taxes on

Table 1.2 Leading Causes of Death in the United States and Related Risk Factors

Rank	Cause	Risk Factors
1	Diseases of the heart	Tobacco use, high blood pressure, elevated serum cholesterol, diet, diabetes, obesity, lack of exercise, alcohol abuse, genetics
2	Malignant neoplasms (cancer)	Tobacco use, alcohol misuse, diet, solar radiation, ionizing radiation, work site hazards, environmental pollution, genetics
3	Chronic lower respiratory disease	Tobacco use
4	Cerebrovascular diseases (stroke)	Tobacco use, high blood pressure, elevated serum cholesterol, diabetes, obesity, genetics
5	Accidents (unintentional injuries)	Alcohol misuse, tobacco use (fires), product design, home hazards, handgun availability, lack of safety restraints, excessive speed, automobile design, roadway design
6	Alzheimer's disease	Age, family history, genetics, head injury, heart health, general healthy aging
7	Diabetes mellitus	Obesity (for type 2 diabetes), diet, lack of exercise, genetics
8	Nephritis, nephritic syndrome, and nephrosis	Infectious agents, drug hypersensitivity, genetics, trauma
9	Pneumonia and influenza	Tobacco use, infectious agents, biological factors
10	Intentional self-harm	

tobacco. Some companies and college campuses are going smoke free. Because these actions have shown decreased rates of smoking in the United States, many advocates suggest applying similar strategies to other health behaviors.

By the end of the twentieth century, life expectancy for men and women was 74.3 and 79.7 years, respectively. Advances in medicine and drug therapy for managing chronic conditions were largely responsible for the increase in life expectancy in the late twentieth century.

Although life expectancy continued to increase, causes of death shifted from infectious diseases in the early half of the century to chronic diseases in the late 1900s and early 2000s. These chronic diseases are the focus of the health promotion field today. Now, the leading causes of death in the United States are primarily chronic disease influenced by risk factors that include personal health choices. Table 1.2 shows the leading causes of death and all related risk factors. Table 1.3 presents the actual causes of death from lifestyle behaviors, comparing 1990 and 2000, specifically the risk factors that advance chronic disease development, and Table 1.4 presents the leading causes of death in the United States.

Table 1.3 Lifestyle Behaviors Related to Disease

	1990		2000	
Actual Cause	**Number**	**%**	**Number**	**%**
Tobacco	400,000	19	435,000	18.1
Poor diet and physical inactivity	300,000	14	365,000	15.2
Alcohol consumption	100,000	5	85,000	3.5
Microbial agents	90,000	4	75,000	3.1
Toxic agents	60,000	3	55,000	2.3
Motor vehicle	25,000	1	43,000	1.8
Firearms	35,000	2	29,000	1.2
Sexual behavior	30,000	1	20,000	0.8
Illicit drug use	20,000	1	17,000	0.7
Total	1,060,000	50	1,124,000	46.7

Sources: For 1990 data, McGinnis & Foege (1993). For 2000 data, Mokdad et al. (2005).

Table 1.4 Number of Deaths for Leading Causes of Death

Heart disease	597,689
Cancer	574,743
Chronic lower respiratory diseases	138,080
Stroke	129,476
Accidents	120,859
Alzheimer's disease	83,494
Diabetes	69,071
Nephritis, nephrotic syndrome, nephrosis	50,476
Influenza and pneumonia	50,097
Intentional self-harm	38,364

Source: Centers for Disease Control (2010).

Health Promotion: An Emerging Field

Health promotion, as a field of study, has a shorter history than public health and health education. The emergence of health promotion was a direct response to the changes in disease patterns in the United States, particularly

health promotion
the process of helping people to move toward a state of optimal health through lifestyle changes

the rise of chronic disease rates beginning in the mid-twentieth century. This rise is attributed primarily to two reasons: the discovery of antibiotics and vaccinations to prevent and treat infectious diseases and the adoption of lifestyle behaviors that increase risk for conditions that lead to chronic diseases.

Although health promotion, public health, and health education overlap to some degree, each is a distinct field of study in and of itself. It is important to understand the distinctions among these three fields, as shown in the following definitions. According to the World Health Organization (WHO Centre for Health Development, 2004), health promotion is

> the process of enabling people to increase control over, and to improve, their health. It moves beyond a focus on individual behaviour towards a wide range of social and environmental interventions. (p. 30)

Dr. Michael O'Donnell (2002), a leading scholar in the field of work site health promotion, offers this definition of health promotion:

> The art and science of helping people discover the synergies between their core passions and optimal health, enhancing their motivation to strive for optimal health, and supporting them in changing their lifestyle to move toward a state of optimal health. Optimal health is a dynamic balance of physical, emotional, social, spiritual, and intellectual health. Lifestyle change can be facilitated through a combination of learning experiences that enhance awareness, increase motivation, and build skills and, most important, through the creation of opportunities that open access to environments that make positive health practices the easiest choice. (p. xx)

Health Education

health education
helping individuals and communities improve their health through learning experiences aimed toward increasing knowledge or influencing attitude

Health education is defined by the World Health Organization (WHO Centre for Health Development, 2004) as

> any combination of learning experiences designed to help individuals and communities improve their health, by increasing their knowledge or influencing their attitudes. (p. 29)

Public Health

Public health, as defined by the World Health Organization (WHO Centre for Health Development, 2004),

> is concerned with the health of the community as a whole. The three core public health functions are: the assessment and monitoring of the

health of communities and populations at risk to identify health problems and priorities; the formulation of public policies designed to solve identified local and national health problems and priorities; and ensuring that all populations have access to appropriate and cost-effective care, including health promotion and disease prevention services, and evaluation of the effectiveness of that care. (p. 48)

public health
organized efforts to promote the health of the community as a whole through measures such as identifying health problems, creating public policies, and ensuring access to cost-effective care

Discussion

These definitions clearly indicate that public health, health education, and health promotion are all working toward the common goal of improving health for individuals and society. However, distinctly different in each definition are the strategies used to address health issues. Green and Kreuter (1999) suggest that

> health promotion draws on the health sciences, programs, practices, and policies that relate to the health of human populations. We must move beyond the tidy boundaries of health institutions, for much of what relates to the health of human populations happens in other sectors, such as schools, industry, social services, and welfare. (p. 2)

The essence of health promotion is to actively promote healthy living by creating a society in which a "culture of health" is evident in places where people live, work, worship, and learn. Health promotion balances individual health behavior choices with creating environments where healthier choices become easier choices. Therefore, health promotion is broader than health education, yet health education is an important component within the field of health promotion. Further, the fields of health promotion and public health are overlapping, yet have distinctly different approaches to addressing the health of society. Public health, as the previous definition demonstrates, is engaged with *monitoring* the health of the public, *formulating* policies, and *ensuring* all citizens have access to health care, all of which are critical to ensuring a healthy society. Health promotion focuses primarily on chronic disease management by *monitoring* health conditions, *assisting* individuals to make healthy choices, and *formulating* policies that create healthy environments.

To illustrate an example of how professionals in the fields of health promotion and public health work together, let's consider the issue of flu vaccines. Each year public health officials work to identify strains of flu that will be a threat to society when flu season arrives. The influenza viruses in the seasonal flu vaccine are selected each year based on surveillance-based forecasts about what viruses are most likely to cause illness in the upcoming season. This work is done primarily by public health epidemiologists and is critically important for the prevention of seasonal flu. The next step is encouraging people to obtain the flu vaccine through health communication campaigns and offering the flu vaccine in places where people frequently visit. It is in these latter steps that health promotion professionals contribute their expertise: understanding their target audience and creating health communication campaigns that trigger individuals to act on the message. In the end both the development of the right flu vaccine and the distribution of the flu vaccine will improve the health of the society.

Determinants of Health

There is no one cause for the increase in behaviors related to chronic disease. We cannot point to one factor or product, such as video games, suburban neighborhoods, or soda, as the singular cause of chronic disease. Therefore, professionals need a comprehensive understanding of the determinants of health and a broad array of strategies to approach these issues. The Department of Health and Human Services (HHS) has guided the development of the determinants of health because they have been at the forefront of establishing strategic goals for the health of the United States citizenry. Since 1979, when the first surgeon general wrote *Healthy People: The Surgeon General's Report on Health Promotion and Disease Prevention*, HHS has guided the development of this overarching document on health indices and goals (US Department of Health, Education, and Welfare, 1980; US Public Health Service, 1979). Healthy People 2020 is considered a strategic document that uses identification, measurement, and tracking to reduce health disparities through a determinants-of-health approach (Koh, 2010).

determinants of health
factors that significantly influence the health of individuals and communities, such as genetic or biological factors, social and physical factors, health services, individual behaviors, and policies

The **determinants of health** are defined as factors that significantly influence or have an impact on the health of individuals and communities. Determinants of health comprise genetic or biological factors, social and physical factors, health services, policies, and individual behaviors. The interrelationship of these factors determines the health of individuals and, collectively, the health of a population (Institute of Medicine, 2001). Understanding how each of these factors contributes to the health of an individual is important; however, the single greatest opportunity to improve health lies in personal health choices. Individual behavior choices account for almost 40% of all deaths in the United States (Mokdad, Marks, Stroup, & Gerberding, 2004).

The types of determinants of health are as follows:

- *Biology and genetics.* These factors relate to family history because individuals can be predisposed to a condition from a parent. Other factors may relate to age; for example, as individuals age they are predisposed to certain physical and cognitive changes.

- *Social and physical factors.* Social determinant of health includes a range of issues that affect the health of people, including education, income, social supports, and quality of schools. Physical factors also affect health by expanding or limiting access to healthy food and opportunities for physical activity. The physical environments where people work and live, including access to grocery stores, safe walking or biking paths, housing, work sites, and exposure to physical hazards, affect health.

- *Health services.* Access to health services and the quality of these health services affect health. Improving access to preventive health services is a primary goal of the Affordable Care Act. However, medical care plays a minor role in preventing premature deaths.

- *Policies.* Policies at the local, state, and national levels, as well as the workplace, affect health. Clean indoor air policies and increased taxes influence the percentage of people who smoke tobacco. More recently, school wellness policies promote healthy school environments for children, although there is little data available to assess the impact of these policies on childhood obesity.

- *Individual behaviors.* Individual behaviors, such as food choices, physical activity, managing stress, or cigarette use, influence the development of chronic health conditions.

Each of these factors contributes to the overall health and well-being of individuals. Health promotion focuses primarily on individual behaviors and recognizes the importance of the physical and social environmental factors and policy formulation and implementation. In the first half of the twentieth century, health advances were made as a result of policies (e.g., improved sanitation practices) and medical care (e.g., discovery of antibiotics). Continued advances in medical procedures and prescription drugs have been important in improving the quality of life for those with chronic disease. However, as we move into the twenty-first century, to address rising health care costs and the health of people, health improvements will be derived from changes in individual health behavior supplemented with environmental supports.

physical environment
the structures, buildings, or services that can either facilitate or hinder healthy behavior

As indicated previously, physical and social environmental factors are critical to achieving successful individual behavior change. The **physical environment** includes the structures, buildings, or services that can either facilitate or hinder healthy behavior. For example, walking paths or lighted streets may encourage more walking in neighborhoods and deter crime; grocery stores may provide improved access to healthy foods and fresh fruits rather than people having to rely only on corner stores in a neighborhood, which traditionally do not stock a wide array of produce. The physical environment creates the opportunity for a person to engage in the behavior, but that alone may not reach everyone.

social environment
the personal relationships or networks that surround people

The **social environment** is the personal relationships or networks that surround people. Social networks establish norms of behavior and these behaviors can facilitate or hinder healthy behavior. Back in the mid-1950s, about half of the country was smoking. Smoking was a very acceptable practice, which may have influenced people to start smoking. Conversely, to help people change behaviors, social support and networks are important for the health behavior change to be realized (Breslow, 1999). For example, if a child is overweight, it is recommended the entire family engage in healthy eating and regular exercise to promote weight management. Work site health promotion programs also rely on social support from employees.

social ecological model
a multilayered approach to health issues that illustrates different spheres that influence individual behavior

Building on the determinants of health, health promotion addresses health issues in a multilayered approach using a **social ecological model**. This model illustrates different spheres that influence individual behavior. Each individual has knowledge, beliefs, or values that will influence his or her health choices. Then there is the family unit and how the family will influence health behaviors. The next sphere is a school or workplace, and because children and adults spend six to eight hours of their day at these places, their programs and policies may influence behavior. The next sphere is the community where people live, and the last area is policy, which includes local, state, and national policies that are related to healthy environments (Sallis, Owen, & Fisher; 2008; Stokols, 1992). This model is presented in figure 1.1 and is furthered discussed in chapter 3 on program planning models. As you read about the different health behaviors in chapters 4 through 8, you will notice the ecological approach to improving each sphere to positively influence health behavior changes.

Important Health Promotion Concepts

Before moving into the chapters discussing the health behaviors that affect chronic disease and the resources, strategies, and models that support health

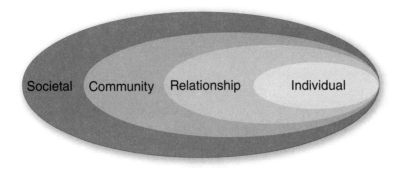

Figure 1.1   Social Ecological Model
Source: Centers for Disease Control (2013).

promotion, this section briefly discusses concepts and terminology relevant in the field.

Risk Factors, Chronic Diseases, and Empowerment

Specific health behaviors are directly associated with chronic disease. These health behaviors are termed **risk factors**. Risk factors may be modifiable or nonmodifiable. **Modifiable risk factors** are those that an individual can change through his or her own actions, such as levels of physical activity or eating habits. **Nonmodifiable risk factors** are those that cannot be changed by the individual, such as age, gender, or family history.

Health promotion focuses on the *modifiable* risk factors that individuals have the ability to change when provided the necessary education, motivation, and a supportive environment. Approaching health from this perspective can empower people to improve their own health status and hence have more control over their well-being. Empowerment of individuals or communities is a key theme in the field of health promotion. When used correctly, empowerment can be a long-term strategy for making permanent changes. Research indicates that small behavior changes in someone's weight status or physical activity patterns can improve health outcomes.

risk factors
specific health behaviors that are directly associated with chronic disease

modifiable risk factors
risk factors that an individual can change through his or her own actions

nonmodifiable risk factors
risk factors that cannot be changed by the individual, such as age, gender, or family history

Health behaviors and choices occur every day in our lives. Stop and consider how many health choices you have made in the last twenty-four hours (brushing your teeth, eating breakfast, wearing a seat belt or bicycle helmet). Each of these choices may exert a strong influence on your health status, although it may be years before the effects of those choices are known. For example, smoking one cigarette will not cause lung cancer but smoking over thirty years of your life will certainly increase your chance of lung cancer.

Prevention Activities: Primary, Secondary, and Tertiary

Health prevention is an important component of managing people's health once a chronic condition develops. Individuals can actively engage in promoting their own health through regular physical activity or managing their stress, but they must also be informed about health prevention activities. Prevention activities are categorized into three levels: primary, secondary, and tertiary. Prevention activities tend to be associated with the health care system.

Primary Prevention

primary prevention
primary prevention aims to prevent the disease from occurring

Primary prevention emphasizes activities to avert illness, injury, or disease conditions. Strategies may be incorporated into an educational situation or a medical visit. For example, elementary school children may have an assembly in which information is shared to discourage them from starting to smoke tobacco or, at the college level, there may be educational programs on the risks of drinking alcohol. During medical visits, primary prevention activities might include scheduled immunizations or appropriate cancer screenings. The Affordable Care Act, described later in this chapter, prioritizes primary prevention activities.

Secondary Prevention

secondary prevention
used after the disease has occurred, but before the person notices that anything is wrong

Secondary prevention emphasizes identifying diseases at their earliest stage and treating the conditions early. Research suggests that when disease is detected early, there is a far greater chance of treatment with a successful outcome. The health care system is sometimes called the "curative" system due to its focus on detecting and treating disease. Examples of secondary prevention abound in the United States because of the number of people with chronic conditions, including high blood pressure or high blood cholesterol. A person with either high blood pressure or blood cholesterol would be prescribed a drug that would help lower either his or her blood pressure or blood cholesterol. Managing chronic conditions by using prescription drugs is a hallmark of the health care system, which has made significant advances in treating chronic conditions.

Tertiary Prevention

tertiary prevention
targets the person who already has symptoms of the disease

Tertiary prevention relies mainly on the health care system and highlights specific medical interventions to limit advancing conditions linked to chronic diseases. If not treated, chronic conditions progress over time and cause further debilitation of the body. Tertiary prevention aims to slow the progression of the chronic condition. Rehabilitation services such as physical or occupational therapy are trademarks of this type of prevention. This type of care is usually considered the most expensive care and is responsible, in part, to driving up health care costs.

Discussion

Secondary and tertiary prevention activities are delivered mainly through the health care system, where the cost is considerably higher as chronic conditions advance. Unfortunately, much less attention is given to preventing the onset of these chronic conditions (primary prevention) until recently. Since about 2000, the US Preventive Services Task Force was established and specifically recommends that managing these conditions begins with lifestyle behavior changes. However, there has been a slow uptake of this approach through the medical system and personal health choices.

Health promotion activities focus on engaging individuals in primary prevention to delay or avoid the onset of chronic conditions. However, health promotion interventions should also be part of secondary and tertiary care as well. Consider someone who is diagnosed with early stages of diabetes and is also overweight and lives a sedentary life. This individual would benefit greatly from losing weight, eating a healthy diet, and slowly beginning an exercise program. The health care system is remarkable at restoring health; however, the cost of this type of care is very high to those who pay the bill, including individuals, organizations, and the federal government. There is a more cost-effective approach to health and disease; health promoters aim to improve the overall wellness of the target audience, which will lead to a decrease in the cost of treating illness and, more important, assist people in living more years free of chronic conditions.

Health Promotion Meets the Health Care System

The United States has an employee-based health care system rather than a government-run system. This means health insurance is offered to employees through the organizations where they work. In some cases, the US government offers health insurance to special segments of the population: people over sixty-five years can enroll in Medicare, military veterans receive care through the Veterans Administration, individuals living below the poverty line and those who are disabled are eligible for Medicaid, and the State Children's Health Insurance Program provides matching funds to states for health insurance to families with children whose incomes are modest but too high to qualify for Medicaid. There are many different health insurance programs in the United States funded by private organizations and the federal and state governments.

The US health care system, whether offered through an organization or through the federal government, has been known as a "restorative" medical system, a system that focuses primarily on treating disease rather than preventing disease. The medical system has made enormous advances in detecting and treating diseases through the use of technology, surgery, and drug treatment. Because of these advances, the United States has a very expensive health care system; however, as a nation, we lag behind other countries on several key health indices, including infant mortality, life expectancy, and rates of chronic disease.

Patient Protection and Affordable Care Act

In 2010, President Barack Obama signed into law the Patient Protection and Affordable Care Act, commonly referred to as the Affordable Care Act (ACA) (Open Congress, 2010). This monumental piece of legislation represents the most comprehensive set of health care reforms in recent US history. One significant component of the ACA was to extend health coverage to citizens in the United States by requiring individuals to have medical coverage; the goal is to have everyone contributing financially into the health care system. As a result of the ACA, it is estimated that an additional thirty-one million Americans will have access to health insurance coverage. One objective of the law is to increase by 2014 the number of quality, affordable, private health insurance plans from which more people are able to choose. By 2014, more than seven million Americans had signed up for health care through the health care exchanges. Access to medical care is an important factor for improving health outcomes; increased access provides more opportunities to promote healthy behavior and offer age-appropriate clinical preventive services.

A second hallmark of the ACA is its emphasis on wellness, health promotion, and prevention. Two parts of the ACA are focused in this area, Title IV, Prevention of Chronic Disease and Improving Public Health, and Title V, Healthcare Workforce. Within these areas is the creation of councils to advance the priority of improving quality of health care through disease prevention and health promotion. Within Title IV, it requires the creation of the National Prevention, Health Promotion, and Public Health Council (the National Prevention Council). This council is tasked with developing the National Prevention Strategy to guide our nation in identifying the most effective and achievable means to improve health and well-being.

The National Prevention Strategy envisions a prevention-oriented society in which all sectors recognize the value of health for individuals, families, and society and work together to achieve better health for all Americans (Fielding, Teutsch, & Koh, 2012; Koh & Sebelius, 2010). Within Title V, the creation of the National Health Care Workforce Commission reviews workforce needs and makes recommendations to the federal government to ensure that national policies are aligned with consumer needs. One initiative under this title is to provide technical assistance to primary care providers about health promotion, chronic disease management, and preventive medicine. These initiatives are focused on the emphasis of health promotion and disease prevention.

The ACA also requires health insurance companies to cover a number of recommended preventive services, such as blood pressure or cancer screenings, without additional costs to patients. This emphasis on early detection of chronic conditions is a critical step to decreasing rates of the leading causes of death in the United States. An independent panel of medical and scientific experts serve on the US Preventive Services Task Force to identify preventive services based on the strength of the scientific evidence documenting their benefits and cost effectiveness. Chapter 8 addresses clinical preventive services and their importance to health promotion and chapter 9 discusses the role of the federal and state governments in health activities.

Discussion

With the new provisions established in the ACA, the nation is experiencing a shift in its approach to health, wellness, and the treatment of illness. For the first time, a greater value is being placed on health promotion and the long-term benefits of preventing disease. By viewing health through this lens, health promoters can reframe the dialogue on many of the chronic diseases and lifestyle risk factors that plague our population. These ACA provisions underscore the value of health promotion and prevention, lending credibility to the field of health promotion.

Positions in the Health Promotion Field

There is an enormous need and demand for the skills of health promotion professionals. Students academically trained in the field will have a scientific understanding of the body, including biology, chemistry, exercise physiology, nutrition and diet, and health psychology. Paired with this science knowledge, health promotion students will also possess a theoretical perspective of program planning and implementation, including assessment, methodology, and evaluation, as well as policy formulation. Chapter 10 provides an extensive discussion on a variety of settings where health promotion is occurring.

Historically, some of the first positions in the field of health promotion were responsible for managing work site health promotion programs. With an employee-based health care system, US corporations share the overall cost of the nation's health care bill; toward the end of the twentieth century, health care costs began to rise significantly. In response to increased costs, many employers established work site health promotion programs.

Beyond work site health promotion programs, which continue to employ a large number of health promotion professionals, the field of health promotion has grown significantly in response to the obesity epidemic and the associated rise in the rates of chronic disease. Health promotion positions are now well established in government and non-governmental agencies, including state and local health departments, health care providers and insurance companies, school districts, commercial gym facilities, and faith-based organizations, as well as companies that supply specialized services related to health promotion, such as social marketing campaigns, health coaching, health screenings, or health education materials.

As students explore different career options within the field of health promotion, interests might focus on a health condition or a life stage. Health issues such as heart disease, osteoporosis, or childhood obesity can frame positions within the field. Another approach is the identification of a specific target population. Health promotion positions address individual behavior at all stages of life, from encouraging healthy prenatal behaviors during pregnancy, to early childhood growth and development, to student health in primary and secondary schools, through the life span in universities, work sites, communities, and assisted living facilities. The nation needs health promotion professionals who are trained to motivate and educate individuals to invest in healthy lifestyles and work with communities and government to build social and physical environments that support healthy living.

Summary

This chapter introduces a number of key terms and the foundation for the emerging field of health promotion. It briefly describes the social and physical changes to the environment from the first half of the twentieth century to the second half. It distinguishes health promotion from public health and health education. Evidence on how the social, behavior, and environmental factors have influenced our behaviors and chronic diseases is described both qualitatively and quantitatively. Understanding the forces that have brought about the changes in these factors is fundamental to the discipline of health promotion.

KEY TERMS

1.   **Life expectancy:** the average number of years that a person from a specific group is projected to live

2.   **Noncommunicable disease:** diseases not passed from one person to another; also known as chronic diseases

3.   **Chronic disease:** a health condition or disease that lasts for a long period of time, usually for longer than three months

4.   **Health promotion:** the process of helping people to move toward a state of optimal health through lifestyle changes

5.   **Health education:** helping individuals and communities improve their health through learning experiences aimed toward increasing knowledge or influencing attitude

6.   **Public health:** organized efforts to promote the health of the community as a whole through measures such as identifying health problems, creating public policies, and ensuring access to cost-effective care

7.   **Determinants of health:** factors that significantly influence the health of individuals and communities, such as genetic or biological factors, social and physical factors, health services, individual behaviors, and policies

8.   **Physical environment:** the structures, buildings, or services that can either facilitate or hinder healthy behavior

9.   **Social environment:** the personal relationships or networks that surround people

10. **Social ecological model:** a multilayered approach to health issues that illustrates different spheres that influence individual behavior

11. **Risk factors:** specific health behaviors that are directly associated with chronic disease

12. **Modifiable risk factors:** risk factors that an individual can change through his or her own actions

13. **Nonmodifiable risk factors:** risk factors that cannot be changed by the individual, such as age, gender, or family history

14. **Primary prevention:** primary prevention aims to prevent the disease from occurring

15. **Secondary prevention:** used after the disease has occurred, but before the person notices that anything is wrong

16. **Tertiary prevention:** targets the person who already has symptoms of the disease

REVIEW QUESTIONS

1. What are the differences and similarities between health promotion and disease prevention?

2. Are promoting health and preventing disease the same thing or different?

3. Why is health promotion framed as an emerging field?

4. How are the determinants of health related to the social ecological model?

5. What is the goal of health promotion?

6. What are chronic disease, risk factors, and levels of prevention?

7. How would you define determinants of health?

8. How would you define "a culture of health"?

STUDENT ACTIVITIES

1. Some researchers have stated that children today will have a shorter life span than their parents. Do you agree or disagree? State your reasons.

2. Draw a graphic showing the intersections of health promotion, public health, and health education.

3. Describe the social and physical environment on your college campus. What areas support health-promoting behaviors and what areas are inconsistent with health-promoting behaviors?

4. Identify an organization that employs health promotion professionals and review the position descriptions.

5. Explain the anticipated shifts in the health care system as a result of the Affordable Care Act.

References

Breslow, L. (1999). From disease prevention to health promotion. *JAMA, 281*(11), 1030–1033.

Centers for Disease Control (CDC). (2010). *Deaths and mortality.* Retrieved from www.cdc.gov/nchs/fastats/deaths.htm

Centers for Disease Control (CDC). (2013). *A framework for prevention.* Retrieved from www.cdc.gov/violenceprevention/overview/social-ecologicalmodel.html

Ellickson, P. B. (2011, April 1). *The evolution of the supermarket industry: From A&P to Wal-Mart.* Simon School Working Paper Series no. FR 11–17. Retrieved from http://ssrn.com/abstract=1814166 or http://dx.doi.org/10.2139/ssrn.1814166

Fielding, J. E., Teutsch, S., & Koh, H. (2012). Health reform and healthy people initiative. *American Journal of Public Health, 102*(1), 30–33.

Green, L. W., & Kreuter, M. W. (1999). *Health promotion planning: An educational and ecological approach* (3rd ed.). Boston: McGraw-Hill.

Keys, A., Alessandro, M., Mariti, J. K., et al. (1986). The diet and 15-year death rate in the Seven Countries Study. *American Journal of Epidemiology, 124*(6), 903–915.

Koh, H. K. (2010). A 2020 vision for healthy people. *New England Journal of Medicine, 362*(18), 1653–1656.

Koh, H. K., & Sebelius, K. G. (2010). Promoting prevention through the Affordable Care Act. *New England Journal of Medicine.* Retrieved from www.nejm.org/doi/full/10.1056/NEJMp1008560.

Institute of Medicine (IOM). (2001). *Health and behavior: The interplay of biological, behavioral, and societal influences.* Washington, DC: Academy Press.

McColloch, M. (1983). *White collar works in transition: The boom years, 1940s–1970s.* Westport, CT: Greenwood Press.

McGinnis, J. M., & Foege, W. H. (1993). Actual causes of death in the United States. *JAMA, 270*(18), 2207–2212.

McKenzie, J. E., Pinger, R. R., & Kotecki, J. F. (1999). *An introduction to community health.* Boston: Jones & Bartlett.

Mokdad, A. H., Marks, J. S., Stroup, D. F., & Gerberding, J. L. (2004). Actual causes of death in the United States, 2000. *JAMA, 291*(10), 1238–1245. doi: 10.1001/jama.291.10.1238

Mokdad, A. H., Marks, J. S., Stroup, D. F., & Gerberding, J. L. (2005). Correction: Actual death in the United States, 2000. *JAMA, 292*(3), 293–294.

O'Donnell, M. P. (2002). *Health promotion at the workplace* (3rd ed.). Albany, NY: Delmar.

Open Congress. (2010). *H.R.3590: Patient Protection and Affordable Care Act.* Retrieved from www.opencongress.org/bill/111-h3590/show#

Sallis, J. F., Owen, N., & Fisher, E. B. (2008). Ecological models of health behavior. In K. Glanz, B. K. Rimer, & K. Viswanath (Eds.), *Health behavior and health education practice: Theory, research, and practice* (4th ed.) (pp. 465–485). San Francisco: Jossey-Bass.

Stokols, D. (1992). Establishing and maintaining healthy environments. Toward a social ecology of health promotion. *American Psychology, 47*(1), 6–22.

US Department of Health, Education, and Welfare. (1980). *Promoting health/ preventing disease: Objective for the nation.* Washington, DC: US Government Printing Office.

US Department of Health and Human Services, National Center for Health Statistics. (2010). Health, United States, 2009: With Special Feature on Medical Terminology. Hyattsville, MD. Report No. 2010–1232.

US Public Health Service. (1979). *Healthy people: The surgeon general's report on health promotion and disease prevention.* Washington, DC: US Government Printing Office.

Weiner, E. (1992). *Urban transportation planning in the United States: A historical overview.* Retrieved from http://ntl.bts.gov/DOCS/UTP.html

WHO Centre for Health Development. (2004). A glossary of terms for community health care and services for older persons. *Ageing and Health Technical Report, 5.* Retrieved from http://whqlibdoc.who.int/wkc/2004/WHO_WKC_Tech.Ser._04.2.pdf

CHAPTER 2

HEALTH BEHAVIOR CHANGE THEORIES AND MODELS

Understanding the Process of Behavior Change

Maura Stevenson

A primary focus of health promotion is to help people limit unhealthy behaviors and, in many cases, replace them with healthy behaviors. Health promotion professionals have long known that it is not enough to simply help people identify unhealthy behaviors in order to eliminate them. Human behavior is far too complex for that to be effective. As such, theories and models that help explain and account for the complexity of human behaviors are often used as the foundation for successful health promotion programs.

Although definitions of theories can be lengthy and complex, Cottrell, Girvan, and McKenzie (2011) offered an applied definition of a theory as it relates to health promotion: "A **theory** is a general explanation of why people act or do not act to maintain and/or promote the health of themselves, their families, organizations, and communities" (p. 100). Failure to understand theories may lead to health promotion initiatives that do not succeed because of inaccurate assumptions about participants' likelihood of successful behavior change.

Imagine an individual given the task of implementing a stop-smoking program. The individual has no knowledge of health behavior theories but establishes a plan to (1) recruit smokers and (2) convince them that smoking is harmful to their health. This individual believes that providing smokers with the knowledge that smoking is harmful to their health will cause them to quit smoking.

LEARNING OBJECTIVES

After reading this chapter, the student will be able to:

* Define the differences between a model and theory.

* Describe the role of models and theories in changing health behavior.

* Identify the constructs in the social cognitive theory, the health belief model, the transtheoretical model of behavior change, and the theory of planned behavior.

* Discuss changes over time and how these models and theories align with changing health behaviors.

theory
an explanation intended to account for the actions that people take or do not take to promote health

Although education is an important part of health behavior intervention and should not be discounted, the likelihood that these two steps alone will achieve success is very limited.

models
theory-based planning framework that helps guide program creation and evaluation

Although theories can help explain why people act or fail to act, **models** help to translate theories into a program planning framework. Models can also be used beyond the planning stage and can serve as a guide for program implementation and evaluation (Glanz & Rimer, 1995). The focus of this chapter will be on behavior change theories; planning models are discussed in chapter 3. It should be noted that two of the four theories presented here include the word *model* in their titles. Although this may be confusing, theories and models are intertwined and not always distinctly separate.

Through the study of theories, one learns that theories are subdivided into elements, generally referred to as *concepts*. Concepts in turn are described in a more concrete form referred to as *constructs*, which in their most applicable form are known as *variables* (figure 2.1). It is the variables that become the basis for assessment of a program (Cottrell, Girvan, & McKenzie, 2011).

Health Behavior Theories

Over the years, a number of theories and models related to health behavior change have been developed. In this chapter, four theories are discussed:

* Social cognitive theory
* Transtheroetical model of behavior change
* Health belief model
* Theory of planned behavior

These are the dominant theories of health behavior and health education based on the frequency of their citation within the health promotion research literature (Glanz, Rimer, & Viswanath, 2008). Each attempts to explain human behavior, motivation, and the processes of personal behavior change.

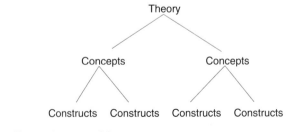

Figure 2.1   Theories, Concepts, and Constructs

Social Cognitive Theory

Social cognitive theory (SCT), developed by Albert Bandura (1986), focuses on not just the psychology of health behavior but on social aspects as well. SCT originated as the social learning theory within a psychological domain; it expanded as concepts studied in sociology and political science were included. SCT embraces the idea that humans do not live in isolation and learn and behave not only according to their own thought processes but also in response to the environments that surround them in terms of the environment of a group (workplace, for example) or the larger society as a whole (Glanz, Rimer, & Viswanath, 2008). Bandura further emphasizes that individuals are not simply products of their environments but help to create those environments. He refers to this concept as **reciprocal determinism** (Bandura, 1986).

> **Social cognitive theory (SCT)**
> theoretical model that frames individual behavior as a response to observational learning from the surrounding environment

SCT explains learning and behavior through a description of constructs (Cottrell, Girvan, & McKenzie, 2011):

> **reciprocal determinism**
> the concept that individuals are a product of their environments and also help to create those environments

- Knowledge of health risks and benefits of various health behaviors

- Perceived self-efficacy of one's ability to control one's own health behaviors

- Outcome expectations related to the consequences of particular health behaviors

- Personal health goals established by individuals

- Perceived facilitators of the desired health behaviors

- Perceived impediments to the desired health behaviors (Bandura, 2004)

Each of these six constructs is described in table 2.1.

Knowledge of Health Risks and Benefits

The knowledge of health risks and benefits associated with particular behaviors serves as the precondition for change (Bandura, 2004). Although not the only factor required for behavior change, knowledge of risks and benefits is the obvious starting point. For example, people smoked for many years with no motivation to stop until it became known that continuing to smoke would bring risks to their health. It followed that stopping smoking would lead to health benefits.

Perceived Self-Efficacy

Perceived **self-efficacy** is referred to as the foundation of behavior change and is described as "people's judgments of their capabilities to organize and execute courses of action required to attain designated types of

> **self-efficacy**
> an individual's perception of his or her capability to execute a course of action necessary to achieve a goal

Table 2.1   Social Change Theory and Application of Constructs

Construct	Sample Application
Knowledge of health risks and benefits	"I'm 50 pounds overweight, which puts me at increased risk for several diseases, including heart attack, stroke, and diabetes. If I lose some weight, those risks will go down."
Perceived self-efficacy	"It's realistic for me to stop eating so many calories each day and get to the gym several times a week to burn some calories."
Outcome expectations	*Physical and material:* "It will be great to fit into some of my clothes again and I will treat myself to a new pair of jeans when I drop two sizes." *Social:* "My boyfriend will be happy if I can slim down." "I won't miss the dirty looks I get when I take a seat next to someone on the bus who thinks I take up too much room."
Personal health goals	"I'm not sure if I'll ever be able to lose fifty pounds, but I can at least try to lose ten pounds."
Perceived facilitators	"I got this great new pedometer that tracks my steps and syncs to my phone so I can make sure I get in enough activity every day." "I found this website that lets me log my food into an online journal and calculates my calorie intake." "My wife also wants to lose some weight so we can do this together."
Perceived impediments	"It's embarrassing to go to the gym and be around all those physically fit people." "I'm going to have to take two different buses to get to the gym." "My friends are not going to want to give up nachos and beer when we go out for Friday night happy hour."

performances" (Bandura, 1986, p. 391). For example, a person who has come to understand the risks associated with his own state of obesity has the precondition to change behaviors that contribute to obesity, but if this individual believes "I've been overweight for all of my life and I'll always be overweight," then the likelihood that the precondition will lead to changed behavior becomes unlikely. Negative self-efficacy stalls the behavior change process in this case. Of key importance for health promotion planners and implementers is the understanding that participants must believe that they have the power to stop performing a negative behavior (smoking, for example) and perform a positive behavior (regular exercise, for example) in order to successfully achieve desired behaviors.

Outcome Expectations

The consequences associated with particular behaviors influence whether or not an individual might engage in the behavior. SCT refers to the consequences as outcome expectations. In particular, an individual may anticipate certain physical and material outcomes and social outcomes to result from changes in behaviors.

Physical and Material Outcomes   A change in an individual's behavior may be expected to result in physical outcomes and sometimes material outcomes associated with those physical outcomes. For example, a woman who enrolls in a stop-smoking program anticipates a reduction in a chronic cough and an improvement in the taste of her food. Additionally, she expects more money in her wallet as a result of no longer purchasing cigarettes or not having to wash her clothes as frequently as a result of no longer smoking cigarettes (Bandura, 2004).

Social Outcomes   Changes in an individual's behavior may also be expected to result in social outcomes, such as approval or disapproval from one's surrounding social groups. For example, the woman who stops smoking may desire to eliminate the disapproval of her behavior by her children that results from her smoking habit. In turn, she desires their approval if she is able to successfully stop smoking. She may also desire to eliminate the disapproval seen on the faces of her nonsmoking coworkers each time she departs the office for a smoke break (Bandura, 2004).

Personal Health Goals

Personal goals surrounding health habits set the course for behavior change. Goals can be viewed as long term or short term. Long-term health behavior change goals can be a challenge given that, for many people, current habits are a far cry from the desired set of habits. These individuals may be overwhelmed by the challenge, which in turn can alter their perceived self-efficacy. SCT encourages short-term goals that are less daunting than longer-term goals (Bandura, 2004). For example, an obese man may have a long-term goal to lose one hundred pounds in order to achieve a healthy body mass index. However, a one-hundred-pound weight loss is daunting; many factors can intervene over the course of the time it takes to lose one hundred pounds. A goal to begin with a ten-pound weight loss within a shorter time frame is likely to be viewed as attainable and success made more likely. Short-term successes can lead to the setting (or resetting) of new goals.

Perceived Facilitators and Perceived Impediments

Last, the perceived facilitators and impediments are important constructs in SCT and directly influence self-efficacy as well (Bandura, 2004). Smokers may perceive that their success in stopping smoking will be facilitated by the use of a nicotine substitute. As such, use of the nicotine substitute increases self-efficacy and boosts confidence in success. An impediment to the successes of would-be ex-smokers might be a fear of weight gain. Moderation of the impact of such an impediment might come in the form of techniques to avoid weight gain during the stop-smoking effort. Smokers may be advised to stock their refrigerator with carrots and celery sticks as they start an effort to stop smoking so as to decrease the likelihood of snacking on less healthy, higher calorie snacks when struck by a craving. An additional example would be a woman who embarks on a new exercise program. She may perceive that her efforts are facilitated by the accompaniment of a friend to the workout facility. An impediment may be lack of transportation to the workout facility or the loneliness of going about it without a friend.

Given the importance of self-efficacy among the constructs of SCT, Bandura (1997) describes methods for increasing self-efficacy in people who desire to change health behaviors:

*   *Observational learning (social and peer modeling)*—people benefit from seeing people similar to themselves achieving successful behavior change. Testimonials from "someone who's been there" fit this category. Consider commercial advertising for stop-smoking and weight-loss programs and note the frequent use of testimonials.

*   *Mastery experience*—practicing a new behavior in small steps, enabling short-term success to be achieved while gradually increasing the challenge.

*   *Improving physical and emotional states*—people attempting behavior change benefit from stress reduction and being well rested, along with enhanced positive emotions about the challenge of behavior change (by avoiding negative terminology and replacing it with positive terms).

*   *Verbal persuasion*—providing strong encouragement in order to boost confidence. Simply telling a person "You can do it!" can help to improve self-efficacy.

Discussion

One can see that understanding the constructs of SCT provides valuable insight for a health promotion professional or health educator. Providing participants with knowledge of health risks and benefits of various health behaviors, enhancing their beliefs in their ability to change behaviors, helping them to establish attainable goals, and providing activities and programming that promote facilitators and limit impediments can lead to a strong foundation for successful outcomes for participants.

The literature is rich with studies of theory-based strategies, including SCT. One example is a program aimed at reducing fat intake and increasing intake of fruits and vegetables (Ammerman, Lindquist, Lohr, & Hersey, 2002). Improvements made were attributed to the constructs of goal setting, along with family and social support strategies. Other studies demonstrate an association between self-efficacy and exercise adherence in adults (Brassington, Atienza, Perczek, DiLorenzo, & King, 2002). Many community-based programs have employed SCT, including impaired driving prevention programs, efforts to prevent adolescent smoking, and heart disease prevention programs.

Transtheoretical Model of Behavior Change

As its name implies, the **transtheoretical model (TTM)** of behavior change integrates principles and processes from several theories of behavior change. Prochaska, DiClemente, and Norcross (1992) proposed TTM after extensive work with smoking cessation and the treatment of drug and alcohol addiction. The model subsequently was adapted for use in a variety of health promotion and health behavior change settings. Using **stages of change**, TTM describes health behavior as a process and notes that at any given time individuals are at varying levels of readiness for change.

TTM differs from SCT in that it assumes that people with problem behaviors are not all beginning at the same stage of readiness to change those behaviors; in fact, one of the TTM stages of change is a stage at which people are not ready for change at all. The practical application of this model for a health promotion professional is to tailor the health promotion message according to each individual's stage of change. Applying a universal health promotion message to a group of individuals assumes that all the individuals in that group are all at the same stage of readiness to make changes in their behavior. Alternatively, matching individual messages with an individual's stage of readiness may be more meaningful and thus more effective (Snelling & Stevenson, 2003).

In TTM, there are six stages of change (see figure 2.2) and ten processes of change. These stages are described in the following.

transtheoretical model (TTM)
theoretical model that describes health behavior as a process characterized by stages of readiness to change

stages of change
varying levels of readiness that a person reaches while changing a health behavior

Stages of Change
Precontemplation   During the precontemplation stage, the individual is not thinking about or intending to eliminate a problem behavior or adopt

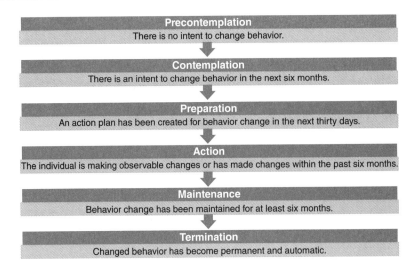

Figure 2.2   Transtheoretical Model: Stages of Change

a healthy behavior in the next six months. Some planners may choose to exclude individuals in the precontemplation phase from programming efforts. However, TTM includes this stage in the model to emphasize that health promotion efforts should not exclude precontemplators. In many cases these individuals lack awareness of the problem behavior or they have regressed to this stage after an unsuccessful attempt to change the behavior (DiClemente, Schlundt, & Gemmell, 2004).

Contemplation   During the contemplation stage, an individual has developed intentions to change a particular behavior within the next six months. Contemplators are aware of the positive benefits of changing their behavior, but are often held back by what are perceived to be negative factors influencing their actions. *Ambivalence* is often a word used to describe this stage; there is a tendency for some individuals to be chronic contemplators (Glanz, Rimer, & Viswanath, 2008). A challenge for program planners is to reduce this ambivalence in order to move contemplators to the next stage: preparation.

Preparation   During the preparation stage, the individual has clear intentions to change a problem behavior or adopt a healthy behavior in the next thirty days. Presumably, the ambivalence of the contemplation stage has been resolved to the point at which the individual believes that the benefits outweigh the negatives. Preparers may have an action plan, often as a result of a prior attempt to change the behavior (DiClemente, Schlundt, & Gemmell, 2004; Glanz, Rimer, & Viswanath, 2008). Many health promotion programs begin at levels appropriate for people in the preparation stage—participants will need to be recruited—but those in the preparation stage are ready enough to sign up for health promotion programs, such as weight-loss or smoking-cessation programs (Glanz, Rimer, & Viswanath, 2008).

Action   During the action stage, an individual is making observable changes in behavior or has made observable changes in behavior within the past six months. According to TTM, an individual in the action stage is halfway through the behavior change process (stage 4 of 6). However, it is worth noting that many other theories or models of health behavior change begin at this stage. It is well established that individuals who change behavior may be likely to relapse and spiral back to a previous stage of readiness. Those who did not experience the efforts that are part of the preparation stage as described in TTM may be particularly vulnerable to relapse due to a lack of preparation (DiClemente, Schlundt, & Gemmell, 2004). According to TTM, this is an important consideration for program planners—the early stages and preparatory steps may be key to successful behavior change.

Maintenance   During the maintenance stage, the individual has successfully changed a behavior and has maintained that change for at least six months. Individuals at this stage are at a lower risk of relapse than those in the action stage but also apply their "change processes" less frequently than those in the action stage (Glanz, Rimer, & Viswanath, 2008). In other words, the strategies employed to help change the behavior in the first place are not used as much during maintenance. For example, individuals stop going to support group meetings or journaling as they did previously. Glanz, Rimer, and Viswanath (2008) described data from the 1990 surgeon general's report that revealed that among people who had refrained from smoking for twelve consecutive months, the rate of relapse to regular smoking was 43%. When individuals abstained from smoking for five consecutive years, the rate of relapse to regular smoking was only 7%. Program planners should consider the importance of the ongoing practice of change processes for those in maintenance (as opposed to a celebration and graduation of sorts that implies that individuals are no longer at risk of relapse).

Termination   Individuals in the termination phase have achieved a complete change in behavior with no risk of relapse. People in the termination stage are said to have 100% self-efficacy and their behavior has become permanent and automatic (Glanz, Rimer, & Viswanath, 2008).

Processes of Change

TTM also describes ten **processes of change** among its constructs. These processes are the activities used by individuals to progress through the six stages of change previously described. Each process is actually a category that includes multiple interventions, methods, and techniques. Understanding the stages of change and how behavior shifts (the processes) is a valuable tool for behavior change programs.

The ten processes are divided into two groups: (1) affective and cognitive experiential processes (thoughts and feelings) and (2) behavioral processes. Each process of change and a description are provided in table 2.2 (Glanz, Rimer, & Viswanath, 2008; Prochaska, DiClemente, & Norcross, 1992).

Additional constructs in the TTM include decision balance and self-efficacy. Decision balance simply refers to the individual's view of the pros and cons of changing a behavior. Self-efficacy in TTM is two pronged: confidence in one's ability to sustain new behaviors across various situations and the temptations to forego new behaviors and relapse to former behaviors.

Discussion

TTM is a robust model with numerous constructs that comprise six stages of change, ten processes of change, and the additional constructs of decision balance and self-efficacy. Glanz, Rimer, and Viswanath (2008) describe several assumptions related to TTM and its application to behavior change intervention programs. Among those assumptions, and perhaps the most directly applicable to health promotion programmers, are these two:

1. A majority of at-risk populations are not prepared for action and will not be served effectively by traditional action-oriented behavior change programs.

2. Specific processes and principles of change should be matched to specific stages to maximize efficacy. (DiClemente, Schlundt, & Gemmell, 2004, p. 103)

There are numerous studies examining TTM interventions. In fact, it has been described as the dominant model of behavior change (Armitage, 2009). TTM has been applied widely to numerous health behaviors including those described in this book's part 2, "Health Behaviors." It is most frequently used in the development and design of smoking-cessation programs (Glanz, Rimer, & Viswanath, 2008). Studies reveal support for

Table 2.2   Processes of Change

Change Process	Description
Experiential Processes	
Consciousness raising	The individual seeks new information to gain understanding about the problem behavior in general and how it affects him or her personally. Actions include feedback, observation, confrontations, interpretations, bibliotherapy (selected reading), and media campaigns.
Dramatic relief	The individual experiences emotions related to behaviors and expresses feelings about the problem behavior and potential solutions. Actions include role-playing, personal testimony, and grieving.
Environmental reevaluation	The individual assesses how personal behavior affects the surrounding physical and social environment as well as the people in it. Actions include empathy training, interventions, testimonials, and public service announcements.
Self-reevaluation	The individual assesses his or her self-image, comparing the image of the self with the unhealthy behavior to an image of self without the unhealthy behavior. Actions include value clarification, imagery, and exposure to health role models.
Social liberation	The individual has access to alternative resources and assistance for behavior change. Resources may be broad such as no-smoking zones or dining areas free of unhealthy choices or may be more specific for particular populations that are sometimes underserved (e.g., minority health initiatives, health promotion for homosexuals, etc.).
Behavioral Processes	
Helping relationships	The individual develops trust, acceptance, and support during attempts to change a problem behavior. Actions include building rapport, therapeutic alliances, and calls to counselors or other support persons.
Self-liberation	The individual makes a commitment to change a problem behavior, including belief in the ability to change. Actions include decision-making therapy, new year's resolutions, public testimony, logotherapy (psychotherapy based on acceptance of self), and commitment-enhancing techniques.
Counterconditioning	The individual replaces problem behaviors with healthy behaviors. Actions include relaxation techniques, desensitization, affirmations, and other forms of positive self-talk.
Reinforcement management	The individual establishes a reward system for successes in behavior change. Actions include rewarding oneself or being rewarded by others for particular achievements in the behavior change process.
Stimulus control	The individual identifies and removes triggers for the problem behavior and replaces those with healthy or nonproblematic prompts. Actions include avoidance, rearrangement of environment, and adding prompts and techniques to cope with temptations.

and criticism of TTM, but making general conclusions is difficult. Many programs have applied only portions of TTM, with minimal consistency regarding which portions are applied. This is contrary to the concept of transtheory.

One review study of TTM (Armitage, 2009) made several conclusions. First, the stages of change may be better collapsed into two phases: motivational and volitional. Second, dividing audiences and targeting them based on which change stage they're in seems preferable to targeting people based on factors such as age or gender. Third, most criticisms of TTM are based on its stages of change; the processes of change may be the more favorable part of TTM, but are less studied. Armitage (2009) examined programs that used processes of change to help smokers to quit, to encourage low-income employees to engage in more physical activity, and to influence members of the public to consume less amounts of alcohol.

Health Belief Model

health belief model (HBM)
theoretical model characterized by value-expectancy theories, which explain that behavior is influenced by values and expectations

Developed in the 1950s, the **health belief model (HBM)** was an attempt by social psychologists at the US Public Health Service to better understand a widespread reluctance of people to access disease prevention services (Snelling & Stevenson, 2003). To describe the origins of HBM, cognitive theorists often identify **value-expectancy theories**, which explain that behavior results from an individual's value of the outcome of the behavior and the expectation that a particular action or actions will lead to the outcome. When applied to health behaviors, it can be assumed that individuals value the avoidance of illness and getting well and expect particular health-related activities lead to improved health and disease prevention (Glanz, Rimer, & Viswanath, 2008).

value-expectancy theories
theories that explain that behavior results from an individual's value of the outcome of the behavior and the expectation that a particular action or actions will lead to the outcome

There are six primary constructs of HBM, each of which is described in the following sections and in table 2.3.

Perceived Susceptibility

Perceived susceptibility refers to an individual's belief that he or she will contract a particular disease or condition. People vary in their feelings of personal vulnerability to a particular condition, depending on a variety of factors, including family history (heart disease, for example), demographics (women and breast cancer, for example), age (Alzheimer's disease, for example), and so on. People who believe they are strongly susceptible to a disease or condition may be more likely to alter behavior to prevent it, whereas those who feel they are not susceptible have little motivation to change a particular behavior (Glanz, Rimer, & Viswanath, 2008; Snelling & Stevenson, 2003).

Perceived Severity

Perceived severity refers to an individual's belief regarding the seriousness of a particular condition or disease and how it would ultimately affect that

Table 2.3   Constructs of the Health Belief Model

Construct	Description
Perceived susceptibility	Individual's belief that he or she will experience negative health outcomes
Perceived severity	Individual's belief about the seriousness of negative health outcomes, physically and socially
Perceived benefits	Individual's belief that behavior change will have a positive impact on health outcomes
Perceived barriers	Individual's belief about the negative impact of making a behavior change (cost, convenience, comfort, etc.)
Cues to action	Triggers that motivate individuals toward a change in behavior
Self-efficacy	Given all conditions and factors, individual's belief that he or she is capable of making the contemplated behavior change

individual's life. Individuals may consider the severity of a condition in terms of its physical consequences (for example, pain, disability, mortality, etc.) and its social consequences (impact on ability to maintain career or impact on family). An example of severity is that people consider developing cancer to be more severe than contracting the flu. Note that perceived susceptibility and severity are often referred to collectively as *perceived threat* (Glanz, Rimer, & Viswanath, 2008; Snelling & Stevenson, 2003).

Perceived Benefits

Perceived benefits refer to an individual's belief that a particular intervention is feasible and efficacious. Individuals who perceive a threat to their health and well-being may not automatically accept any and all recommended interventions; rather, they must believe that a particular action reduces the threat. Aside from personal health benefits, individuals may also consider other benefits of a changed behavior (for example, cost savings, increased approval from friends and family, etc.) (Glanz, Rimer, & Viswanath, 2008; Snelling & Stevenson, 2003).

Perceived Barriers

Perceived barriers are those actions or outcomes that the individual perceives are potentially negative aspects of a health intervention. Individuals often consider interventions in terms of cost, time commitment, convenience, side effects, and their agreeableness.

Cues to Action

Cues to action are described as the triggers that motivate individuals toward action to change behavior. Perhaps a personal health scare or that of a loved one could trigger an interest in changing a behavior associated with the health condition. Although early versions of HBM included cues to action as a construct, referring to such things as "bodily events" (Glanz, Rimer, & Viswanath, 2008, p. 49) or outside events such as a public service announcement, Glanz, Rimer, and Viswanath (2008) have noted that this construct is not well studied and is difficult to study. It remains a construct in HBM and, again, can refer to techniques to activate readiness to change.

Self-Efficacy

Self-efficacy in HBM is defined in the same way it is defined in social cognitive theory: the "conviction that one can successfully execute the behavior required to produce the outcomes," as described by Bandura (1997). In relation to other constructs of HBM, individuals may perceive a threat to their health (perceived susceptibility and severity) and must believe that a particular intervention will help them reduce the threat without unacceptable cost (benefit minus barriers). However, they must perceive that they are personally capable (self-efficacious) of overcoming identified barriers to yield the desired outcome.

Rosenstock (1974) described the first four constructs in conjunction with one another as follows: *perceived* threat (*susceptibility* and *severity*) serves as the motivation to do something, whereas the *perceived benefits* of an intervention minus the *barriers* help to guide the individual toward a particular action (see figure 2.3).

Discussion

To better understand HBM, consider the following scenarios in which some but not all of the necessary constructs are in place for an individual to change an unhealthy behavior.

• A smoker perceives a threat to his health and thinks that a smoking-cessation program will offer sufficient benefit to his health. He

| Perceived threat (susceptibility plus severity) | =======================> | Motivation to change |
| Perceived benefits minus perceived barriers | =======================> | Guide efforts toward making the change |

Figure 2.3   Health Belief Model in Summary

perceives that the barriers to participating in the program are out-weighed by the benefits. However, the individual has tried to stop smoking before, potentially several times. The recall of the failed past attempts to stop smoking can jeopardize his self-efficacy in this case.

- A sedentary person has sufficient perceived threats to motivate her behavior change to become more active. Her path is to join the local YMCA at the start of the new year in order to participate in a regular exercise program. Perhaps she has underestimated the barriers; in January, it is cold and dark when she leaves work in the evening and the weather may not be conducive to making the trip to the YMCA on a regular basis, or she is going to the YMCA on her own and wonders who will miss her if she skips?

There is widespread availability of research that uses HBM to study health behaviors and examines HBM interventions to change behaviors. These studies include examinations of breast cancer screenings, colonos-copies, AIDS-related behaviors, risky sexual behaviors, eating behaviors, stop-smoking interventions, and calcium intake and exercise, to name a few (Carpenter, 2010; Glanz, Rimer, & Viswanath, 2008).

Over time, there have been proposals to increase the complexity of HBM (including cues to action and self-efficacy) and potentially improve its effectiveness in predicting successful behavior change across a wide area of health issues. Although some early reviews of the utility of HBM were supportive of its use (Glanz, Rimer, & Viswanath, 2008), more recent reviews of HBM in its simplest form (not always including cues to action and self-efficacy) have not been as supportive. The reviews, however, do make a case for increasing its complexity through the addition of self-efficacy or combin-ing it with other models in order to improve its utility (Carpenter, 2010).

Theory of Planned Behavior

The **theory of planned behavior (TPB)** was developed from theory of reasoned action (TRA), which essentially states that behaviors result from intentions (Ajzen, 1985). In turn, a person's intention to engage in a particular behavior is a function of (1) the individual's personal attitude toward the behavior, whether it is positive or negative, and (2) the individual's perception of **subjective norms** related to the behavior, the social pressures to perform or not perform a particular behavior. It follows that an individual is more likely to perform a behavior when it is viewed positively by that individual and also when the individual believes that others whom they value approve of that performance (Ajzen, 1985).

theory of planned behavior (TPB)
theory in which an individual's intention to engage in a behavior is influenced by personal attitude toward the behavior and the individual's perception of subjective norms related to the behavior

subjective norm
a factor of normative beliefs, that is, what valued others think about the behavior to be performed or eliminated and how motivated is the individual to seek approval from those valued others

Glanz, Rimer, and Viswanath (2008) reported that TRA was effective in explaining and predicting behavior when that behavior was considered to be under volitional control of the individual. Because it was less clear that the TRA components would be similarly effective when behaviors were less volitionally controlled by an individual, Ajzen and others added the construct of *perceived control* over a behavior and, in turn, expanded TRA into TPB (Ajzen, 1985, 1991; Glanz, Rimer, & Viswanath, 2008).

TPB then has three primary constructs:

• Personal attitude

• Subjective norm

• Perceived control

TPB allows that the intended behavior is a goal established by an individual, but explains that there are factors beyond the control of the individual that may interfere with the goal being pursued. Each of the three described constructs has underlying factors; the individual's beliefs about each construct are among those factors (see figure 2.4).

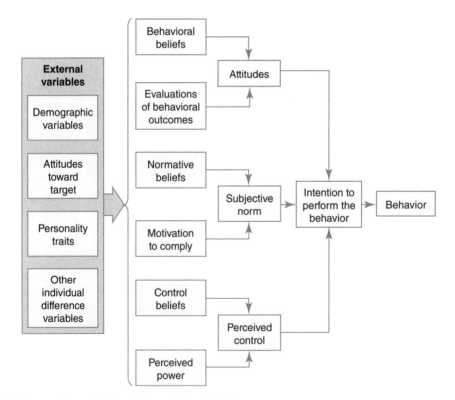

Figure 2.4   Theory of Reasoned Action and Theory of Planned Behavior

Attitude

The construct of attitude toward the behavior is a function of the individual's behavioral beliefs about the behavior and his or her evaluation of the results of performing the behavior. Individuals who believe that favorable, important outcomes will result if a behavior is performed are considered to have a positive attitude toward that behavior. A negative attitude results if an individual believes that negative valued outcomes would result from performance of the behavior (Glanz, Rimer, & Viswanath, 2008).

For example, an individual may believe that smoking is a harmful behavior. The individual evaluates the outcomes of not smoking and determines that one outcome would be weight gain. Because the individual values not being overweight, the individual may have a negative attitude toward quitting smoking in this case, which in turn affects his or her intent to stop smoking.

Subjective Norm

The construct of subjective norm is a factor of normative beliefs, that is, what do valued others think about the behavior to be performed or eliminated and how motivated is the individual to seek approval from those valued others. A positive subjective norm occurs when an individual believes that valued others approve of a particular behavior and the individual is motivated to seek approval from those others (Glanz, Rimer, & Viswanath, 2008).

For example, a young man may consider smoking to be harmful and views a positive outcome from quitting. However, the young man may have a parent who not only smokes but also has a view that "we are all going to die anyway, so why bother quitting?" The young man then has a negative subjective norm that influences his intention to stop smoking.

Perceived Control

The original TRA was based only on the described constructs of attitude and subjective norms. That theory potentially infers that performing a behavior is under volitional control. As previously described, **perceived control** was added as a construct to TRA as it developed into TPB (Ajzen, 1985; Glanz, Rimer, & Viswanath, 2008). The perceived control construct is influenced by the individual's control beliefs, those beliefs that facilitate or inhibit factors that exist related to the behavior and the individual's perception of the power of these factors to facilitate the behavior or impose a barrier to it (Glanz, Rimer, & Viswanath, 2008).

perceived control
refers to people's perceptions of their ability to perform a given behavior

Volitional control represents a very important part of TPB in that it is the construct that sets it apart from TRA. As such, it is important to consider the factors that influence an individual's volitional control over a particular intended behavior. Those factors are classified as either internal factors or external factors.

internal factors
perceived possession of personal characteristics that influence an individual's ability to control his or her behavior

Internal factors   **Internal factors** include the very general perceived possession of personal characteristics that influence an individual's ability to control his or her behavior, as well as the specific factors listed in the following (Ajzen, 1985):

Information, Skills, and Abilities

* A woman may intend to participate in regular exercise. However, if she lacks knowledge about resources, safe ways to begin an exercise program, how to strength train, and so on, then volitional control is reduced.

Willpower

* A man may intend to abstain from tobacco use, but is unable to say no when his best buddies, who are smokers, insist that he join them for a tailgate party at which a significant amount of smoking will take place.

Emotions

external factors
situational and environmental factors that influence an individual's ability to control his or her behavior, including opportunity and time and dependence on others

* A recently divorced woman intends to abstain from alcohol use, but finds herself extremely sad on her first Christmas Eve alone. Overwhelmed by her emotions, she may turn to the very behavior she seeks to avoid.

External Factors   There are two major categories of **external factors**, described in the following (Ajzen, 1985).

OPPORTUNITY AND TIME

A woman signs up for a week-long weight loss camp at a location that requires her to travel via plane. If a hurricane takes place and the flight is canceled, none of the other factors of her intention to lose weight are changed, but the opportunity to engage in weight loss behaviors is affected by circumstances beyond her control. Alternatively, perhaps her job situation has changed such that she no longer has the time to go to the camp as she had intended. In either case, the likelihood that she still intends to lose weight is great and the behavior may occur with a different opportunity or more time.

DEPENDENCE ON OTHERS

The more any behavior depends on other people, the less there is volitional control for the individual. For example, two college roommates sign up for a safe sex workshop hosted by their campus health center. If one roommate decides she is unable to go, the other is unlikely to go. If the instructor of the workshop cancels the session, neither roommate will go.

For time and opportunity and dependence on others, such barriers may result in only temporary changes in the intentions of individuals to engage in particular behaviors. In the best case, performance of the behavior may be only delayed. However, if factors beyond an individual's control are numerous and repeated, it can ultimately result in more permanent changes in intentions (Ajzen, 1985).

TPB describes a structure for interventions to improve health behaviors for target populations. Through the identification of behavioral beliefs, normative beliefs, and control beliefs, interventions are designed to adjust those beliefs in turn to adjust attitude, subject norms, and perceived control in such a way that individuals' intentions to perform healthy behaviors are favorably oriented (Glanz, Rimer, & Viswanath, 2008).

There is evidence that TPB has been successfully used in health promotion settings in which smoking, exercise, mammography, and sexually transmitted disease prevention were the targets (Glanz, Rimer, & Viswanath, 2008). Glanz, Rimer, and Viswanath (2008) noted the strength of perceived behavioral control, in particular, as a predictor of behavior change, and has recommended its consideration during the design of health promotion interventions.

Historical Perspective

In the 1980s, the health science community initiated a concerted effort to identify interventions that might help people alter behaviors associated with particular diseases (Institute of Medicine, 1982). The early interventions were largely in the form of public education campaigns and targeted at individuals. Numerous publications referred to HBM and TRA-TPB as the foundation of such efforts (Glanz, Rimer, & Viswanath, 2008).

In 1964, the US surgeon general released America's first report on smoking and health. Many health education campaigns ensued and many people stopped smoking. Eventually, these came to be considered initial gains. The focus of HBM and TRA-TPB on raising awareness about risks of unhealthy behaviors and benefits of changing those behaviors seemed to require additional constructs to better reach larger numbers of people and affect a wider variety of health behaviors. To be sure, the role of health knowledge in shaping attitudes and beliefs was necessary, but perhaps not sufficient to make initial gains become lasting behavior changes (Orleans & Cassidy, 2008).

Bandura's SCT (1986) identified knowledge of health risks as a construct, similar to HBM and TPB, but added external determinants of behavior and offered perceived facilitators and perceived impediments as constructs. Described as the dominant behavior change theory or model even today, SCT helped shift the focus from *why* change unhealthy behaviors toward the *how* to change those unhealthy behaviors and replace them with healthy ones. With this expanded focus came suggestions for modifying one's surrounding environments so as to reduce temptation and relapse, improving self-efficacy for behavior change.

A similar shift also took place with regard to the target of behavior change interventions. Early efforts targeted individuals. Later models targeted populations. The stages of change model served as a way to avoid a one-size-fits-all approach that inevitably results when targeting populations. The model's recognition that behavior change is a process with recognizable steps enabled tailoring of interventions; it is said to have had a significant impact on how health behavior intervention programs are designed and implemented (Orleans & Cassidy, 2008). As noted previously in this chapter, the tendency of some programs to begin at the action stage, assuming that all participants are indeed ready to change behaviors, can be problematic, particularly in the case of individuals who relapse to problem behaviors. Those individuals would not have had the benefit of completing preparation for behavior change and thus would not necessarily re-prepare for another attempt, understanding that relapses are not necessarily failures, but part of the behavior change process.

Summary

This chapter provided an introduction to four theories of behavior, along with evidence of the application of those theories in health behavior change settings. A visual of the constructs associated with these theories is found in table 2.4. Some aspects of the theories are similar, and others are unique. Additional theories also exist; however, the four described are considered the dominant theories in the field at this time.

Perhaps the most significant construct that stretches across the four dominant theories is self-efficacy—a person's belief in his or her own ability to be successful in a given situation. It would follow that interventions

Table 2.4   Presented Theories and Their Constructs

SCT	TTM	HBM	TPB
Knowledge of health risks and benefits	Stages of change:	Perceived susceptibility	Perceived attitude
Perceived self-efficacy	• Precontemplation	Perceived severity	Subjective norms
Outcome expectations	• Contemplation	Perceived benefits	Perceived control
Personal health goals	• Preparation	Perceived barriers	Internal:
Perceived facilitators	• Action	Cues to action	• Information, skills, and abilities
Perceived impediments	• Maintenance	Self-efficacy	• Willpower
	• Termination		• Emotions
	Processes of change:		External:
	• Consciousness raising		• Opportunity and time
	• Dramatic relief		• Dependence on others
	• Environmental reevaluation		
	• Self-reevaluation		
	• Social liberation		
	• Helping relationships		
	• Self-liberation		
	• Counterconditioning		
	• Reinforcement management		
	• Stimulus control		
	• Decision balance (pros and cons)		
	• Self-efficacy		

targeting people with strong senses of self-efficacy are more likely to succeed than those targeting people with weak senses of self-efficacy. As such, behavior change theories include various other constructs designed to help planners of interventions boost the self-efficacy of people involved in behavior change intervention.

Knowledge and understanding of behavior change theories is but the first step in the program planning process in a health promotion setting. A health promotion program planner must decide which theory or theories are most applicable to a particular setting. Glanz, Rimer, and Viswanath (2008) asserted that the strength of health promotion interventions will be enhanced through the application of multiple theories but warn that health promoters should take care to avoid redundancy, overlap, and difficulty in interpretation.

Although chapter 3 describes program planning based on theory, it should be emphasized that prior to targeting program participants and customizing health behavior interventions, understanding the contributing factors of behavior and the impact of the environment are critical.

KEY TERMS

1. **Theory:** an explanation intended to account for the actions that people take or do not take to promote health

2. **Models:** theory-based planning framework that helps guide program creation and evaluation

3. **Social cognitive theory (SCT):** theoretical model that frames individual behavior as a response to observational learning from the surrounding environment

4. **Reciprocal determinism:** the concept that individuals are a product of their environments and also help to create those environments

5. **Self-efficacy:** an individual's perception of his or her capability to execute a course of action necessary to achieve a goal

6. **Transtheoretical model of behavior change (TTM):** theoretical model that describes health behavior as a process characterized by stages of readiness to change

7. **Stages of change:** varying levels of readiness that a person reaches while changing a health behavior

8. **Processes of change:** the covert and overt activities that people use to progress through the six stages of change

9. **Health belief model (HBM):** theoretical model characterized by value-expectancy theories, which explain that behavior is influenced by values and expectations

10. **Value-expectancy theories:** theories that explain that behavior results from an individual's value of the outcome of the behavior and the expectation that a particular action or actions will lead to the outcome

11. **Theory of planned behavior (TPB):** theory in which an individual's intention to engage in a behavior is influenced by personal attitude toward the behavior and the individual's perception of subjective norms related to the behavior

12. **Subjective norm:** a factor of normative beliefs, that is, what valued others think about the behavior to be performed or eliminated and how motivated is the individual to seek approval from those valued others

13. **Perceived control:** refers to people's perceptions of their ability to perform a given behavior.

14. **Internal factors:** perceived possession of personal characteristics that influence an individual's ability to control his or her behavior

15. **External factors:** situational and environmental factors that influence an individual's ability to control his or her behavior, including opportunity and time and dependence on others

REVIEW QUESTIONS

1. Why do we need to study health behavior theories?

2. What are the different theories and models described in the chapter and how do you identify their differences?

3. How are these theories applied to behavior change programs?

STUDENT ACTIVITIES

1. For each of the stages within the stages of change construct, what type of information would be part of a behavior change program? For example, in the precontemplation stage you might consider a social marketing campaign that uses an emotional appeal.

2. For each of the process of change within the transtheoretical model, translate each change process into a short phrase, for example, consciousness raising—just get people thinking about the behavior.

3. Identify one or two constructs that appear in each of the theories or models for behavior change.

4. Which of the approaches to behavior change resonates with you and why?

References

Ajzen, I. (1985). From intentions to actions: A theory of planned behavior. In J. Kuhl & J. Beckman (Eds.), *Action-control: From cognition to behavior* (pp. 11–39). Heidelberg, Germany: Springer.

Ajzen, I. (1991). The theory of planned behavior. *Organization Behavior and Human Decision Processes, 50,* 179–211.

Ammerman, A. S., Lindquist, C. H., Lohr, K. N., & Hersey, J. (2002). The efficacy of behavioral interventions to modify dietary fat and fruit and vegetable intake: A review of the evidence. *Preventive Medicine, 35*(1), 25–41.

Armitage, C.J.I. (2009). Is there utility in the transtheoretical model? *British Journal of Health Psychology, 14,* 195–210.

Bandura, A. (1986). *Social foundations of thought and action: A social cognitive theory.* Englewood Cliffs, NJ: Prentice-Hall.

Bandura, A. (1997). *Self-efficacy: The exercise of control.* New York: W. H. Freeman.

Bandura, A. (2004). Health promotion by social cognitive means. *Health Education & Behavior, 31*(2), 143–164.

Brassington, G. S., Atienza, A. A., Perczek, R. E., DiLorenzo, T. M., & King, A. C. (2002). Intervention-related cognitive versus social mediator of exercise adherence in the elderly. *American Journal of Preventive Medicine, 23*(2 Supplement), 80–86.

Carpenter, C. J. (2010). A meta-analysis of the effectiveness of health belief model variables in predicting behavior. *Health Communication, 25,* 661–669.

Cottrell, R., Girvan, J. T., & McKenzie, J. (2011). *Principles and foundations of health promotion and education* (5th ed.). Upper Saddle River, NJ: Benjamin Cummings.

DiClemente, C. C., Schlundt, D., & Gemmell, L. (2004). Readiness and stages of change in addiction treatment. *American Journal on Addictions, 13*(2), 103–119.

Glanz, K., & Rimer, B. K. (1995). Theory at a glance: A guide for health promotion. In G. G. Gilbert & R. G. Sawyer, *Health education: Creating strategies for school and community health education* (pp. 79–81). Boston: Jones & Bartlett.

Glanz, K., Rimer, B. K., & Viswanath, K. (Eds.). (2008). *Health behavior and health education: Theory, research and practice.* San Francisco: Jossey Bass.

Institute of Medicine. (1982). *Health and behavior: Frontiers of research in the biobehavioral sciences.* D. A. Hamburg, G. R. Elliott, & D. L. Parron (Eds.) Washington, DC: National Academies Press.

Orleans, C. T., & Cassidy, E. F. (2008). Health-related behavior. In A. R. Kovner & J. R. Knickman (Eds.), *Health care delivery in the United States* (9th ed.) (pp. 267–297). New York: Springer.

Prochaska, J. O., DiClemente, C. C., & Norcross, J. C. (1992). In search of how people change: Applications to addictive behaviors. *American Psychiatrist, 47,* 1102–1114.

Rosenstock, I. M. (1974). The health belief model and preventive health behavior. *Health Education Monographs, 2*(4), 354–386.

Snelling, A. M., & Stevenson, M. O. (2003). Using theories and models to support program planning. In *ACSM's worksite health promotion manual: A guide to building and sustaining healthy worksites*. Columbus, MO: Human Kinetics.

CHAPTER 3

PROGRAM PLANNING MODELS

Anastasia Snelling

Health promotion programs that initiate and sustain health behavior change do not happen by chance but are a result of a systematic approach to understanding the factors that influence change in individuals and groups. To develop effective programs, program planners must use a framework or model that ensures that the intended results will be achieved. This chapter presents the most recognized and respected program planning model, the PRECEDE-PROCEED model, as well as four other program planning models. Two of these models are based on the social ecological theory of planning, two are considered consumer-based planning models, and the fifth is considered a community-level program planning model.

These health promotion program models share many of the same elements, but the steps may be different or the models may emphasize different aspects of the planning process. Regardless of which planning model is selected as the basis of a health promotion program, the use of a model is critical. The use of an established model prompts program planners to consider all phases of program planning and ensures a comprehensive, well-designed program. More advanced practitioners may successfully identify the model that best meets the needs of a specific program, population, or setting through review of prior experiences.

LEARNING OBJECTIVES

After reading this chapter, the student will be able to:

- Describe the purpose of program planning models.

- Explain the social ecological model and how it relates to program planning.

- Identify key elements of the PRECEDE-PROCEED model.

- Discuss key elements of the MATCH model.

- Define the elements of health communication planning models.

- Explain the similarities and differences between program planning models and health communication models.

- Summarize why these models are an important step to successful health promotion programs.

Effective Health Promotion Planning

The goal of health promotion program planning is to "intervene" to improve the health of individuals or communities. Hence, program planning centers on gathering assessment information and designing an intervention that will improve the health of populations or decrease the risk of illness, disability, or death.

Different from the health behavior change theories presented in chapter 2 that focus on why and how people make health behavior changes, program planning models serve to guide the development, implementation, and evaluation of a specific health promotion program. A **planning model** is a blueprint for building and improving programs (Crosby & Noar, 2011). Ultimately, in order to address a target behavior and population, program planners must incorporate behavior change theories into program planning models when designing and implementing the intervention.

planning model serves to guide the development, implementation, and evaluation of a specific health promotion program; a blueprint for building and improving programs

Effective planning ensures that practitioners can accomplish the following:

- Understand the health issue the program will be addressing

- Identify the population the program will target

- Identify the policy and educational approaches necessary to bring about or support the desired changes

- Establish a logical program development process

- Set priorities and goals

- Establish objectives to achieve goals

- Assess progress

- Measure impact and outcomes

Often in organizations time is limited; under the pressure of deadlines and demands, there may be a tendency to skip the planning stage. However, following a program planning model process saves health promotion practitioners time in the long run. There may not be one perfect model; however, effective models should be sequential, be adaptable to different populations, and ultimately lead to the intended outcomes of improved health (Glanz, Rimer & Viswanath, 2008).

Social Ecological Model

The twenty-first century has brought a shift from individual-oriented programs to those that encompass environmental strategies. As noted in chapter 1, the determinants of health have expanded our understanding of how and why people make health behavior choices. Health promotion professionals recognize that by making the healthy choice the easy choice in the places people live, work, and learn, people will be more likely to live healthier lives. Further, by extending health promotion programs beyond the individual approach, there is an opportunity to reach a larger population, especially those individuals who are in the precontemplation stage of behavior change. The program planning models included in this chapter reflect a shift from an individual-focus approach to an environment- and community-oriented approach. Chapter 2 presented the social cognitive theory, emphasizing the role of environment and behavior change. An ecological approach is one that considers the role of the environment on the target audience, along with health status, behavior, and skills.

The **social ecological model of planning** is based on the interrelationships of human beings and their environments (Stokols, 1996), recognizing that within the environment there are physical, social, economic, and cultural forces that have the potential to alter health outcomes. The environment is important but not to the exclusion of the individual. This theory includes individual attributes such as genetics, behaviors, and knowledge. Other social and environmental factors are also acknowledged in the theory, such as environmental settings, sectors of influence, and norms and cultures within society (figure 3.1). The social ecological model has made an important contribution to the field of health promotion, particularly with regards to the design of interventions to improve health behaviors. No longer are programs designed only with the individual in mind; they must assess other factors that may either hinder or facilitate the behavior change process.

Figure 3.1 provides a graphic representation of an ecological model for physical activity and healthy eating designed for the United States Department of Agriculture's Dietary Guidelines for Americans. The social ecological model is evident in the PRECEDE-PROCEED model as well as all of the models presented in this chapter.

social ecological model of planning
a planning model based on the interrelationships of human beings and their environments, recognizing that within the environment there are physical, social, economic, and cultural forces that have the potential to alter health outcomes

PRECEDE-PROCEED Model

The **PRECEDE-PROCEED model** is considered the most popular and well-respected model in the field for health promotion program planning. The model was designed in the 1970s and has been widely used by planners and practitioners to guide program design, implementation, and evaluation for a variety of diverse health promotion programs. This model uses an ecological approach to program planning and is considered by many to be the gold standard in health promotion planning due to the extensive assessments that are required prior to any program development is initiated.

PRECEDE-PROCEED model
a nine-phase logic model, using an ecological approach, applied in health promotion program planning

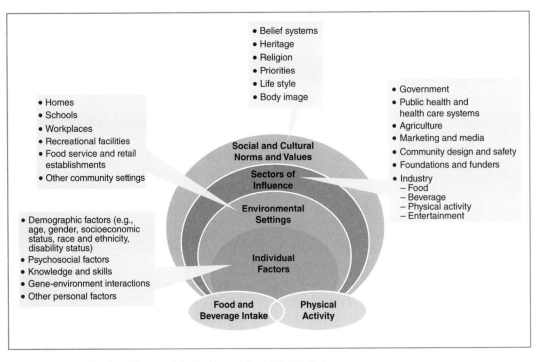

- Belief systems
- Heritage
- Religion
- Priorities
- Life style
- Body image

- Government
- Public health and health care systems
- Agriculture
- Marketing and media
- Community design and safety
- Foundations and funders
- Industry
  - Food
  - Beverage
  - Physical activity
  - Entertainment

- Homes
- Schools
- Workplaces
- Recreational facilities
- Food service and retail establishments
- Other community settings

- Demographic factors (e.g., age, gender, socioeconomic status, race and ethnicity, disability status)
- Psychosocial factors
- Knowledge and skills
- Gene-environment interactions
- Other personal factors

Social and Cultural Norms and Values

Sectors of Influence

Environmental Settings

Individual Factors

Food and Beverage Intake

Physical Activity

Figure 3.1   A Social Ecological Framework for Nutrition and Physical Activity Decisions
Source: US Department of Agriculture and US Department of Health and Human Services (2010).

There is a strong emphasis on gaining a thorough understanding of the health issue, the target audience, and the environment prior to implementing a policy or program. In addition, the model encourages community involvement to ensure community buy in and support, which is essential for sustaining behavior change. Thousands of research studies have examined PRECEDE-PROCEED and numerous articles have been published regarding the model, its applications, and professional commentaries.

The nine-phase logic model is subdivided into two phases: PRECEDE and PROCEED. PRECEDE is an acronym for **p**redisposing, **r**einforcing, and **e**nabling **c**auses in **e**ducational **d**iagnosis and **e**valuation (phases 1 through 4). PROCEED is an acronym for **p**olicy, **r**egulatory, and **o**rganizational **c**onstructs in **e**ducational and **e**nvironmental **d**evelopment (phases 5 through 9).

Phase 1: Social Assessment

In phase 1, social assessment involves an investigation into the quality of life of the target population to accurately understand it. This is best accomplished by involving community members. General quality-of-life information regarding measurable social factors such as unemployment rates, poverty, crime, and population density can be obtained through government offices or other sources. Beyond these statistics, it is critical to engage community members to voice their needs, wants, and desires. Using a combination of statistical data and community voices and opinions results in a more comprehensive and complementary approach to understanding the social factors of a community.

Phase 2: Epidemiological Assessment

In phase 2, epidemiological assessment involves the identification of health issues and associated goals. **Epidemiology** is the study of the distribution and determinants of health-related conditions or events in defined populations and the application of findings to control health problems. In this phase, planners must identify the health issue and the population that is affected by the health issue. Gathering this information and answering relevant questions can be done using health statistics collected by local, state, and national governments or other health organizations. In addition, data from community members themselves, as they explore what health issues are most pressing for their community, should be collected during this phase.

epidemiology
the study of the distribution and determinants of health-related conditions or events in defined populations and the application of findings to control health problems

Phase 3: Behavioral and Environmental Assessment

In phase 3, behavioral and environmental assessment includes the identification of the health behaviors that are associated with the health issue selected in phase 2 and the identification of the key environmental influences that may be promoting or hindering health behavior. Behavioral indicators include factors such as consumption patterns, preventive actions, self-care, and use. Environmental indicators include medical services and economic and community gauges. This type of information can be found in departments of health at the local or state level or through the CDC. Another source for this information could be nonprofit advocacy groups focused on the health status of people in a general area. The environmental indicator data may be available at local or state health offices, or reports may be available at advocacy organizations.

Phase 4: Educational and Ecological Assessment

In phase 4, educational and ecological assessment occurs to identify the factors that will facilitate changes in individual behavior and the environmental context. These types of factors are called *predisposing, enabling,* and *reinforcing.*

- *Predisposing factors* occur at the cognitive level and include knowledge, self-efficacy, attitudes, skills, and beliefs. These antecedents to behavior provide the motivation for the behavior.

- *Enabling factors* help individuals act on the motivation to change behavior. Examples include the presence of walking paths, skills to cook healthy foods, community resources, and laws.

- *Reinforcing factors* are the continuing rewards or incentives to repeat the behavior.

These factors can be concrete or abstract and may come from self, family, coworkers, or peers. These factors can help health promotion planners identify and better understand health-compromising behaviors and health-enhancing behaviors.

Phase 5: Administrative and Policy Assessment

In phase 5, administrative and policy assessment involves the identification of organizational and administrative opportunities and barriers for developing and implementing a program. Opportunities might include local community sentiment or organizational support, financial support, or available staff to support the program. Policy assessment involves identifying existing policies and regulations that either support or discourage the behavior changes that are being advanced. Policies can be found in organizations, local communities, schools, or government. Regardless of where the program is being implemented, it is critical to review the regulations and policies that govern that setting to clearly understand how they will influence the program.

Phase 6: Program Implementation

In phase 6, the program is implemented based on the assessment and planning processes identified in phases 1 through 5. Program implementation can vary based on the results of the assessments and the desires of the target audience. In the early days of health promotion, educational programs were the intervention of choice. Now interventions might include a citywide policy to limit secondhand smoke or a social marketing campaign to encourage physical activity or a text message program to limit drunk driving. It is in this stage that understanding best practices for behavior change meets creative and innovative thinking.

Phases 7, 8, and 9: Evaluation Phases

Phases 7, 8, and 9 are the evaluation phases that comprise three types of evaluation: process, impact, and outcome.

- *Process evaluation* (phase 7) collects information regarding program implementation. Is the program being implemented according to the developed protocol? Were changes to initial plans made and why? Is the program having the reach that was originally anticipated? Process evaluation is valuable for program improvement and replication purposes but does not examine any resulting behavior changes.

* *Impact evaluation* (phase 8) measures the impact of the program. Specifically, what are the measurable changes in predisposing (knowledge, skills, or attitudes), enabling (physical environment or policies), and reinforcing (positive or negative feedback) factors?

* *Outcome evaluation* (phase 9) measures the actual change in health and social benefits or the quality of life for the target participants. This evaluation determines the effect the program had on the community and if the program reached its intended goals.

See table 3.1 for a description of the PRECEDE-PROCEED model components and figure 3.2 for a graphical representation.

Multilevel Approach to Community Health (MATCH)

The **multilevel approach to community health (MATCH) model**, similar to PRECEDE-PROCEED, is considered an ecological model of program planning. The MATCH framework focuses on assessing population health and working with communities to help them identify opportunities for improving community health and to find and implement evidence-based programs and policies to address the identified health issues. As may be seen through the phases identified in table 3.2, less time is dedicated to assessment compared to the PRECEDE-PROCEED model. The emphasis of this model is on program implementation, with more time devoted to intervention planning, program development, and program implementation. Understanding the population and health issue may help health promotion planners decide which of these two models is more appropriate to guide the planned intervention. Figure 3.3 provides a graphic representation of the MATCH model.

Consumer-Based Planning Models for Health Communication

Health communication and social marketing campaigns have become key components of health promotion for a number of reasons. **Consumer-based planning models** focus on the consumer or intended audience, borrowing concepts from the business marketing field and applying those concepts to health promotion. Understanding behavior change through a business marketing approach recognizes that consumers have choices to

multilevel approach to community health (MATCH) model an ecological model of program planning focusing on assessing population health and working with communities to help them identify opportunities for improving community health and to find and implement evidence-based programs and policies that address the identified health issues

consumer-based planning models models that focus on the consumer or intended audience, borrowing concepts from the business marketing field and applying those concepts to health promotion

Table 3.1   PRECEDE-PROCEED Model

Phase	Title	Description
1	Social assessment	Assessment in both objective and subjective terms of high-priority problems for the common good, defined for a population by economic and social indicators and by individuals in terms of their quality of life.
2	Epidemiological assessment	Identification of the extent, distribution, and causes of a health problem in a defined population.
3	Behavioral and environmental assessment	Identification of the specific health-related actions that will most likely cause a health outcome. A systematic assessment of the factors in the social and physical environment that interacts with behavior to produce health effects or quality-of-life outcomes.
4	Educational and ecological assessment	Assessment of the factors that predispose, enable, and reinforce a specific behavior. A predisposing factor is any characteristic of a person or population that motivates behavior prior to the occurrence of the behavior. An enabling factor is any characteristic of the environment that facilitates action and any skill or resource required to attain a specific behavior. A reinforcing behavior is any reward or punishment following or anticipated as a consequence of a behavior, serving to strengthen the motivation for or against the behavior.
5	Administrative and policy assessment	An analysis of the policies, resources, and circumstances prevailing in an organization to facilitate or hinder the development of the health promotion program.
6	Implementation	The act of converting program objectives into actions through policy changes, regulation, and organization.
7	Process evaluation	Assessment of the program including number of individuals reached by the program or the feedback of the program from participants.
8	Impact evaluation	Assessment of program effects including changes in predisposing, enabling, and reinforcing factors, as well as behavioral and environmental changes.
9	Outcome evaluation	Assessment of the effect of a program, including changes in health and social benefits or quality of life.

Source: Green and Kreuter (2005).

make when selecting health behaviors. If a health promotion program is to achieve success, program planners need to consider their "competition" and apply applicable business marketing concepts to promote, or "sell," health behavior change. In business marketing there is a financial exchange for the customer between money and a product; in health marketing, the "product" is a health behavior and improved health outcomes, and the "cost" to the customer is time, effort, and motivation for a change.

Effective communications campaigns raise awareness of and share information about health issues to large audiences and are usually considered the first step in the behavior change process. Also, effective campaigns may motivate individuals to act. Consistent messaging over a period of time

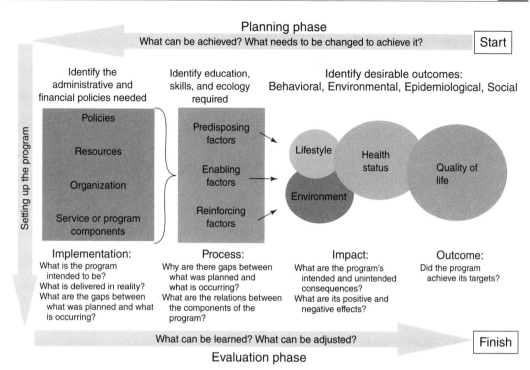

Figure 3.2   PRECEDE-PROCEED Model

Source: Green (2009).

Table 3.2   MATCH Phases and Steps

Phase	Name	Activities
1	Goal selection	Select health status goals
		Select high-priority population(s)
		Identify health behavior goals
		Identify environmental factor goals
2	Intervention planning	Identify the targets of the intervention
		Select intervention objectives
		Identify mediators of the intervention objectives
		Select intervention approaches
3	Program development	Create program units or components
		Select or develop curricula and create intervention guides
		Develop session plans
		Create or acquire instructional materials, projects, and resources
4	Implementation preparations	Facilitate adoption, implementation, and maintenance
		Select and train individuals to implement the program
5	Evaluation	Conduct process evaluation
		Measure impact
		Monitor outcomes

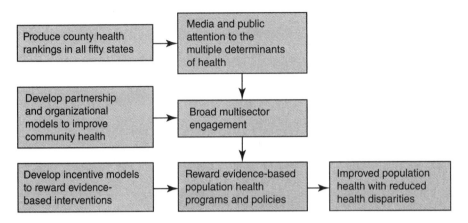

Figure 3.3   MATCH Model
Source: Kindig, Booske, and Remington (2010).

sustains the message to the target audience. As technology and communication tools develop and change, health promotion messages can be more diverse and targeted to broader or more specific audiences. With the recent, significant increase in social marketing to promote healthy behavior among populations, health communication campaigns have become an important strategy in health promotion activities.

Health promotion messages are communicated through numerous methods that can be categorized by the following:

- Mass media (e.g., television, radio, billboards)

- Small media (e.g., brochures, posters)

- Social media (e.g., Facebook, Twitter, web logs)

- Interpersonal communication (e.g., one-on-one or group education)

The Community Preventive Services Task Force (www.communityguide.org) is an independent, nonfederal, unpaid body, appointed by the director of the CDC. It is composed of sixteen members who represent a broad range of research, practice, and policy expertise in community preventive services, public health, health promotion, and disease prevention. The task force was established in 1996 by the US Department of Health and Human Services to provide evidence-based recommendations regarding community preventive services, programs, and policies that are effective in saving lives, increasing longevity, and improving Americans' quality of life. This group recommends health communication campaigns that use multiple channels to facilitate adoption and maintenance of health-promoting behaviors (e.g., increased physical activity through pedometer distribution combined with walking campaigns).

The two most prominent health communication models are CDCynergy, developed by the CDC, and *Making Health Communication Programs Work,* developed by the National Cancer Institute. These models are similar to one another and are described in the following sections.

CDCynergy

CDCynergy (www.cdc.gov/healthcommunication/CDCynergy) was developed by the Office of Communication at the CDC. The steps or phases of this model closely resemble those of the PRECEDE-PROCEED model, although CDCynergy clearly emphasizes marketing and business communication concepts that include population feedback, segmentation principles, and targeted communication strategies.

The CDCynergy model emphasizes a process that involves the following actions:

CDCynergy
a planning model developed by the CDC that emphasizes marketing and business communication concepts that include population feedback, segmentation principles, and target communication strategies

- Using research to describe and determine the causes of the health issue

- Describing the audience affected by the health issue

- Exploring a range of strategies to address the issue or problem

- Developing a comprehensive communication plan that includes audience research, pretesting, production, and launch

- Planning for and conducting evaluation activities throughout the entire process

Phase 1: Understanding the Problem

Phase 1 is identifying and fully understanding the problem, determining who is being affected by the problem, and assessing the factors that will affect the direction of the project. During this phase health promotion planners use descriptive epidemiological data and conduct a strengths, weaknesses, opportunities, and threats (SWOT) analysis.

Phase 2: Problem Analysis

Phase 2 involves problem analysis to identify the factors that contribute to the health problem, the population groups affected by it, and a list of the potential partners. During this phase goals are written to guide the strategy. Phase 2 relies on analytic epidemiologic methods to delineate the causes of the problem identified in the previous phase. Based on this analysis, program planners then identify and select intervention activities that strike at the root of the problem determinants. Also in phase 2, it is recommended that program planners solidify partners and consider the program budget.

Phase 3: Communication Planning

Phase 3 is communication program planning, the center of CDCynergy. During this phase, communication planning begins in earnest. Health promotion planners decide whether communication will be used as a dominant intervention or to support other intervention activities. Based on this determination, audiences are identified and segmented, communication goals and objectives are formulated, and formative research is conducted. Formative evaluation is a method of judging the program components while the program is being developed. The results of the formative research in this phase will be used to develop a creative brief. The creative brief is used to inform the development of messages and the testing and selection of settings, channel-specific activities, and materials that will be used to disseminate the messages to intended audiences.

Channel-specific activities include the following:

* Interpersonal channels (e.g., physicians, friends, family members, counselors, parents, clergy, and coaches of the intended audiences)

* Group channels (e.g., brown bag lunches at work, classroom activities, neighborhood gatherings, and club meetings)

* Organizations and community groups (e.g., advocacy groups)

* Mass media channels (e.g., radio, network and cable television, magazines, direct mail, billboards, transit cards, newspapers)

* Interactive digital media channels (e.g., Internet websites, bulletin boards, newsgroups, chat rooms, CD-ROMs, kiosks)

Phase 4: Program and Evaluation Development

Phase 4 focuses on program and evaluation development and involves pretesting the communication concepts, messages, and materials that were developed in phase 3. Ideally, pretesting is done by engaging a sample of the target audience to assess how they respond to the selected strategy. In this phase, planners use the brief developed in the previous phase to guide the process of testing and selecting concepts, messages, settings, channel-specific activities, and materials. The decisions made during these activities culminate in a communication plan that lays out who will do what, when, where, and how often in executing health promotion communication activities.

Phase 5: Program Implementation and Management

Phase 5 is described as program implementation and management. The purpose of this phase is to provide guidance on how to systematically conceptualize, plan, execute, and provide meaningful and timely feedback on an evaluation.

Phase 6: Evaluation

Phase 6 is the overall feedback or evaluation phase for the program planners to identify key findings that resulted from the program. During this phase program practitioners evaluate the communication plan, modify the program based on feedback, and disseminate lessons learned.

Making Health Communication Programs Work

Originally printed in 1989, **Making Health Communication Programs Work** is a guide to communication program planning developed by the Office of Cancer Communications (OCC, now the Office of Communications) of the National Cancer Institute (NCI). During the twenty-five years that NCI has been involved in health communication, ongoing evaluation of its communication programs has affirmed the value of using specific communication strategies to promote health and prevent disease (Parvanta & Freimuth, 2000). The *Making Health Communications Programs Work* model is considered a practical guide for planning and implementing a health promotion effort. The Health Communication Program Cycle (see figure 3.4) is supported by the National Cancer Institute and can be accessed on their website, called *Making Health Communication Programs Work* (www.cancer .gov/cancertopics/cancerlibrary/pinkbook/page1).

Making Health Communication Programs Work a guide to communication program planning developed by the National Cancer Institute

As displayed in figure 3.4, this model identifies a four-step process to effective health communication planning. The stages constitute a circular process in which the last stage feeds back to the first as health promoters work through a continuous loop of planning, implementation, assessment, and improvement. Similar to the CDCynergy model, this model focuses on consumers, engaging them in the assessment of the health issue and the design of the communication plan or intervention to address the health issue. Table 3.3 describes activities for each of the CDCynergy model phases.

Health Promotion Planning Model for Community-Level Programs

As the need for increased health promotion activities and programs at the community level has grown since the new millennium, new models have

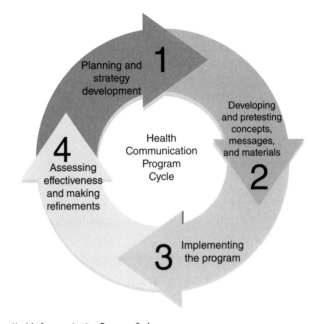

Figure 3.4 Health Communication Program Cycle

Source: National Cancer Institute (nd).

Table 3.3 CDCynergy Program Planning Model

Phase	Title	Activities
1	Planning and strategy development	Identify how the organization can use communication to effectively address a health issue.
		Identify the intended audiences; use consumer research to craft a communication strategy.
		Design an evaluation plan.
2	Developing and pretesting concepts, messages, and materials	Develop relevant messages.
		Draft messages.
		Pretest messages with intended audiences.
3	Implementing the program	Communicate with partners and clarify involvement.
		Activate communication and distribution.
		Document procedures and compare progress to time lines.
		Refine the program continuously.
4	Assessing effectiveness and making refinements	Assess the degree to which the target population is receiving the program.
		Assess the immediate impact on the target population and refine the programs as necessary.
		Ensure that program delivery is consistent with protocol.
		Analyze changes in the target population.

been developed to focus on the unique nature of community-level health intervention programs. Although the PRECEDE-PROCEED and MATCH models are applicable to community-level programs, the mobilizing for action through planning and partnerships (MAPP) model was designed with the interrelationships of communities in mind.

The MAPP model emphasizes the importance of successful partnerships in the development of activities and solutions to address health issues. For example, as communities begin to address rising obesity rates, the issue of access to healthy food has been identified as a potential barrier to combatting obesity. This community-level model is very useful in communities that want to address the issue of food deserts and the reliance on corner stores, providing the right steps for a community to address the issue of access to healthy foods for its residents.

Mobilizing for Action through Planning and Partnerships (MAPP)

The **mobilizing for action through planning and partnerships (MAPP) model** was created by the National Association for County and City Health Officials (NACCHO) to assist local health departments and local health coalitions with program planning that specifically targets community health issues. MAPP is a community-driven strategic planning process for improving community health. Using an interactive process, the framework helps communities apply strategic thinking to prioritize public health issues and identify resources to address them (Kindig, Booske, & Remington, 2010; Minkler & Wallerstein, 2005).

mobilizing for action through planning and partnerships (MAPP) model
a planning model developed by the National Association of County and City Health Officials to assist local health departments and local health coalitions with program planning that specifically targets community health issues

Phase 1: Organizing for Success and Partnership Development

This first phase centers on two critical and interrelated activities: organizing the planning process and developing partnerships. The purpose of this phase is to structure a planning process that builds commitment, engages participants as active partners, uses participants' time well, and results in a plan that can be realistically implemented.

Phase 2: Visioning

This phase provides focus, purpose, and direction to the MAPP process so that participants collectively achieve a shared vision for the future. A shared community vision provides an overarching goal for the community.

Phase 3: Assessments

This phase focuses on conducting four assessments: (1) community themes and strengths, (2) the capacity of the local public health system, (3) the community health status based on epidemiological data, and (4) the focus of where change needs to or should occur. These assessments provide important information, unique to that community, for improving community health outcomes.

Phase 4: Identify Strategic Issues

During the fourth phase, planning participants work together to prioritize the most important issues facing the community. Once these issues are recognized, strategic solutions are identified or developed by exploring the results of the previous assessments and determining how those issues affect the achievement of the shared vision.

Phase 5: Formulate Goals and Strategies

This phase builds on the strategic issues that were identified and involves the formulation of goal statements related to those issues. Planning participants then pinpoint strategies for addressing issues and achieving goals related to the community's vision.

Phase 6: The Action Cycle

During this phase, planning, implementing, and evaluating occur. The local public health system or other health promotion coalition develops and implements an action plan for addressing priority goals and objectives. Further evaluation is emphasized to identify what activities are having the most impact on changing the targeted health issue.

MAP-IT

When Healthy People 2020 was launched, the Department of Health and Human Services also launched MAP-IT, a framework for creating, implementing, and evaluating programs. The acronym MAP-IT stands for mobilize, assess, plan, implement, and track.

This framework is similar to the steps identified in other program planning models. What makes this framework different is that it is on the Healthy People 2020 website. Healthy People 2020 is the strategic plan for health improvement of Americans and is discussed in chapter 9. The MAP-IT framework helps all types of health professionals create programs to promote healthy communities. Table 3.4 presents some key questions to use for each stage of the MAP-IT framework.

Table 3.4 Key Questions for Each Stage of MAP-IT

Mobilize	Assess	Plan	Implement	Track
What are the vision and mission of the coalition?	Who is affected and how?	What is our goal? What do we need to do to reach our goal?	Are we following our plan? What can we do better?	Are we evaluating our work? Did we follow the plan?
Why do I want to bring people together?	What resources do we have?	Who will do it? How will we know when we have reached our goal?		What did we change? Did we reach our goal?
Who should be represented?	What resources do we need?			
Who are the potential partners (organizations and businesses) in my community?				

Connecting Health Behavior Theories to Program Planning Models

Chapter 2 and this chapter contain the building blocks for creating programs that will sustain behavior change. The constructs, theories, phases, and models are a health promotion professional's tools of the trade and, when used correctly, programs will more likely create success for individuals, organizations, and communities. Knowing and applying these theories and models will distinguish your skill set from other professionals and, most important, will demonstrate that practice-based evidence is a key to helping health-promoting change to reverse the behaviors linked to chronic disease.

The next five chapters discuss behaviors that promote healthful living. As you read and discuss the chapters, keep in mind the content of these first two chapters and begin to apply the constructs of how people change behaviors and how programs must collect and use data on the target audience to design a program specifically tailored for that population.

Summary

This chapter introduced the process by which program planners develop, implement, and evaluate health promotion programs. To ensure that a program achieves the intended results, the identification and use of a program planning model is an important first step. This chapter describes two ecological models, two health communication models, and one community model. Although these models are most commonly accepted in the health promotion field, there are many other program planning models available to health promotion practitioners. The most important factor is to identify a model that is appropriate for the project and use that model as a guide for program development. Program planning may seem "instinctual" to some, but using a model that provides a step-by-step guide ensures that a thorough assessment and planning process guides the implementation of the program.

KEY TERMS

1. **Planning model:** serves to guide the development, implementation, and evaluation of a specific health promotion program; a blueprint for building and improving programs

2. **Social ecological model of planning:** a planning model based on the interrelationships of human beings and their environments, recognizing that within the environment there are physical, social, economic, and cultural forces that have the potential to alter health outcomes

3. **PRECEDE-PROCEED model:** a nine-phase logic model, using an ecological approach, applied in health promotion program planning

4. **Epidemiology:** the study of the distribution and determinants of health-related conditions or events in defined populations and the application of findings to control health problems

5. **Multilevel approach to community health (MATCH) model:** an ecological model of program planning focusing on assessing population health and working with communities to help them identify opportunities for improving community health and to find and implement evidence-based programs and policies that address the identified health issues

6. **Consumer-based planning models:** models that focus on the consumer or intended audience, borrowing concepts from the business marketing field and applying those concepts to health promotion

7. **CDCynergy:** a planning model developed by the CDC that emphasizes marketing and business communication concepts that include population feedback, segmentation principles, and target communication strategies

8. **Making Health Communication Programs Work:** a guide to communication program planning developed by the National Cancer Institute

9. **Mobilizing for action through planning partnerships (MAPP) model:** a planning model developed by the National Association of County and City Health Officials to assist local health departments and local health coalitions with program planning that specifically targets community health issues

REVIEW QUESTIONS

1. At which stage in the program planning model will you use the theories of behavior change?

2. How will using a program planning model save time in the long run?

3. How are the models similar and how are they different?

4. What issues might arise if you do not use a program planning model?

5. The PRECEDE-PROCEED model has five assessment phases. What sources could you use to obtain the data for each phase?

STUDENT ACTIVITIES

1. Many health promotion practitioners enjoy the implementation phase of program planning. Identify key reasons why the assessment and evaluation phases are critical to the success of any program.

2. Identify a social marketing campaign, its message, the target audience, what behavior change theory it is employing, and what recommendations you would suggest to improve it, and why.

3. Identify one article in the literature that exemplifies each of the program planning models.

4. Describe the ecological model and relate it to program planning.

References

Crosby, R., & Noar, S. M. (2011). What is a planning model? An introduction to PRECEDE-PROCEED. *Journal of Public Health Dentistry, 71*, S7–S15.

Glanz, K., Rimer, B. K., & Viswanath, K. (Eds.). (2008). *Health behavior and health education: Theory, research and practice* (4th ed.). San Francisco: Jossey-Bass.

Green, L. W. (2009). *PRECEDE-PROCEED model.* Retrieved from www.lgreen.net /precede.htm

Green, L. W., & Kreuter, M. W. (2005). *Health program planning: An educational and ecological approach* (4th ed.). Boston: McGraw-Hill.

Kindig, D. A., Booske, B. C., & Remington, P. L. (2010). Mobilizing action toward community health (MATCH): Metrics, incentives, and partnerships for population health. *Preventing Chronic Disease, 7*(4), A68. Retrieved from www.cdc.gov/pcd /issues/2010/jul/10_0019.htm

Minkler, M., & Wallerstein, N. (2005). Improving health through community organization and community building: A health education perspective. In M. Minkler (Ed.), *Community organizing and community building for health* (2nd ed.) (pp. 26–50). New Brunswick, NJ: Rutgers University Press.

National Cancer Institute. (nd). *Pink book—Making health communication programs work.* Retrieved from www.cancer.gov/cancertopics/cancerlibrary/pinkbook/page4

Parvanta, C. F., & Freimuth, V. (2000). Health communication at the Centers for Disease Control and Prevention. *American Journal of Health Behaviors, 24*(1), 18–25.

Stokols, D. (1996). Translating social ecological theory into guidelines for community health promotion. *American Journal of Health Promotion, 10*(4), 282–298.

US Department of Agriculture and US Department of Health and Human Services. (2010). Helping Americans make healthy choices. *Dietary guidelines for Americans 2010* (p. 56). Washington, DC: US Government Printing Office.

PART TWO

HEALTH BEHAVIORS

Chapters 4 through 8 present a short history of personal behaviors that are related to promoting health and preventing disease. These behaviors are closely linked to the onset and progression of chronic disease and the aim of health promotion professionals to help individuals and communities to modify these behaviors. Tobacco use, eating, physical activity, and emotional health have evolved as a result of changes in our social and physical environments. Clinical preventive services have evolved due to advances in medicine for early detection. These chapters provide a comprehensive discussion of the health behaviors that influence the onset of chronic disease in our country and how and why these behaviors have changed over time. Chapter 8 highlights the important role clinical preventive services have on also promoting health by monitoring chronic disease development and overall health status; hence, preventive services (immunizations and age-appropriate screenings) available through the medical community need to be understood and promoted. Collectively, these behaviors have the potential to dramatically reduce the incidence of chronic disease and improve the quality of people's lives throughout the United States.

These chapters examine how changes in our environment and society over the past several decades have impacted behaviors, and how those changed behaviors impact health and disease. By studying the historical perspective of each of these behaviors, health promotion professionals will gain a richer context for their work, understanding that multiple forces have shaped and continue to affect the health of individuals and our society. Health behavior change is complex; in order to advance innovative solutions, it is critical that health promoters fully understand the history of these behaviors. Within each chapter, examples of policies and programs that exemplify health promotion in action are provided.

Chapter 4 introduces students to tobacco use, which is the leading cause of preventable death in the United States. It has been fifty years since the first surgeon general's report on smoking was published and there has been a significant reduction in the number of people who smoke in addition to increased restrictions to where smoking is allowed. But more needs to be done because other forms of tobacco, such as e-cigarettes, are practiced as alternatives to smoking cigarettes. Many health advocates view the war on tobacco as a prototype for addressing other behaviors such as eating and physical activity.

Eating practices are related to four of the leading causes of death in the United States, yet everyone needs to eat to survive. Chapter 5 provides an extensive review of the relationship of food and chronic disease, food guides, shifts in the eating patterns, and multiple examples of policy and program efforts that are underway to encourage healthy eating practices. The cost of food has decreased over time but the real cost of poor dietary habits occurs years later when chronic disease occurs. This cost is then shifted to the health care system, which provides procedures, medicine, and ongoing management of the chronic condition. A less tangible cost is the person's quality of life is changed as a result of chronic disease.

Exercise will be the most widely prescribed medicine in the United States (a trend that is predicted in chapter 12). Chapter 6 brings together research and practice to highlight the importance of being physically active on a regular basis. Changes in our physical environment have engineered physical activity out of our lives, so the goal of health promotion professionals is to identify how individuals and communities can make being physically active enjoyable and rewarding. The Affordable Care Act highlights the importance of physical activity and as a result new initiatives at the local, state, and federal levels are promoting this behavior.

Stress is all around us, but it is how we react to a situation that will trigger the stress response in our bodies. Chapter 7 details the physiological response to stress and how life stress is related to illness. Different from the other behaviors, stress is a perception and hence there is great variability from one person to the next. Although there are challenges to linking stress and disease, there is a plethora of strategies, activities, and programs to assist individuals of all ages to manage their stress.

Promoting health through proper eating and regular exercise is a large part of the role of health promotion professionals. Yet, these behaviors may not protect us from all diseases; therefore, we must responsibly advocate for clinical preventive services. Chapter 8 introduces us to preventive services from vaccinations to age-specific screenings. A large part of the Affordable Care Act is to promote clinical preventive services and to decrease the barriers to accessing these services. Outlined in this chapter are the government agencies that monitor and recommend these services.

It is important to note that there are numerous other health behaviors that can affect a person's quality of life and well-being. Alcohol abuse, sexual health, and even environmental health are part of the scope of health promotion. There is no set hierarchy of health behaviors; it is very much dependent on your interests and how you see yourself helping people to live a healthier lifestyle. Health promotion is a broad field and the concepts learned in chapters 2 and 3 can be applied to many health behaviors.

CHAPTER 4

TOBACCO USE

Trends, Health Consequences, Cessation, and Policies

Laurie DiRosa

Since 1964, when Surgeon General Luther L. Terry first published the definitive report that smoking caused lung cancer in men, the culture of smoking has dramatically changed for the better (US Department of Health and Human Services, 2014). We see the impact of these changes daily as smokers huddle in obscurely located "smoking areas" outside of office buildings, malls, hospitals, and other public establishments. As of April 1, 2014, thirty-six states and the District of Columbia had enacted comprehensive smoke-free laws banning smoking in all workplaces, restaurants, and bars. This equals 81.3% of the US population currently living under a ban on smoking (American Nonsmokers' Rights Foundation, 2014).

This culture is much different from the one a short fifty years ago when smoking was permitted everywhere, including on airplanes and in doctors' offices. Before conclusive evidence linked smoking to lung cancer, approximately 42% of the US population smoked. Today, we have cut that in half: approximately 20% of the US population smokes tobacco (CDC, 2011b). Government bans on smoking did not begin until the 1990s; in 1995, California became the first state to enact a statewide smoking ban, and in 1998, the US Department of Transportation banned smoking on all commercial passenger flights (CDC, 2012a). Although smoking rates are much improved, the United States is still short of the Healthy People 2020 goal of only 12% of the US population smoking (Healthy People, 2012). Smoking is not only

LEARNING OBJECTIVES

After reading this chapter, the student will be able to:

- Describe the trends of tobacco use over the past several decades.

- Discuss the effects tobacco has on the human body.

- Identify the barriers to tobacco cessation programs.

- Summarize best practice for tobacco cessation.

- Restate the policies that have been enacted to limit tobacco use.

- Explain the impact that Clean Indoor Air has had on smoking rates.

hazardous to our health but it also affects our culture and economy; government policies have been established to control the spread of its addictive capacity.

Just as smoking has a pervasive effect on the organs and cells throughout our body, it also has a pervasive effect on our society. Those in the health promotion field continue to work to encourage current smokers to quit and to discourage adolescents and others from starting the habit. This chapter discusses general tobacco-related statistics, the chronic diseases related to smoking, smoking trends and changes in the United States related to smoking, and effective cessation programs.

Tobacco Use

Tobacco use is the single most preventable cause of death and disease in the United States (CDC, 2011c). Despite ongoing efforts by health promotion professionals, people continue to smoke, putting their bodies at risk for cancer, cardiovascular disease, pulmonary disease, and reproductive and developmental effects. Figure 4.1 identifies many different cancers and chronic diseases that are causally linked to mainstream smoking and also identifies additional illnesses and cancers that occur through secondhand smoke exposure.

Tobacco Use Statistics

Data from 2011 indicate that 19% of US adults smoke, with more men smoking than women. Of those who smoke, almost 80% smoke every day. The proportion of those who smoke more than thirty cigarettes per day is 9%, whereas the proportion of those who smoke one to nine cigarettes per day is 22% (CDC, 2011a).

The person most likely to smoke is between fifteen and forty-four years old, living below the poverty level, and of low education (GED or no high school diploma). The ethnic group with the highest rate of smoking is American Indian at 31.5%, followed by multiple race at 27.4%, and Caucasian at 20% (CDC, 2011c). It is more common for those with a disability to smoke compared to individuals without disabilities (25.4% versus 17.9%) (CDC, 2011b).

Adolescents

In 2012, the surgeon general published a report specifically focused on adolescent tobacco use (US Department of Health and Human Services, 2012). This is a vulnerable population that deserves special attention when it

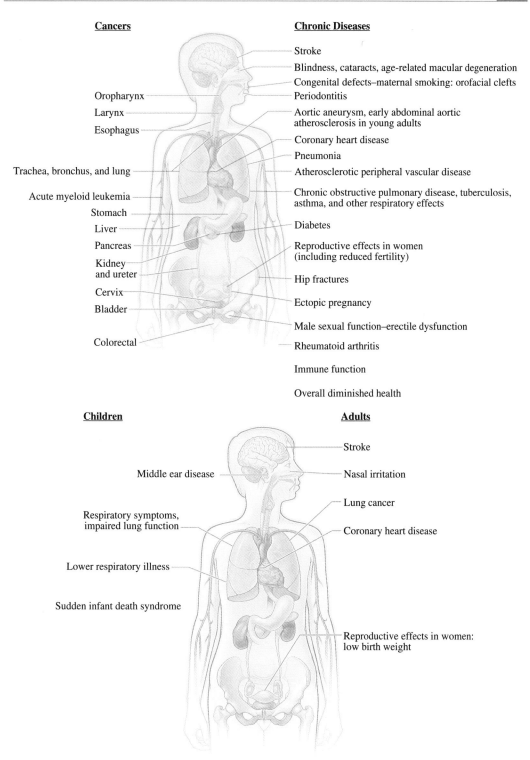

Cancers

Oropharynx
Larynx
Esophagus

Trachea, bronchus, and lung

Acute myeloid leukemia

Stomach
Liver
Pancreas
Kidney
and ureter
Cervix
Bladder

Colorectal

Chronic Diseases

Stroke
Blindness, cataracts, age-related macular degeneration
Congenital defects–maternal smoking: orofacial clefts
Periodontitis
Aortic aneurysm, early abdominal aortic
atherosclerosis in young adults
Coronary heart disease
Pneumonia
Atherosclerotic peripheral vascular disease
Chronic obstructive pulmonary disease, tuberculosis,
asthma, and other respiratory effects
Diabetes
Reproductive effects in women
(including reduced fertility)
Hip fractures
Ectopic pregnancy
Male sexual function–erectile dysfunction
Rheumatoid arthritis
Immune function
Overall diminished health

Children

Middle ear disease

Respiratory symptoms,
impaired lung function

Lower respiratory illness

Sudden infant death syndrome

Adults

Stroke
Nasal irritation
Lung cancer
Coronary heart disease

Reproductive effects in women:
low birth weight

Figure 4.1   The Health Consequences Causally Linked to Smoking and Exposure to Secondhand Smoke

Note: The condition in gray is a new disease that has been causally linked to smoking in this report.

Source: US Department of Health and Human Services (2004, 2006, 2012).

comes to smoking because they are more susceptible to tobacco marketing and are also easily influenced by peers and social pressure to try smoking. Research indicates that 80% of adult smokers begin by age eighteen and 99% of all first-time tobacco use occurs before age twenty-six—this is alarming, yet provides hope. Health promotion professionals can significantly reduce the number of smokers overall if they can successfully prevent first use at a young age. The health risks of beginning to smoke at a young age are particularly high; becoming addicted to nicotine as a minor promotes longer lifetime use and greater chances of heart and lung damage (US Department of Health and Human Services, 2012). Research shows the presence of atherosclerosis in young smokers, which can lead to reduced lung growth and function in later years (US Department of Health and Human Services, 2012).

Although the percentage of adolescents who smoke decreased from 2005 (24%) to 2011 (19%), adolescent tobacco use is still considered to be at an epidemic level. One out of every four high school seniors smokes, one in five white adolescent males uses smokeless tobacco, and one in ten young adults smokes cigars. Alarmingly, adolescents also report the use of multiple tobacco products: over 50% of male adolescents report the use of cigarettes, smokeless tobacco, and cigars (US Department of Health and Human Services, 2012).

Smokeless Tobacco

According to 2010 data from the Substance Abuse and Mental Health Services Administration (SAMHSA) (2011), an estimated 3.1% of US adults over age twenty-six use smokeless tobacco. This is an increase from 2005, when only 2.3% of adults reported using smokeless tobacco. The prevalence of smokeless tobacco use is highest among young adults aged eighteen to twenty-five years (6.4%), adults with less than a high school education, and adults living in states with a high cigarette smoking prevalence. The states with the highest smokeless tobacco use are Wyoming (9.1%), West Virginia (8.5%), and Mississippi (7.5%) (CDC, 2010). No state comes close to the Healthy People 2020 goal of 0.3% use of smokeless tobacco (Healthy People, 2012).

Although the prevalence rate of smokeless tobacco use is not nearly as high as cigarette smoking levels, the rise of the use of smokeless tobacco is cause for concern. It is hypothesized that the increased use may be related to the more prevalent bans on smoking in public, increased excise taxes on cigarettes, and the misconception that using smokeless tobacco is less of a health risk than smoking cigarettes. In truth, an individual using smokeless tobacco eight to ten times a day is absorbing the same amount of nicotine as one would absorb from smoking sixty cigarettes a day.

Smoking-Related Deaths and Illnesses

A total of 443,000 US adults die from smoking-related illness each year. It is predicted that half of all long-term smokers will eventually die from the use of tobacco. For every eight smokers who die from tobacco use, one nonsmoker will die from passive smoking. For every person who dies from tobacco use, twenty more people suffer from at least one serious tobacco-related illness. It is estimated that secondhand smoke exposure causes approximately 3,000 deaths from lung cancer, 46,000 deaths from heart disease, and 430 newborn deaths from sudden infant death syndrome (SIDS) annually (US Department of Health and Human Services, 2006). Most significantly, smoking could kill eight million people each year by 2030 worldwide if prevalence rates remain constant (World Health Organization, 2012).

As shown in figure 4.1, cigarette smoking has been causally linked to cancer of the larynx, esophagus, trachea, bronchus, lungs, blood, stomach, pancreas, kidney, bladder, ureter, and cervix. Additionally, the chronic diseases of coronary artery disease, vascular disease, periodontitis, blindness, pneumonia, chronic obstructive pulmonary disease, asthma, and reduced fertility and incidences of stroke and aneurysms are also causally linked to smoking. Smokeless tobacco use leads to nicotine addiction as often as cigarette smoking does and has been linked to cancer of the mouth and gums, periodontitis, and tooth loss. Studies also suggest a relationship between smokeless tobacco use and precancerous oral lesions, oral cancer, and cancers of the kidney, pancreas, and digestive system, as well as death from cardiovascular and cerebrovascular disease (US Department of Health and Human Services, 2010). An estimated eight thousand people die each year because of smokeless tobacco use (CDC, 2012c).

Tobacco-Related Costs

The economic burden of tobacco use is calculated through direct and indirect costs. **Direct costs** include health care expenditures required to address smoking-related illness. **Indirect costs** include lost earnings due to premature death (mostly due to lung cancer, ischemic heart disease, and chronic obstructive pulmonary disease). Experts calculate that cigarette smoking costs the United States $96 billion annually in direct costs and $97 billion indirectly through losses in productivity, based on 5.1 million years of potential life lost. It should be noted, however, that this number likely underestimates costs; lost productivity related to disability and

direct costs
in managed care, the costs of labor, supplies, and equipment to provide direct patient care services

indirect costs
resources forgone as a result of a health condition

employee absenteeism and disease morbidity and mortality attributed to secondhand smoke were not included in the calculation. It is estimated that the effects of exposure to secondhand smoke cost the United States $10 billion per year. In the most recent surgeon general's report on the economic effect of tobacco on the economy, it was reported that "smoking and exposure to tobacco smoke continue to increase and now approach $300 billion annually, with direct medical costs of at least $130 billion and productivity losses of more than $150 billion a year" (US Department of Health and Human Services, 2014).

Smoking Tobacco and Chronic Disease

There is no risk-free level of exposure to tobacco smoke. When tobacco smoke is inhaled, the toxic compounds in the smoke are transferred from the lungs to the bloodstream. This enables the toxins to travel throughout the body, affecting nearly every organ. As noted previously in this chapter, there is clear evidence linking smoking to cancer, cardiovascular disease, pulmonary disease, and reproductive and developmental effects. In fact, smoking is the cause of 30% of all cancer deaths and nearly 80% of all deaths from chronic obstructive pulmonary disease (COPD). This section will review the biological basis of how smoking causes these diseases.

Cancer

cancer
a term used for diseases in which abnormal cells divide without control and are able to invade other tissues

The National Cancer Institute defines **cancer** as uncontrolled cell growth in any part of the body. Depending on where in the body the cell growth occurs, these cells can form tumors and affect the tissues surrounding them. Normally, DNA produces genes that keep cell growth under control. However, sometimes DNA becomes damaged and creates mutated genes that no longer control cell growth and natural cell death.

carcinogens
a cancer-causing substance or agent

   Carcinogens are toxic compounds that can damage DNA and lead to this cancerous growth of cells. Cigarette smoke contains the potent carcinogens polycyclic aromatic hydrocarbons, N-nitrosamines, aromatic amines, 1,3-butadiene, benzene, aldehydes, and ethylene oxide. These particular carcinogens are proven to have a significant role in changing cellular pathways and the genetic processes that foster the growth and development of cancer (Hecht, 1998). As shown in figure 4.2, these carcinogens can cause cancer through three different pathways. The most common pathway of cancer formation is when carcinogens are not detoxified but rather activated, damaging DNA and the coding process. The miscoded DNA produces mutated genes that are not able to control cell growth, resulting in cancerous cell growth. Alternatively, co-carcinogens and tumor promoters

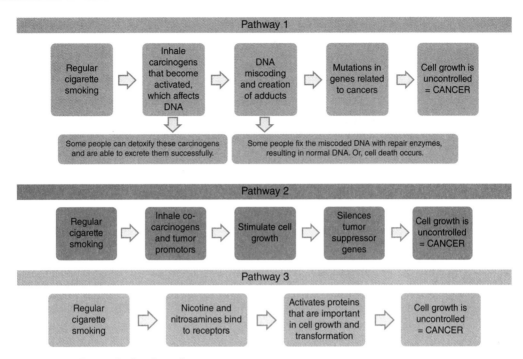

Figure 4.2   How Cigarette Smoking Causes Cancer

Source: US Department of Health and Human Services (2010), chapter 5.

are activated through regular cigarette smoking, which stimulate cell growth and at the same time silence tumor suppressor genes. Third, nicotine and nitrosamines can bind to receptors, activating proteins that are important in cell growth and transformation. All of these pathways lead to uncontrolled cell growth and cancer.

Of course, not everyone who smokes will get cancer, although the risk for cancer among smokers is higher than among nonsmokers. Cancer occurrence varies based on each individual's ability to detoxify carcinogens, repair damaged DNA, and, if need be, kill damaged cells.

Cardiovascular Disease

A primary risk factor of **cardiovascular disease (CVD)** is smoking. In the United States, more than one-third of all deaths from CVD can be attributed to smoking. In addition to being an independent risk factor for CVD, smoking also has a significant effect on other CVD risk factors, specifically high blood pressure, diabetes mellitus, and high blood lipids. The surgeon general warns that a smoker who also presents with two additional risk factors will have eight times the risk of CVD as compared to a nonsmoker with no other risk factors. There is no safe level of smoke exposure. CVD risk occurs at low levels of use, including infrequent smoking and exposure

cardiovascular disease (CVD)
refers to conditions that involve narrowed or blocked blood vessels that can lead to a heart attack, chest pain (angina), or stroke

to secondhand smoke. Therefore, smoking fewer cigarettes each day does not reduce the risk of CVD; only smoking cessation reduces the risk of CVD.

The cardiovascular system moves blood and lymph throughout the body to deliver oxygen and nutrients to the cells and pick up cellular waste. This circulation of materials relies on healthy, flexible, and strong arteries and veins to properly move these fluids through the system. CVD occurs when arteries that deliver blood to the heart become clogged, the valves of the heart are damaged, or the heart does not pump effectively. Also, arteries can become clogged, harden, and weaken, or blood clots can form that stop the flow of blood to the heart or brain, causing death.

Cigarette smoke causes CVD through various mechanisms; nicotine, carbon monoxide, and oxidizing chemicals are most responsible for damage to the cardiovascular system. Nicotine is a drug that continually stimulates the nervous system, increasing the resting heart rate, which is a possible risk for CVD. Carbon monoxide binds with hemoglobin the same way that oxygen does; however, it is more powerful at doing so. Therefore, smokers are left with less oxygen released to cells. In the long term, in order to compensate for the loss of hemoglobin to carbon monoxide, the body produces more red blood cells to deliver oxygen. The negative effect is thicker blood, which is not as easy to pump through the arteries and veins.

The presence of oxidizing chemicals (e.g., free radicals) in cigarette smoke reduces the amount of antioxidants found in the body naturally. Fewer antioxidants available to combat toxins, specifically the antioxidant vitamin C, leads to inflammation, the inner linings of blood vessels not functioning properly, oxidation of low-density lipoproteins, and the activation of platelets. This cascade of ill effects ultimately leads to blood clots, which can cause death if they lodge in the heart or lungs.

In summary, cigarette smoking causes damage to the interior linings of arteries, increases heart rate, increases blood pressure, reduces oxygen and nutrients to the heart, and reduces blood flow to the heart. These conditions may cause stroke, aortic aneurysm, peripheral arterial disease, coronary heart disease (CHD), or sudden death due to a heart attack.

Pulmonary Disease

In a typically functioning **lung**, when a person inhales, **oxygen** travels down the trachea to tubes that eventually branch off into smaller tubes called bronchioles. At the end of these bronchioles, gas exchange occurs as oxygen is absorbed and carbon dioxide is released in the tiny air sacs called alveoli. The bronchioles and alveoli are elastic and increase and decrease in size with every inhale and exhale.

---

lung
one of the usually paired compound saccular thoracic organs that constitute the basic respiratory organ of air-breathing vertebrates; the lungs remove carbon dioxide from and bring oxygen to the blood and consist essentially of an inverted tree of intricately branched bronchioles communicating with thin-walled terminal alveoli swathed in a network of delicate capillaries where the actual gaseous exchange of respiration takes place

oxygen
the odorless gas that is present in the air and necessary to maintain life; patients with lung disease or damage may need to use portable oxygen devices on a temporary or permanent basis

Each day, adults inhale approximately ten thousand liters of air. This necessitates a system for removing inhaled particles (such as pollen and road dust) and repairing damage to the lungs due to the particles. Some of the respiratory system's mechanisms for removing potentially damaging particles include creating mucous, coughing, sneezing, blocking with nasal hair, and using alveolar macrophages to destroy carcinogens.

When a smoker inhales on a cigarette, the smoke travels the same path as oxygen does from the mouth, through the trachea, to the upper lungs, and ultimately to the alveoli where gas exchange occurs. Along this path, the carcinogens present in cigarette smoke damage the respiratory system. Although there are mechanisms to repair the damage, the large volume and large size of the toxic particles present in cigarette smoke causes repairs to fall behind, ultimately leading to pulmonary disease.

Acrolein, formaldehyde, nitrogen oxides, cadmium, and hydrogen cyanide found in cigarette smoke damage the lungs. Together, these carcinogens damage the cilia in the lungs, impair lung defenses, irritate the membranes, and create oxidative stress. Research indicates that with chronic cigarette smoking, nearly 60% of the inhaled particles from cigarette smoke are not removed and remain in the lower lung. Additionally, up to 20 mg of tar per day is deposited in the lungs per cigarette smoked. The presence of these particles and tar create inflammation, which in turn creates oxidative stress from an immune response to the carcinogens. This inflammation and response is the hallmark of pulmonary disease. The diseases specifically caused by the carcinogens in smoke are chronic obstructive pulmonary disease (COPD) and asthma.

COPD is a progressive condition that includes the diseases of chronic bronchitis and emphysema. With COPD, airflow is diminished due to either alveoli losing their elasticity, the walls between alveoli being destroyed, airway walls becoming thick and inflamed, or excess mucous being created and clogging airways.

Chronic bronchitis is defined as a specific set of symptoms—that of a productive cough for three months in each of two successive years where other causes of productive chronic cough have been excluded. Emphysema is a condition defined by a certain pattern of lung damage in which the lung's elasticity is damaged and airspaces are permanently enlarged. This does not allow the lungs to properly inflate and deflate with air, making victims feel as if they are always out of breath.

Asthma is a chronic inflammatory disease of the airways that is characterized by airflow obstruction; symptoms include wheezing, breathlessness, chest tightness, and cough in response to a stimulus, in this case cigarette smoke. Immediate treatment is necessary to remove the symptoms and increase airflow.

Reproductive and Developmental Effects

The female and male reproductive systems rely on healthy blood flow, appropriate hormone levels, and undamaged DNA to create new human life and for women to carry the fetus to full-term delivery. The toxic compounds found in smoke, specifically carbon monoxide, nicotine, cadmium, lead, mercury, and polycyclic aromatic hydrocarbons, are associated with adverse reproductive outcomes, such as infertility, miscarriage, and congenital abnormalities.

Among women, research indicates that 13% of infertility may be attributed to smoking. Follicle-stimulating hormones (necessary for ovulation), as well as estrogen and progesterone (necessary for normal menstruation), are adversely affected by the toxins in cigarette smoke and nicotine. Additionally, carcinogens can diminish oviduct functioning, making fertilization difficult when the egg is not able to travel to the uterus to be fertilized by sperm. Among men, evidence links smoking to chromosome changes and DNA damage in sperm, which affects pregnancy viability and may cause anomalies in offspring.

Smoking prior to conception and throughout pregnancy can have damaging effects on the fetus, including congenital abnormalities and miscarriage. Damage to the fetus is primarily due to the presence of carbon monoxide, which binds to hemoglobin and decreases oxygen flow to the fetus. Additionally, placental abnormalities are also possible, leading to fetal loss, preterm delivery, or low birth weight.

smokeless tobacco
a tobacco product that is not smoked but rather placed directly in the mouth, cheek, or lip to be sucked or chewed; the saliva is either swallowed or spit out and is commonly referred to in the United States as *dip*, *chew*, or *snuff*

Smokeless Tobacco and Chronic Disease

Smokeless tobacco is a tobacco product that is not smoked but rather placed directly in the mouth, cheek, or lip to be sucked or chewed; the saliva is either swallowed or spit out and is commonly referred to in the United States as *dip*, *chew*, or *snuff*.

In addition to loose tobacco that has been on the market for many years, a new product, "snus," has been released in recent years by the R. J. Reynolds and Philip Morris. Snus is particularly popular among adolescents because it does not require the user to spit and can therefore be concealed from parents and teachers. Similar to chewing tobacco, this form of moist tobacco is placed between the upper gum and lip—the difference is that it is sold in a small packet rather than loose tobacco (Boon, 2012).

Another new smokeless tobacco product, dissolvable tobacco, hit the test market in 2011. This is sold as pellets, flat strips, or sticks, and is designed to look like nontobacco products. For example, the pellet shape resembles Tic Tacs, the flat sheets look similar to breath strips, and the sticks look like toothpicks. The user ingests this tobacco orally; spitting is not required for the use of the product.

Other, less popular smokeless tobacco products available in the United States include loose-leaf chewing tobacco, which is sold in small strips of leaves and flavored with sugar or licorice, plug chewing tobacco, which is sold in oblong blocks and sweetened, and nasal snuff, which is sold as a fine tobacco powder that is sniffed through the nostrils by the user.

In addition to these more traditional smokeless tobacco products, gaining in popularity are e-cigarettes. **E-cigarettes** are devices that vaporize a mixture of water, propylene glycol, nicotine, and flavorings. They are battery powered and cost anywhere from $70 to $90 for a starter pack that includes the device, chargers, and nicotine cartridges. Each cartridge costs approximately $2 and equals a pack of cigarettes in terms of "puffs." It looks like a cigarette, and users inhale on it just as they would a cigarette through a mouthpiece. Studies have shown that the amount of nicotine provided per e-cigarette is approximately 8 to 16 mg, similar to regular cigarettes. As of this writing, e-cigarettes are not regulated by the FDA so it is unclear whether or not the actual ingredients pose significant health risks. However, because it contains nicotine, it is still an addictive product and does not encourage complete abstinence from tobacco use.

e-cigarettes
devices that vaporize a mixture of water, propylene glycol, nicotine, and flavorings; battery powered and cost anywhere from $70 to $90 for a starter pack that includes the device, chargers, and nicotine cartridges

Health promotion professionals are particularly concerned about smokeless tobacco and newer products on the market. Because users no longer need to spit out tobacco-filled saliva, smokeless tobacco use can easily be concealed, deterring cessation and prevention efforts among adolescents. Youth may be more inclined to experiment with this type of tobacco, because the risk of being seen is reduced. Additionally, smokeless tobacco and e-cigarettes are often marketed toward adult smokers trying to quit as a safer, healthier alternative. These adults may switch to these products instead of quitting, further enabling their nicotine addiction rather than curtailing use.

Harm Reduction

Nicotine is the primary ingredient in smokeless tobacco and is a highly addictive drug. However, nicotine itself is not the primary cause of diseases related to cigarette smoking. This has created a very heated scientific debate

nicotine
a colorless, poisonous alkaloid derived from the tobacco plant and used as an insecticide; the substance in tobacco to which smokers can become addicted

over whether or not smokeless tobacco is as harmful as previously reported (Grimsrud, Gallefoss, & Løchen, 2012). Discussions regarding whether or not health professionals should promote the use of smokeless tobacco to those who are unwilling or unable to quit smoking are starting to occur. This strategy of "harm reduction" has gained popularity in other countries, such as the United Kingdom (Rodu, 2011). However, the United States does not endorse this strategy. Although it is clear that compared to the health effects of cigarette use, the health risks of smokeless tobacco are significantly less, they still exist (Scientific Committee on Emerging and Newly-Identified Health Risks, 2008). Therefore, it remains the recommendation to abstain from all tobacco use. Chronic diseases associated with smokeless tobacco use are described in the following sections.

Cancer

There are twenty-eight known carcinogens in smokeless tobacco, including N-nitrosamino acids, volatile N-nitrosamines, polycyclic aromatic hydro-carbons, volatile aldehydes, hydrazine, metals, and radioactive polonium. Tobacco-specific nitrosamines (TSNAs) are carcinogens considered to be the most important because of their abundance in smokeless tobacco. Although TSNAs are also found in products not related to smoking (such as food and beer), there are one hundred to one thousand times higher levels in smokeless tobacco products. Studies indicate that these TSNAs are the main cause of oral cancer in smokeless tobacco users. The specific aspects of the mechanism remains unclear; however, in general the metabolic activation of TSNAs (specifically NNK and NNN) lead to the formation of DNA adducts, which lead to uncontrolled cell growth and cell death (Boffetta et al., 2008).

In 2007, a monograph published by the World Health Organization and the International Agency for Research on Cancer Working Group on the Evaluation of Carcinogenic Risks to Humans stated that smokeless tobacco use is carcinogenic to humans, causing oral and pancreatic cancer. More recently, additional meta-analyses completed in 2008, 2009, and 2011 have shown that there is no increased risk for pancreatic cancer (Bertuccio et al., 2011; Lee & Hamling, 2009; Sponsiello-Wang, Weitkunat, & Lee, 2008). The risk for oral cancer remains as previously documented.

Cardiovascular Disease

The amount of nicotine that a smokeless tobacco user will take in is similar to that of a cigarette smoker, although the nicotine from smokeless tobacco is absorbed at a much slower rate than from a cigarette. Nicotine affects receptors in the brain that activate the release of epinephrine, a hormone that increases heart rate and blood pressure. Nicotine also constricts coronary arteries and other blood vessels. The additives found in smokeless tobacco (such as licorice and sodium) also increase the blood pressure of the user. Therefore, smokeless tobacco use results in a chronic state of increased heart rate and blood pressure.

According to some studies, the long-term effects of smokeless tobacco can include greater risk of fatal heart attack and fatal stroke because users have a reduced chance of survival after such events. In 2010, the American Heart Association (AHA) released a policy statement, based on data from two large studies in the United States and Sweden, that smokeless tobacco use did not increase the incidence or prevalence of high blood pressure, the risk of nonfatal or fatal heart attack, or biochemical risk factors for cardiovascular disease (Heidenreich et al., 2011). However, the statement indicated that the use of smokeless tobacco results in an elevated risk of death from stroke. The AHA does not endorse the use of smokeless tobacco, despite the results of the report, but firmly recommends abstaining from use.

Pregnancy

Similar to smoking cigarettes, using smokeless tobacco poses serious risks to the developing fetus. Research indicates that the nicotine in smokeless tobacco increases the risk of stillbirth, premature delivery, and possibly preeclampsia, which is a dangerous state of high blood pressure, among other symptoms. The only way to cure preeclampsia is to deliver the baby, even if it is very early in the pregnancy. Mothers who use smokeless tobacco have a higher risk of giving birth to a low-birth-weight baby, putting the baby at risk for many complications such as problems fighting infection, difficulty eating and gaining weight, breathing problems, bleeding in the brain, intestinal diseases, and SIDS.

Oral Complications

According to the CDC, smokeless tobacco is linked to cancer of the mouth and gums, gum disease (periodontal disease and gingivitis), and tooth loss. The constituents of smokeless tobacco cause the cells of the mouth to not grow properly, creating tumors. These tumors can either remain in the mouth or the cancer cells can dislodge and travel to other parts of the body. They can attach to lymph nodes and other organs, causing metastatic cancer that is only treatable through chemotherapy, radiation, and surgery. Oral cancer is associated with a high death rate; the five-year survival rate is only 50% and much lower in minority populations.

Smokeless tobacco also causes gum disease, which is when the gums pull away from the teeth and form pockets that become infected with bacteria. The body recognizes this infection and attempts to remove the infected area, but results in destroying the bone and tissue that hold the teeth in place. This results in painful chewing and eventual tooth loss.

Secondhand Smoke Exposure and Chronic Disease

secondhand smoke
the mixture of the smoke produced by a lit cigarette and smoke exhaled by the smoker; more than fifty carcinogens are present in secondhand smoke

Secondhand smoke is the mixture of the smoke produced by a lit cigarette and smoke exhaled by the smoker. The smoke of a lit cigarette, termed sidestream smoke, tends to have higher concentrations of the carcinogens than cigarette smoke inhaled by the smoker. More than fifty carcinogens are present in secondhand smoke. Research indicates that secondhand smoke, also called involuntary smoking, can result in premature death and disease in children and adults, primarily through the same mechanisms by which smoking causes disease in smokers.

Exposure to secondhand smoke has decreased by about half since the late 1980s. Previously, 88% of those greater than four years old were exposed to tobacco smoke. Today, that number has decreased to 43% (US Department of Health and Human Services, 2006). Most of this exposure occurs in the home and the workplace, despite the trend toward banning smoking in public places. Lower-income children are more likely to be exposed to smoke in their homes compared to other populations. As stated previously, it is estimated that secondhand smoke exposure causes approximately three thousand deaths from lung cancer and forty-six thousand deaths from heart disease.

The 2006 surgeon general's report, *The Health Consequences of Involuntary Exposure to Tobacco Smoke* (US Department of Health and Human Services, 2006), concluded that secondhand smoke causes the following:

1. *Immediate adverse effects on the cardiovascular system and coronary heart disease.* Secondhand smoke causes platelet and endothelial dysfunction, which leads to 25% to 35% increase of CHD. There is an increased risk of stroke; however, there is no causal relationship established to date. One thousand seventeen hundred excess deaths of nonsmokers from CHD can be attributed to secondhand smoke due to exposure in the workplace.

2. *Lung cancer.* Similar to the causal effect of smoking on lung cancer, secondhand smoke exposure causes genetic changes that lead to lung cancer (see figure 4.2). Studies show a 20% to 30% increase in the risk of lung cancer for those living with someone who smokes regularly. More

than fifty studies have addressed the association between exposure and lung cancer among a diversity of populations (more than twenty countries represented); all but eight studies indicated causal effects.

3. *Increased risk for SIDS, acute respiratory infections, ear problems, and more severe asthma in children.* Although the biological basis for all SIDS cases is still unclear, research is sufficient to associate SIDS with exposure to secondhand smoke. The smoke that the infant breathes in affects the brain's ability to regulate breathing and to properly respond to hypoxia. Nerve cell development and function are also affected by the presence of the carcinogens in the smoke. Approximately 10% of all SIDS cases can be attributed to exposure. It is also estimated that annually, because of secondhand smoke exposure, between 24,300 and 71,900 low birth weight–preterm babies are born, 202,300 asthma cases are diagnosed, and 789,700 ear infections are reported.

4. *Slowed lung growth and respiratory symptoms in children who live with parents who smoke.* Adverse effects to the lungs begin with exposure of the fetus to secondhand smoke from the mother and other smokers in the house. The components in secondhand smoke reduce airway size and change lung properties (e.g., reduces elasticity) by affecting the hormones that speed lung maturation but inhibit their growth. As the child grows into late adolescence, coughing and wheezing occur in response to the nerves that control reflex response in the lungs being stimulated and irritated.

Political and Cultural History of Tobacco Use

Significant changes have occurred in US culture and government policy with regards to smoking, which may have seemed unimaginable fifty years ago. During the second half of the twentieth century, US culture went from accepting smoking to avoiding it. This change in attitude, which was heavily influenced at the beginning by the 1964 surgeon general's report that showed smoking caused lung cancer in men, was then continuously influenced by the large volumes of research disseminated in the following years on the wide spectrum of ill effects of smoking, and resulted in policy changes at the state and federal levels to reduce the incidence of secondhand smoke and protect citizens from big tobacco advertising schemes. These policy changes started in the 1990s, when California passed the first Clean Indoor Air Act and the Master Settlement Agreement was signed. Subsequently, state and federal policies, such as the Family Smoking Prevention and Tobacco Control Act of 2009, began to further change the culture of smoking.

Historically, records indicate that as early as 1914 local governments may have acted to limit or control tobacco use. That year Houston, Missouri, prohibited the sale of tobacco to minors, and in 1936, Milwaukee, Wisconsin, prohibited smoking on buses.

Most of the changes we are familiar with today started to take place around 1970 and reached their height in 1998 with the Master Settlement Agreement.

Warning Labels

In 1966, the United States began to require warning labels on cigarettes. The message was simple and cautionary: "Cigarette Smoking May be Hazardous to Your Health." From 1970 to 1985, with evidence supporting its statement, the message became a warning: "The Surgeon General Has Determined that Cigarette Smoking is Dangerous to Your Health." The warning labels that we are familiar with today were required beginning in 1985. One of the following four labels is required to be on a cigarette pack:

* Smoking Causes Lung Cancer, Heart Disease, Emphysema, And May Complicate Pregnancy

* Quitting Smoking Now Greatly Reduces Serious Risks to Your Health

* Smoking By Pregnant Women May Result in Fetal Injury, Premature Birth, And Low Birth Weight

* Cigarette Smoke Contains Carbon Monoxide

Although the United States was the first nation to require warning labels on cigarette packaging, these labels are now the smallest and most inconspicuous labels compared to those in other developed countries. In 2009, a federal policy was enacted to change these labels to a more colorful, prominent, graphic label. However, because of lawsuits filed by "big tobacco," these changes are still pending (Wilson, 2011). This topic is addressed in further detail later in the chapter.

2009 Tobacco Control Act

includes more than twenty provisions, rules, and regulations; targeting adolescents, there are specific provisions that restrict the sale of cigarettes and smokeless tobacco and restrict tobacco product advertising and marketing

Starting in 2010, as part of the **2009 Tobacco Control Act**, smokeless tobacco products were required to show a warning label. One of the following four labels is required to be on the two principle sides of the package and cover at least 30% of each side:

* This product can cause mouth cancer.

* This product can cause gum disease and tooth loss.

* This product is not a safe alternative to cigarettes.

* Smokeless tobacco is addictive.

Purchasing Restrictions

Age restrictions on who can purchase cigarettes have existed in the United States since 1992. The average legal age for purchasing is eighteen years old. In four states (Alabama, Alaska, New Jersey, and Utah) the age is nineteen years old. However, there is no state or federal law that prohibits the *use* of tobacco, just the purchase of the tobacco products. In other words, there is no penalty for smoking tobacco at younger than eighteen years of age.

Taxation

Tobacco has a long history of taxation in the United States. In 1862, the federal government instituted the first tobacco tax. By 1969, all states and the District of Columbia had instituted additional state tobacco taxes. The largest federal tobacco tax increase occurred in 2009, when the tax was increased by 62 cents to $1.01 per pack. This particular increase in tax may have resulted in the 8.3% decrease in cigarette sales in 2009.

Increasing tobacco taxes is an important step in decreasing the number of tobacco users in the United States. Research indicates that for every 10% increase in price, youth smoking decreases 7% and overall smoking decreases by approximately 4%. Epidemiologic estimates predict that increasing the cost of cigarettes could lead to the prevention of two million adolescents from starting to smoke, help one million adults quit, prevent nine hundred thousand smoking-caused deaths, and save $44.5 billion in long-term health care costs.

Each state has the ability to set its own tax rate in regards to cigarette sales. Since 1999, only three states have not increased cigarette taxes (California, North Dakota, and Missouri). All others have increased these taxes at least once in that time frame. Currently, the average tax is $1.48 per pack, with a significant gap between levels of taxation in tobacco states (states that grow tobacco) and nontobacco states. Tobacco states impose average taxes of 48.5 cents, whereas nontobacco states impose taxes averaging $1.61. New York has the highest tax rate of $4.35 per pack. The CDC estimates that for each pack sold, $10.47 is spent on health costs and productivity losses. Therefore, even the highest tax rate does not cover the direct and indirect costs of smoking.

1998 Master Settlement Agreement

The **Master Settlement Agreement (MSA)** is a joint lawsuit that was settled by forty-six states in November 1998 (National Association of Attorneys General, 1998). During the mid-1990s, the attorney generals of forty-six states sued Philip Morris, Inc., R. J. Reynolds, Brown &

Master Settlement Agreement (MSA) a joint lawsuit that was settled by forty-six states in November 1998; during the mid-1990s, the attorneys general of forty-six states sued Philip Morris, Inc., R. J. Reynolds, Brown & Williamson, and Lorillard, commonly referred to as the four "big tobacco" companies, for damages and health care costs to states that resulted from tobacco use by state residents; the settlement payout is $246 billion over twenty-five years; each state is awarded a yearly payment

Williamson, and Lorillard, commonly referred to as the four "big tobacco" companies, for damages and health care costs to states that resulted from tobacco use by state residents. The settlement payout is $246 billion over twenty-five years; each state is awarded a yearly payment. There are more specific provisions of the agreement, with a number that specifically affect public health by moving "big tobacco" away from an industry that freely advertised to youth using cartoons and promotions to one that is restricted in their advertising markets and no longer permitted to obscure or dilute the health risks of tobacco use. Practically speaking, as a student reading this text, you may not have experienced the days when "Joe Camel" was more recognized by children than Mickey Mouse, when smokers redeemed their "Marlboro Miles" for free products with Marlboro logos (lighters, hats, shirts, and various household items), or when sporting events sponsored by big tobacco were household names (e.g., "Winston Cup" NASCAR premier race). The MSA is responsible for establishing this new antitobacco culture and may have played a key role in the 21% decrease in cigarette sales since the settlement was announced. Table 4.1 lists the specific provisions of the MSA.

Table 4.1 Provisions of the Master Settlement Agreement

• Prohibition of youth targeting	• Limitations on lobbying
• Ban on use of cartoons	• Restrictions on advocacy concerning settlement proceeds
• Limitation of tobacco brand name sponsorship	• Dissolution of the Tobacco Institute, Inc., The Council for Tobacco Research—USA, Inc., and the Center for Indoor Air Research, Inc.
• Elimination of outdoor advertising and transit advertising	• Regulation and oversight of new tobacco-related trade associations
• Prohibition of tobacco payments related to tobacco products and media	• Prohibitions on agreements to suppress research
• Ban on tobacco brand-name merchandise	• Prohibition on material misrepresentations
• Ban on youth access to free samples	• Granting public access to documents
• Ban on gifts to underage persons based on proof of purchase	• Establishing tobacco control and underage use laws
• Limitation of third-party use of brand names	• Establishment of a national foundation (Legacy—responsible for the Truth campaign)
• Ban on tobacco brand names	
• Minimum pack size of twenty cigarettes	
• Corporate culture commitments related to youth access and consumption	

Recent Efforts to Reduce Tobacco Use

In general, US public opinion regarding smoking has changed. According to the 2011 Gallup poll on smoking bans, a majority of Americans (59%) are in favor of a smoking ban and clean indoor air for all (Newport, 2011). This is a significant change from the 2001 poll, when only approximately 39% were in favor of a smoking ban.

As public opinion has shifted since the new millennium, major federal, state, and local initiatives have further discouraged smoking in the United States. These initiatives include the expansion of the authority of the Food and Drug Administration (FDA) to regulate the sales, advertising, and ingredient content of all tobacco products, an increase in the federal tobacco excise tax to $1.01 per pack, and the passage of comprehensive statewide smoke-free laws in thirty states. In addition, workplace and school policies and community programs have been effective in discouraging smoking among adults and adolescents.

National Policy

Federal antitobacco policies and laws have been enacted since the 1990s to discourage smoking, protect citizens from big tobacco advertising schemes, protect citizens from secondhand smoke, and prevent adolescent tobacco use. It is a federal law that all domestic and international flights departing from the United States be smoke free. Also, federal law inhibits smoking in agencies that receive federal funding to serve youth (e.g., schools). In 1998, an executive order was passed stating that all buildings owned, rented, or leased by the federal government must be smoke free. The most recent federal law to be passed is the Family Smoking Prevention and Tobacco Control Act of 2009.

Family Smoking Prevention and Tobacco Control Act of 2009

In June 2009, President Barack Obama signed into law the Family Smoking Prevention and Tobacco Control Act (Tobacco Control Act). The main goal of this law is to prevent and reduce tobacco use by adolescents under the age of eighteen. It is well established that most first-time use of tobacco occurs at a young age; only 1% of the smoking population reports first cigarette use after the age of twenty-six, with 88% initiating before the age of eighteen. The law gives the FDA the authority to regulate the marketing, sales, and development of all tobacco products, new and old. It is appropriate to grant the FDA this regulatory authority because the agency's purpose is to protect the public's health by ensuring the safety and security of consumable products—including but not limited to the food supply, human drugs and medical devices, cosmetics, and dietary supplements. In order to oversee full implementation of the Tobacco Control Act, the FDA established the Center for Tobacco Products and the Tobacco Products Scientific Advisory Committee.

The Tobacco Control Act includes more than twenty provisions, rules, and regulations. Targeting adolescents, it has specific provisions that restrict the sale of cigarettes and smokeless tobacco, and restricts tobacco product advertising and marketing. For example, proof of age (over eighteen) is required to purchase cigarettes and smokeless tobacco, and face-to-face sales (no vending machines) are required unless in certain adult-only facilities. Also, tobacco companies are not permitted to sponsor sporting or entertainment events or distribute free samples of cigarettes and brand-name promotional items (e.g., Marlboro gym bags). The Tobacco Control Act prohibits the use of reduced harm claims such as "light," "low," or "mild" unless approved by the FDA, requires the tobacco industry to submit marketing documents for FDA approval, and requires certain standards for tobacco products. Marketing orders (permission from FDA to market the new product) are now also required for new products and those that are claiming the product "reduces harm" compared to cigarette smoking (e.g., e-cigarettes and smokeless tobacco) (US Food and Drug Administration, 2012).

Also under the Tobacco Control Act, the tobacco industry is required to disclose research findings regarding the health effects of tobacco use and information about the ingredients and constituents in tobacco products. There are more than seven thousand chemicals in tobacco and tobacco smoke, termed harmful and potentially harmful constituents (HPHCs). HPHCs are chemicals or chemical compounds that cause or may cause health problems. The FDA created a list of twenty HPHCs that are easy to test their presence in tobacco products and are representative of the full list of seven thousand HPHCs. The list of the amount of HPHCs in specific products is available on the FDA website (www.fda.gov/TobaccoProducts /GuidanceComplianceRegulatoryInformation/ucm297786.htm). However, the ingredient list will not be labeled on the box. Consumers will need to access the list via the Internet or through printed documents. For the list of HPHCs required to be disclosed in cigarettes and smokeless tobacco, see table 4.2.

The Tobacco Control Act also requires more prominent warning labels for cigarettes and smokeless tobacco products. This provision is stirring heated debate. The new labels were required to cover the top 50% of the front and rear panels of each cigarette package, with font colors limited to black and white. (See figure 4.3.)

Table 4.2   List of Harmful and Potentially Harmful Constituents (HPHCs) in Cigarette Smoke and Smokeless Tobacco

Cigarette Smoke	Smokeless Tobacco
Acetaldehyde	Acetaldehyde
Acrolein	Arsenic
Acrylonitrile	Benzo[a]pyrene
4-Aminobiphenyl	Cadmium
1-Aminonaphthalene	Crotonaldehyde
2-Aminonaphthalene	Formaldehyde
Ammonia	Nicotine (total and free)
Benzene	4-(methylnitrosamino)-1-(3-pyridyl)-1-butanone
Benzo[a]pyrene	N-nitrosonornicotine
1,3-Butadiene	
Carbon monoxide	
Crotonaldehyde	
Formaldehyde	
Isoprene	
Nicotine (total)	
4-(methylnitrosamino)-1-(3-pyridyl)-1-butanone	
N-nitrosonornicotine	
Toluene	

Lawsuits against these label requirements were filed in August 2011 by five tobacco companies (Lorillard, R. J. Reynolds, Commonwealth Brands, the Liggett Group, and Santa Fe Natural Tobacco), claiming that the labels violate the First Amendment protections for commercial speech. A decision in August 2012 by the federal appeals court (divided decision) was that the FDA needed to immediately revise the law and the required and proposed labels will not be used. Judge Janice Brown wrote that the "FDA failed to present any data—much less the substantial evidence required under the federal law—showing that enacting their proposed graphic warnings will accomplish the agency's stated objective of reducing smoking rates. The rule thus cannot pass muster" (Mears, 2012). The legal question was whether the new labeling was purely factual and accurate in nature or was designed to discourage the use of

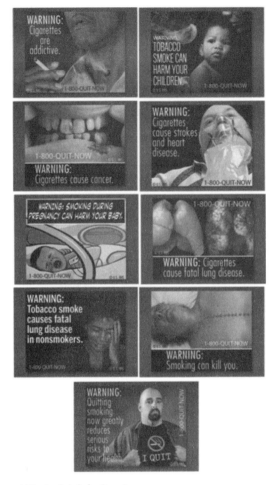

Figure 4.3   Proposed Warning Labels for Cigarettes
Source: US Food and Drug Administration.

the products. It appears that the FDA may have underestimated the impact of the labels in reducing smoking. The court did not allow the labeling because the FDA did not present compelling evidence that the graphic labels would make an impact (Huang, Chaloupka, and Fong, 2013).

State Policy

State antitobacco policies and programs focus primarily on restricting smoking in public places and preventing adolescent smoking initiation.

Smoking Bans

Many states have implemented the Clean Indoor Air Act by banning smoking in certain locations and under certain circumstances, with varying provisions. The Clean Indoor Air Act typically prohibits smoking in enclosed public places, including bars and restaurants. They do not typically prohibit smoking in private workplaces; however, many workplaces are voluntarily going smoke free. Some states allow exemptions for certain facilities, such as tobacconists, cigar bars, casinos, and private clubs. Violations are typically enforced by the health department and are considered civil infractions. Multiple violations may result in multiple fines or business license suspensions.

According to the American Nonsmokers' Rights Foundation, 81.3% of the US population lives under a ban on smoking prohibited by state, commonwealth, or local laws. As of December 2012, only ten states did not have a general statewide smoking ban on nongovernment properties: Alabama, Alaska, Kentucky, Mississippi, Missouri, Oklahoma, South Carolina, Texas, West Virginia, and Wyoming. These states permit separate smoking and nonsmoking sections with signage to designate these areas.

Master Settlement Agreement State Initiatives

The MSA is now in its fifteenth year, with mixed results in terms of how it has affected tobacco use. One of the downsides of the agreement is that states are not required to use the annual settlement money for antitobacco initiatives. Each state may use the money at its own discretion; during the recent economic downturn, states were using the money to fill gaps in budgets rather than to address tobacco use.

Research suggests that antitobacco programs are successful at increasing cessation rates. The CDC recommends a certain level of antitobacco initiative spending based on state population. The recommended level is the amount deemed necessary to affect changes in tobacco use rates. As of 2012, the CDC reported that only two states funded tobacco control programs at the recommended level (Alaska and North Dakota), whereas twenty-nine states and the District of Columbia funded tobacco control programs at less than 25% of this level. Unfortunately, in 2013 there are four states that will not use any of their settlement funding for tobacco control (New Hampshire, New Jersey, North Carolina, and Ohio). In fiscal year 2013, settlement and tobacco tax income will total $25.7 billion; however, it is projected that states will only spend 1.8% of this money (equaling 2 cents of every dollar) on prevention and cessation programs (Campaign for Tobacco Free Kids, 2012).

Local Policy

Most successful statewide smoking bans started with grassroots efforts of local municipalities implementing smoke-free legislation. In order to be considered 100% smoke free, municipalities must ban smoking in all workplaces (including offices, factories, and warehouses) and all restaurants and bars (no separate smoking section or ventilated room is allowed). According to the American Nonsmokers' Rights Foundation, as of April 2014 there are 627 local municipalities that are 100% smoke free. In total, 3,671 municipalities across the United States restrict smoking in some way. Common restrictions include bans on smoking in outdoor areas, near (fifteen to twenty feet) entrances and windows of enclosed places, public outdoor places such as beaches and parks, outdoor stadiums, and other sports and entertainment venues (American Nonsmokers' Rights Foundation, 2014). Although not required or typically covered under a municipal policy, approximately 1,182 universities and colleges have implemented a voluntary smoke-free campus policy (American Nonsmokers' Rights Foundation, 2014). This is a significant change compared to ten years ago, when no campuses were smoke-free.

Effective Programs That Discourage Tobacco Use

In order to further decrease the percentage of people smoking, effective tobacco control programs need to be implemented by employers, in communities, in schools, and for individuals. As stated previously, the proportion of adult smokers has decreased from 42.4% in 1965 to 19.0% of the population in 2011. However, despite this victory, the United States is still short of its Healthy People 2020 goal of 12%.

Healthy People 2020

Healthy People is a federal interagency work group that sets ten-year agendas for improving the health of Americans. These agendas are used by health promotion professionals to guide decisions regarding what types of programs should be provided and to whom. The Healthy People 2020 tobacco-related goal is to reduce illness, disability, and death related to tobacco use and secondhand smoke exposure. There are twenty specific objectives to meet to attain this goal, which includes reducing smoking among adults and adolescents, increasing quit attempts and success among all types of smokers (adult, adolescent, and pregnant), and reducing smoking initiation. For a full list of these objectives, see table 4.3. Chapter 9 explores other state and federal government activities.

The good news is that smokers do make attempts to quit—research suggests that more than half of smokers (51.8%) make a quit attempt for longer than one day each year. Additionally, the majority of smokers quit

Table 4.3   Healthy People 2020 Objectives Related to Tobacco Use

Category	Objective
Tobacco use	Reduce tobacco use by adults
	Reduce the initiation of tobacco use in children, adolescents, and young adults
	Reduce tobacco use by adolescents
Tobacco cessation	Increase smoking cessation attempts by adult smokers
	Increase recent smoking cessation success by adult smokers
	Increase smoking cessation during pregnancy
	Increase smoking cessation attempts by adolescent smokers
	Increase comprehensive Medicaid insurance coverage of evidence-based treatment for nicotine dependency in the states and the District of Columbia
Health system changes	Increase tobacco screening in health care settings
	Increase tobacco cessation counseling in health care settings
	Reduce the proportion of nonsmokers exposed to secondhand smoke
	Increase the proportion of persons covered by indoor work site policies that prohibit smoking
	Establish laws in the states, District of Columbia, territories, and tribes on smoke-free indoor air that prohibit smoking in public places and work sites
	Increase the proportion of smoke-free homes
Social and environmental changes	Increase tobacco-free environments in schools, including all school facilities, property, vehicles, and school events
	Eliminate state laws that preempt stronger local tobacco control laws
	Increase the federal and state taxes on tobacco products
	Reduce the proportion of adolescents and young adults in grades 6 through 12 who are exposed to tobacco advertising and promotion
	Reduce the illegal sales rate to minors through enforcement of laws prohibiting the sale of tobacco products to minors
	Increase the number of states and the District of Columbia, territories, and tribes with sustainable and comprehensive evidence-based tobacco control programs

without using specific treatments (e.g., quit "cold turkey"). However, smokers who quit successfully are more likely to remain smoke free if they use an evidence-based approach. There are a variety of effective programs available to help smokers quit.

Population-Based Strategies

Population-based strategies have been shown to be effective in helping smokers quit. For example, in a systematic review of fifty studies, data indicate that smoke-free laws for workplaces and public places are effective in reducing active smoking rates and reducing exposure to secondhand smoke (Callinan et al., 2010). This resulted in decreased hospital admissions for heart attacks, a significant accomplishment. Research also shows that health warning labels with graphic images have short-term effects on adult smokers, including those with low health literacy, a population that is typically difficult to reach (Thrasher et al., 2012). Antitobacco media campaigns featuring graphic personal stories have been shown to be effective in increasing quitting and reducing smoking prevalence, as shown in a review of eleven national and international campaigns. The most effective programs were those that were part of a comprehensive tobacco control program that offer individual assistance for quitting (e.g., telephone quit lines) that last after the campaign has ended.

Effective Examples of Population-Based Strategies

Multimedia interventions are most likely to be successful in reducing smoking rates if they are part of a complex set of interventions; for example, one component of a state tobacco control program. In a systematic review of multimedia interventions, over half of the studies reported an increase in abstinence from smoking (Secker-Walker et al., 2002). The campaigns with longer duration, more intense advertising, and part of a larger comprehensive tobacco control plan were most likely to be successful. A few examples of effective campaigns are provided in the following sections.

Truth

One provision of the 1998 Master Settlement Agreement was the establishment of a national foundation, the Legacy Foundation, focused on anti-tobacco messaging and preventing adolescents from initiating tobacco use. Funded by the MSA, the Legacy Foundation has implemented multimedia campaigns and programs to meet this goal. The "Truth" campaign aims to empower youth to decide not to smoke. It is an ongoing publicity campaign that advertises on television, the Internet, social networking sites, and promotes in-person events and grassroots outreach programs. The most recent successful advertising initiative was "The Sunny Side of Truth," which in 2008 used sarcasm in a Broadway-style theme to promote the truth of the hazards of smoking. Research suggests that 22% of the overall decline in youth smoking is attributable to the Truth campaign, resulting in three hundred thousand fewer youth smokers (Matthew et al., 2005). Additionally, exposure to the campaign results in more accurate perceptions of peer smoking, which has been shown to deter initiation (Davis, Nonnemaker, & Farrelly, 2007).

Tips from Former Smokers

"Tips" was the first federally funded mass media campaign to reduce smoking rates. It is a $54 million campaign funded through the Prevention and Public Health Fund of the Patient Protection and Affordable Care Act (ACA). The CDC ran the campaign for twelve weeks starting in March 2012. It consisted of thirty-second radio and TV ads, print media, billboards, videos on YouTube, and Facebook and Twitter posts. The target audience was eighteen to fifty-four, and the short-term goal was to prompt people to quit and raise awareness of free government resources to help smokers quit. The ads ran in English and Spanish and featured real people telling stories of how it feels to have a tobacco-related disease and how they finally quit for good. The diseases featured include Buerger's disease (blocking of blood vessels, which leads to infection in the limbs and results in multiple amputations), heart disease and stroke, cancer, and asthma due to secondhand smoke. The campaign successfully raised awareness (reached 80% of smokers), as shown by tripled hits to the website and double the amount of calls to the quit line (Rigotti & Wakefield, 2012). Long-term results of the campaign indicate that there was a 12% increase in quit attempts during the campaign, with 1.6 million additional smokers making a quit attempt. It is estimated that two hundred thousand smokers remained smoke free at the end of the campaign and at least one hundred thousand of these will stay smoke free long term. Based on these estimates, the CDC reports that this will add one-third to a half a million quality-adjusted life years to the US population (McAfee et al., 2013).

EX

From March 2008 to September 2008, the National Alliance for Tobacco Cessation sponsored a mass-media campaign entitled "EX." The target audience was smokers who were open to quitting but did not know how to successfully quit. Advertisements ran on cable TV, with 68% of the ads running in the first three months of the campaign. The message was simple and relayed in an empathic voice from smoker to smoker: relearn life without cigarettes. The ads prompted viewers to go to their website for support (www.becomeanEX.org). Research showed that the campaign was effective in increasing quit attempts (Vallone et al., 2011). Although the campaign is no longer running, the website is active with virtual online support, connections to Facebook and Twitter, and a mobile platform.

Work Site Initiatives

According to the CDC, an employer can expect to save nearly $3,500 annually for each employee who successfully quits using tobacco (CDC, 2006). The savings is derived from decreased health care costs and increased productivity. The primary objectives of work site smoking programs are to decrease the number of smokers and reduce employee exposure to second-hand smoke. A workplace smoking ban is the most effective strategy to achieve these objectives. Research indicates that bans can reduce exposure by an average of 72%. At minimum, it is recommended that a workplace smoking ban prohibit smoking in the building and within fifteen to twenty feet of all entrances, windows, and ventilation intakes. Companies can take it a step further and deem their property a smoke-free campus, which would require employees to leave company property to smoke (discouraging smoke breaks) (CDC, 2012b).

smoking cessation programs
interventions, such as counseling and quit lines, designed to help individuals quit smoking

Some employers offer **smoking cessation programs** for employees. These programs include counseling and quit lines and are most effective when offered on-site for easy employee access. Companies that are large enough may hire a health educator or a tobacco cessation counselor to provide individual or group counseling. It is recommended that employees participate in more than four sessions lasting more than ten minutes with a counselor. Implementing a workplace smoking ban with referral services to smoking cessation programs is ideal. It is well established that a combination of intensive counseling, over-the-counter (OTC) nicotine replacement therapy (nicotine patch, gum, or lozenge), and prescription medications (buproprion SR, varenicline tartrate, nicotine spray or inhaler) is the most effective individual treatment. Employee health benefits should provide full coverage of these treatments. A combination of all these strategies provides a comprehensive tobacco cessation program that is more effective than any single program alone (US Office of Personnel Management, 2013).

Practical Examples of Work Site Initiatives

Quest Diagnostics

Quest Diagnostics provides diagnostic testing services to 151 million patients annually. They employ approximately forty-one thousand employees and are located worldwide. Their in-house health promotion program, called HealthyQuest, is focused on improving the health of their employees as well as creating an overall culture of health. Their smoking cessation program is part of HealthyQuest and is provided by an outside vendor. In-house, however, Quest has more than six hundred employees who volunteer to be leaders on the health promotion team. Most of the leaders are either former smokers or those trying to quit. The duties of the leaders are to educate employees on the long-term health effects of smoking on themselves as well as the effects on those around them. They also champion corporate smoking events (such as the Great American Smokeout) and support tobacco-free corporate guidelines by implementing them in their business units. They encourage their fellow employees to join the smoking cessation program that is provided free of charge and serve as mentors and as resource persons.

After implementation of HealthyQuest, the quit rate was 35% and the overall prevalence of smoking decreased 2% (Partnership for Prevention, 2008). The company reported the following tips for large corporations interested in adding a smoking cessation program: (1) don't be judgmental, (2) be sure the health promotion teams are compassionate and committed, (3) encourage employee testimonials, because this will drive others to join, (4) create program specific to the corporate culture, not one that is cookie cutter, (5) and collect objective data to inform leadership on the effectiveness of the program as well as resource allocation needs.

Union Pacific Railroad

Union Pacific Railroad is the largest railroad serving twenty-three states west of the Mississippi, with fifty thousand employees. It has been in business for more than 150 years and has a large percentage of fifth-generation employees. Its health promotion program, HealthTrack, has a tobacco program wrapped into it titled Butt Out and Breathe. For the program, employees are asked to assess their stage of change (readiness to quit) and, based on their stage, are given a tailored intervention. The interventions range from covered pharmacologic treatment (including OTC nicotine replacement therapy), individual health coaching, online services, to self-help guides. Employees are given progress reports every three, six, and twelve months as well as multiple-year progress reports if applicable.

Union Pacific Railroad has successfully created a culture that is reflective of a tobacco-free environment. The key initiatives the company has undertaken are (1) integrating nonsmoking as a safety rule within its safety structure, because it found that smoking is a risk for getting injured on the job, (2) a hiring policy that does not hire job candidates who smoke (in the states where it is legal to ask the question), (3) advocating for the city of Omaha to be smoke free, and (4) writing into managers' job agreements the provision that they will support the smoke-free initiatives of the company. The success of the program has been dramatic—in the early

1990s, its smoking rate was 40%; currently, it is 17% (which is lower than the national average).

School Initiatives

Various methods have been used in schools to prevent smoking initiation among adolescents. Information-giving curricula teach students about the prevalence, incidence, and risks of tobacco use. Social competence programs teach students cognitive behavioral skills and self-management personal and social skills to resist media and interpersonal influences to initiate smoking. Social influence programs teach students refusal skills; increase awareness of media, peer, and family influences; and encourage public commitments not to smoke. All three of these methods may also be used in combination, enabling a more comprehensive approach. Some multimodal programs combine curricular programs with community-based initiatives and policy changes on the taxation, sale, and availability of tobacco.

In a review of ninety-four randomized controlled trials that used one or more of the previously mentioned interventions, results indicated that information given alone is less effective or no different from other models. Social competence interventions had some positive short-term results, as did social influence programs, although neither did in the long term (Thomas & Perera, 2006). Programs that combine social competence and influence showed success in the short term; however, there is insufficient evidence to make a definitive determination if a combined model is more effective than social influence programs alone. Last, of four studies that tested the impact of social influence and competence programs in the context of larger community initiatives, three showed positive results. In sum, information-only programs have not been shown to be effective, social influence programs can be effective in the short term, and adding components such as community involvement may improve effectiveness.

The CDC's guideline on school health programs, developed by numerous agencies and based on existing research and practice, lists seven recommendations to prevent tobacco use among school-aged students. These comprise: (1) school policies that ban smoking and tobacco advertising on school grounds, (2) requiring instruction on avoiding tobacco use, (3) providing K–12 tobacco prevention education, (4) teacher training, (5) involving parents and families, (6) providing cessation programs for students and staff, and (7) regularly evaluating the program for effectiveness (CDC, 2008).

Practical Examples of School Initiatives

West Virginia Schools

In collaboration with state and community agencies and using the strategies discussed previously, West Virginia was successful in reducing its high school smoking rate from 28% to 22% in two years. Its efforts were widespread, starting with a state mandate that all students receive instruction on tobacco and potential health hazards from tobacco use in grades K–12. It also developed a Regional Tobacco Prevention Specialist Network, which resulted in tobacco prevention initiatives in all fifty-five school districts in the state. At the school level, the state developed a teen smoking cessation program titled Not-On-Tobacco (N-O-T) that is conducted in all West Virginia secondary schools. In collaboration with the American Lung Association of West Virginia, the state also created an antitobacco youth movement called Raze, which involves more than seven thousand students (CDC, 2011d).

South Carolina Schools

In a collaborative effort among school boards and state agencies, South Carolina was successful in increasing the number of school districts adopting its model, comprehensive, tobacco-free school policy from 22% to 35% two years later. Its success was due to the implementation of the community roundtable model to promote and train school administrators on the comprehensive program and the employment of a school health policy coordinator. The program includes policies regarding use of tobacco on school property, procedures for enforcement, education for tobacco prevention, cessation programs, and information about tobacco industry advertising (CDC, 2011d).

Community Initiatives

According to the CDC (2014, p. 22), a **community** "encompasses a diverse set of entities, including voluntary health agencies; civic, social, and recreational organizations; businesses and business associations; city and county governments; public health organizations; labor groups; health care systems and providers; health care professionals' societies; schools and universities; faith communities; and organizations for racial and ethnic minority groups." In a review of the current literature on effective community-based interventions, the CDC developed a best practices guideline for health promotion professionals at the state and community levels to implement effective treatment and cessation programs. In summary, community-based

community
"encompasses a diverse set of entities, including voluntary health agencies; civic, social, and recreational organizations; businesses and business associations; city and county governments; public health organizations; labor groups; health care systems and providers; health care professionals' societies; schools and universities; faith communities; and organizations for racial and ethnic minority groups" (CDC)

interventions should focus on changing social norms related to smoking by advocating and initiating policy changes at the state level (US Department of Health and Human Services, 2007). For example, communities may offer educational programs or quit line support that is advertised through mass media campaigns run by the state encouraging adults to quit smoking. The main goal is to have state and community agencies work together in order to increase the reach of smaller, individual-based clinical and educational interventions.

These recommendations are based on the evidence that community-based interventions alone do not affect prevalence of smoking. A systematic review of thirty-seven studies showed that although programs were successful in increasing the knowledge of health risks, changing attitudes toward smoking, increasing quit attempts, and providing better environmental and social support for quitting, community-level smoking rates did not decrease. In the best designed trial, the US COMMIT study, there was disappointingly no difference in prevalence. However, the authors point out that the studies that were included in the systematic review had measurement issues; therefore, health promotion professionals should make greater efforts to use sound methodologies to evaluate their programs. Also, they should consider the following:

- Use community members to staff coalitions and task forces and supervise implementation.

- Allow several years to realize the results of interventions and provide readily available resources throughout the community.

- Use mass media to change social norms.

- Provide referral services to health professionals specifically trained in tobacco cessation techniques.

- Provide nicotine replacement therapy and prescription medications at little or no cost.

Individual Programs

The individual-based treatments that have been shown to be effective in helping people quit smoking cigarettes are brief clinical interventions from a doctor; individual, group, or telephone counseling; behavioral counseling; intensive one-on-one counseling; and OTC and prescription medications (Fiore et al., 2008). OTC medications include nicotine replacement products such as the nicotine patch, gum, and lozenges. Prescription medications include nicotine inhalers, nasal spray, bupropion SR (Zyban), and varenicline tartrate (Chantix). Research indicates that successful, sustained quitting results from a combination of intensive counseling and some sort of medication, be it OTC or prescription (or a combination of both) (US Department of Health and Human Services, 2008).

For smokeless tobacco cessation, a systematic review of twenty-five randomized controlled trials revealed that the best intervention is behavioral intervention, followed by telephone counseling and oral examination with feedback on effects of smokeless tobacco use. Prescription drugs such as buproprion SR (Wellbutrin) and OTC nicotine replacement products are not shown to be effective (Ebbert et al., 2011). Varenicline (Chantix) is effective for increasing abstinence among snus users, according to a single study.

Challenges to Reducing Smoking

Significant health promotion challenges to reducing smoking are discussed in this section.

Access to Treatment

Getting access to treatment methods and supports is the first step to quitting smoking. According to Healthy People 2020, only five states have comprehensive Medicaid insurance coverage of evidence-based tobacco treatment. Given that 36% of those enrolled in Medicaid are smokers (significantly more than the general population), this creates a challenge for this demographic to obtain much needed tobacco cessation services (CDC, 2004). The Tobacco Use and Dependence Guideline Panel (2008) recommends a systems approach to identifying and treating patients who use the health care system. However, data show that only 20% of visits to office and hospital-based ambulatory care settings offer tobacco cessation services or order treatments. The Healthy People 2020 goal is to increase this percentage by at least 10%.

In response to the overwhelming evidence that tobacco cessation treatment is effective and cost-saving, managed care plan coverage of comprehensive tobacco treatment has increased significantly to 90%. However, employers, who are purchasers of insurance coverage, are still not offering tobacco cessation programs to their employees. Research shows that only 20% of employers offer these services free of charge through their insurance coverage—even though employers rank the impact and value of tobacco cessation services as very high. Additionally, of these 20%, only 4% offer optimal services (Bondi et al., 2006), which should include brief advice from a physician, three hundred minutes of behavioral counseling from a multidisciplinary team over eight sessions, and at least one form of medication. This type of program costs about $1,500 per smoker, a cost that employers may not be willing to pay, even though the return on investment can be up to $5.45 per dollar spent (O'Donnell & Roizen, 2011).

Research indicates that when smokers do not have to pay for treatment, there is an increase in the number of smokers attempting to quit, use of evidence-based treatments, and success in quitting (Reda et al., 2012).

Addictive Property of Nicotine

According to the *International Classification of Diseases,* tenth revision (ICD-10) (CDC, 1999), a person is considered to be dependent on a substance if he or she exhibits any of the following three criteria in a twelve-month period:

- Increased tolerance
- Physical withdrawal at times
- Strong desire to take drug
- Difficulty controlling use
- Persistent use despite harmful consequences
- Higher priority given to drug use than to other activities and obligations

It is clear that tobacco users display these behaviors on a regular basis due to the presence of the drug nicotine in tobacco leaves. It has been reported that nicotine causes addiction much the same as heroin and cocaine, making cessation difficult. Nicotine affects the body by affecting the ventral tegmental area of the brain and dopamine neurotransmitters. Dopamine levels are increased by nicotine because it directly stimulates and excites several nicotinic acetylcholine receptors (nAChRs). These nAChRs are present in several systems, but the most extensively researched are the dopamine, glutamate (an excitatory neurotransmitter), and GABA (an inhibitory neurotransmitter) systems. When dopamine is increased through these systems, the tobacco user feels good and thus becomes addicted to the substance.

The addictive property of nicotine is a unique challenge. Unlike changing other health behaviors, such as increasing physical activity or using sunscreen, quitting smoking involves overcoming physical withdrawal symptoms. These symptoms can be painful and are easily cured by smoking a cigarette or chewing tobacco. Health promotion professionals should be mindful of this when assisting someone in the quitting process and should encourage the use of OTC and prescription nicotine replacement therapies to lessen the withdrawal symptoms.

Common withdrawal symptoms can include feeling depressed, irritable, anxious, restless, hungry; having trouble thinking clearly; difficulty concentrating; sleep issues; and a slower heart rate.

Tobacco Industry Practices

The tobacco industry is well aware of the addictive property of their products and understands the difficulty in quitting. They understand that by getting adolescents addicted, they have a lifetime consumer. They also know that chronic use of their product will end with the death of the customer, so they need to consistently attract new, young lifetime users. In order to accomplish this task in the wake of the MSA, which limits direct marketing to adolescents, the tobacco industry has several practices in place. They regularly lobby against tobacco tax increases, the implementation of local and state Clean Indoor Air acts, graphic cigarette warning labels, and restrictions to selling to adolescents. The evidence is clear that these types of initiatives decrease the number of adult and adolescent smokers. They also develop new products that are specifically geared to attract adolescent users—such as the new dissolvable tobacco that looks like breath strips and Tic Tacs and do not require spitting. Adolescents can use these products in places cigarettes are not allowed, giving full access to the addictive product. Additionally, the new e-cigarettes, which have yet to be included in Clean Indoor Air acts, allow adolescents to smoke these in any environment, again giving full access. They also appeal to adolescents' fascination with new technology and electronics, reducing the focus of the product as a cigarette per se and more as an innovative electronic device.

Summary

This chapter reviewed the general statistics related to tobacco use in the United States; discussed the chronic diseases related to tobacco use and their biological basis; considered the social, political, and economic changes in the United States, along with how the culture, policies, and environment changes related to tobacco use. Further, it provided a discussion on the evidence-based and practice-based prevention and cessation programs for general and specific populations. Tobacco use has a profound influence on the health of Americans. Health promotion professionals need to be aware of the information provided herein in order to develop and implement effective programs to decrease the number of tobacco users in this country.

KEY TERMS

1. **Direct costs:** in managed care, the costs of labor, supplies, and equipment to provide direct patient care services

2. **Indirect costs:** resources forgone as a result of a health condition

3. **Cancer:** a term used for diseases in which abnormal cells divide without control and are able to invade other tissues

4. **Carcinogens:** a cancer-causing substance or agent

5. **Cardiovascular disease (CVD):** refers to conditions that involve narrowed or blocked blood vessels that can lead to a heart attack, chest pain (angina), or stroke

6. **Lung:** one of the usually paired compound saccular thoracic organs that constitute the basic respiratory organ of air-breathing vertebrates; the lungs remove carbon dioxide from and bring oxygen to the blood and consist essentially of an inverted tree of intricately branched bronchioles communicating with thin-walled terminal alveoli swathed in a network of delicate capillaries where the actual gaseous exchange of respiration takes place

7. **Oxygen:** the odorless gas that is present in the air and necessary to maintain life; patients with lung disease or damage may need to use portable oxygen devices on a temporary or permanent basis

8. **Smokeless tobacco:** a tobacco product that is not smoked but rather placed directly in the mouth, cheek, or lip to be sucked or chewed; the saliva is either swallowed or spit out and is commonly referred to in the United States as *dip, chew,* or *snuff*

9. **E-cigarettes:** devices that vaporize a mixture of water, propylene glycol, nicotine, and flavorings; battery powered and cost anywhere from $70 to $90 for a starter pack that includes the device, chargers, and nicotine cartridges

10. **Nicotine:** a colorless, poisonous alkaloid derived from the tobacco plant and used as an insecticide; the substance in tobacco to which smokers can become addicted

11. **Secondhand smoke:** the mixture of the smoke produced by a lit cigarette and smoke exhaled by the smoker; more than fifty carcinogens are present in secondhand smoke

12. **2009 Tobacco Control Act:** includes more than twenty provisions, rules, and regulations; targeting adolescents, there are specific provisions that restrict the sale of cigarettes and smokeless tobacco and restrict tobacco product advertising and marketing

13. **Master Settlement Agreement (MSA):** a joint lawsuit that was settled by forty-six states in November 1998; during the mid-1990s, the attorneys general of forty-six states sued Philip Morris, Inc., R. J. Reynolds, Brown & Williamson, and Lorillard, commonly referred to as the four "big tobacco" companies, for damages and health care costs to states that

resulted from tobacco use by state residents; the settlement payout is $246 billion over twenty-five years; each state is awarded a yearly payment

14. **Smoking cessation programs:** interventions, such as counseling and quit lines, designed to help individuals quit smoking

15. **Community:** According to the CDC, "encompasses a diverse set of entities, including voluntary health agencies; civic, social, and recreational organizations; businesses and business associations; city and county governments; public health organizations; labor groups; health care systems and providers; health care professionals' societies; schools and universities; faith communities; and organizations for racial and ethnic minority groups"

REVIEW QUESTIONS

1. What are the health concerns for smoking tobacco and using smokeless tobacco?

2. What are the definitions of direct and indirect costs associated with smoking?

3. What are the three pathways of how smoking can cause cancer?

4. What is the prevalence of smoking now versus fifty years ago? What do you think had the most influence in changing the prevalence?

5. What is the prevalence of smokeless tobacco?

6. What are the new tobacco products on the market today? What effect do you think these new products will have on adolescent use?

7. What does the term *secondhand smoke* mean and what are the associated health risks?

8. What is the Master Settlement Agreement (MSA)? What are the provisions of the MSA? What effect do you feel the agreement had on the way smoking is viewed today?

9. Identify the warnings currently used on cigarette packs. Do you feel that graphic warnings are more effective than the current text-only warnings? If they are more effective, in what way would they be—to deter new users or to stop current users?

10. What are current local, state, and federal policies on smoking?

11. Do you think the e-cigarette should be considered part of Clean Indoor Air acts? Why or why not?

12. What are the implications of tobacco industry practices to develop new products that are specifically geared toward adolescents?

STUDENT ACTIVITIES

1. Create a social marketing campaign for the following groups:

   a. African American high school students in the precontemplation stage

   b. New parents in the contemplation stage

   c. Nursing or medical students in the preparation stage

2. Conduct a literature search on the cost of a pack of cigarettes in Ohio and Massachusetts. If the cost is different, discuss who and what contributes to the pricing of a pack of cigarettes.

3. Debate whether a company should be allowed to hire or not hire smokers.

References

American Nonsmokers' Rights Foundation. (2014). *Smokefree lists, maps, and data.* Retrieved from www.no-smoke.org/pdf/SummaryUSPopList.pdf

Bertuccio, P., et al. (2011). Cigar and pipe smoking, smokeless tobacco use and pancreatic cancer: An analysis from the International Pancreatic Cancer Case-Control Consortium (PanC4). *Annals of Oncology.* doi: 10.1093/annonc/mdq613

Boffetta, P., Hecht, S., Gray, N., Gupta, P., & Straif, K. (2008). Smokeless tobacco and cancer. *Lancet Oncology, 9,* 667–675.

Bondi, M. A., Harris, J. R., Atkins, D., French, M. E., & Umland, B. (2006). Employer coverage of clinical preventive services in the United States. *American Journal of Health Promotion, 20*(3), 214–222.

Boon, A. (2012, June 15). *Smokeless tobacco in the United States.* Retrieved from www.tobaccofreekids.org/research/factsheets/pdf/0231.pdf

Callinan, J. E., Clarke, A., Doherty, K., & Kelleher, C. (2010). Legislative smoking bans for reducing secondhand smoke exposure, smoking prevalence and tobacco consumption. *Cochrane Database of Systematic Reviews, 4,* CD005992. doi: 10.1002/14651858.CD005992.pub2

Campaign for Tobacco Free Kids. (2012, December 6). *Broken promises to our children: The 1998 state tobacco settlement fourteen years later.* Retrieved from www.tobaccofreekids.org/content/what_we_do/state_local_issues/settlement /FY2013/1.%202012%20State%20Report%20-%20Full.pdf

Centers for Disease Control and Prevention. (1999). International classification of diseases. Retrieved from www.cdc.gov/nchs/icd/icd10cm.htm

Centers for Disease Control and Prevention. (2004). State Medicaid coverage for tobacco-dependence treatments—United States, 1994–2002. *Morbidity and Mortality Weekly Report, 53*(03), 54–57.

Centers for Disease Control and Prevention. (2006). *Save lives, save money: Make your business smoke-free*. Atlanta: US Department of Health and Human Services, Centers for Disease Control and Prevention, National Center for Chronic Disease Prevention and Health Promotion, Office on Smoking and Health.

Centers for Disease Control and Prevention. (2008). *School health guidelines to prevent tobacco use, addiction, and exposure to secondhand smoke*. Atlanta: Centers for Disease Control and Prevention.

Centers for Disease Control and Prevention. (2010). State-specific prevalence of cigarette smoking and smokeless tobacco use among adults—United States, 2009. *Morbidity and Mortality Weekly Report, 59*(43), 1400–1406.

Centers for Disease Control and Prevention. (2011a). Current cigarette smoking prevalence among working adults—United States, 2004–2010. *Morbidity and Mortality Weekly Report, 60*(38), 1305–1309.

Centers for Disease Control and Prevention. (2011b). Current cigarette smoking among adults—United States, 2011. *Morbidity and Mortality Weekly Report, 61*(44), 889–894.

Centers for Disease Control and Prevention. (2011c). Vital signs: Current cigarette smoking among adults aged ≥ 18 years—United States, 2005–2010. *Morbidity and Mortality Weekly Report, 60*(35), 1207–1212.

Centers for Disease Control and Prevention, Division of Adolescent and School Health. (2011d). *Success stories: State, local, and nongovernmental organization examples*. Retrieved from www.cdc.gov/healthyyouth/stories/pdf/ss_booklet_1011.pdf

Centers for Disease Control and Prevention. (2012a, July 24). *History of the surgeon general's reports on smoking and health*. Retrieved from www.cdc.gov/tobacco/data_statistics/sgr/history/index.htm

Centers for Disease Control and Prevention. (2012b, August 30). *Workplace health promotion: Tobacco-use cessation*. Retrieved from www.cdc.gov/workplacehealthpromotion/implementation/topics/tobacco-use.html

Centers for Disease Control and Prevention. (2012c, December 18). *Smokeless tobacco facts*. Retrieved from www.cdc.gov/tobacco/data_statistics/fact_sheets/smokeless/betel_quid/index.htm

Centers for Disease Control and Prevention. (2014). Best practice for comprehensive tobacco control programs. Atlanta: US Department of Health and Human Services, Centers for Disease Control and Prevention, National Center for Chronic Disease Prevention and Health Promotion, Office on Smoking and Health. Retrieved from www.cdc.gov/tobacco/stateandcommunity/best_practices/pdfs/2014/comprehensive.pdf

Davis, K., Nonnemaker, J., & Farrelly, M. (2007). Association between national smoking prevention campaigns and perceived smoking prevalence among youth in the United States. *Journal of Adolescent Health, 41*(5), 430–436.

Ebbert, J., Montori, V., Erwin, P., & Stead, L. (2011). Interventions for smokeless tobacco use cessation. *Cochrane Database of Systematic Reviews, 2*, CD004306. doi: 10.1002/14651858.CD004306.pub4

Fiore, M., Bailey, W., Cohen, S., et al. (2008). *Treating tobacco use and dependence: 2008 update.* Rockville, MD: US Department of Health and Human Services, Public Health Service.

Grimsrud, T., Gallefoss, F., & Løchen, M.-L. (2012). At odds with science? *Nicotine & Tobacco Research, 15*(1), 302–303.

Healthy People. (2012, October 30). *Healthy people 2020 summary of objectives: Tobacco use.* Retrieved from www.healthypeople.gov/2020/topicsobjectives 2020/pdfs/TobaccoUse.pdf

Hecht, S. (1998). Biochemistry, biology, and carcinogenicity of tobacco-specific N-nitrosamines. *Chemical Research in Toxicology, 11*(6), 559–603.

Heidenreich, P. A., Trogdon, J. G., Khavjou, O. A., Butler, J., Dracup, K., Ezekowitz, M. D., . . . & Woo, Y. J. (2011). Forecasting the future of cardiovascular disease in the United States; a policy statement from the American Heart Association. *Circulation, 123*(8), 933–944.

Huang, J., Chaloupka, F., & Fong, G. (2013). Cigarette graphic warning labels and smoking prevalence in Canada: A critical examination and reformulation of the FDA regulatory impact analysis. Tobacco Control. doi: 10.1136/tobaccocontrol-2013-051170.

Lee, P., & Hamling, J. (2009). Systematic review of the relation between smokeless tobacco and cancer in Europe and North America. *BMC Medicine, 7,* 36.

Matthew, C., Farrelly, K., Davis, M., Haviland, L., Messeri, P., & Healton, C. (2005). Evidence of a dose–response relationship between "truth" antismoking ads and youth smoking prevalence. *American Journal of Public Health, 95*(3), 425–431.

McAfee, T., Davis, K., Alexander, R., Pechacek, T., & Bunnell, R. (2013). Effect of the first federally funded US antismoking national media campaign. *Lancet.* doi: 10.1016/S0140–6736(13)61686–4

Mears, B. (2012, August 8). *Federal appeals court strikes down FDA tobacco warning label law.* Retrieved from www.cnn.com/2012/08/24/justice/tobacco -warning-label-law/index.html

National Association of Attorneys General. (1998). *The master settlement agreement.* Retrieved from www.naag.org/backpages/naag/tobacco/msa/msa-pdf

Newport, F. (2011, July 15). *For first time, majority in U.S. supports public smoking ban.* Retrieved from www.gallup.com/poll/148514/first-time-majority-supports -public-smoking-ban.aspx

O'Donnell, M., & Roizen, M. (2011). The SmokingPaST framework: Illustrating the impact of quit attempts, quit methods, and new smokers on smoking prevalence, years of life saved, medical costs saved, programming costs, cost effectiveness, and return on investment. *American Journal of Health Promotion, 1*(26), e11–e23.

Partnership for Prevention. (2008). *Advanced care management: Diabetes, obesity, weight management and smoking cessation programs.* Washington, DC: Third Employer Health & Human Capital Congress.

Reda, A., Kotz, D., Evers, S., & van Schayck, C. (2012). Healthcare financing systems for increasing the use of tobacco dependence treatment. *Cochrane Database of Systematic Review, 6,* CD004305. doi: 10.1002/14651858.CD004305.pub4

Rigotti, N., & Wakefield, M. (2012). Real people, real stories: A new mass media campaign that could help smokers quit. *Annals of Internal Medicine, 156*(12), 907–910.

Rodu, B. (2011). The scientific foundation for tobacco harm reduction, 2006–2011. *Harm Reduction Journal, 8*(19), 1–22.

Scientific Committee on Emerging and Newly-Identified Health Risks (SCENIHR). (2008). *Scientific opinion on the health effects of smokeless tobacco products.* Brussels, Belgium: Health & Consumer Protection DG, European Commission. Retrieved from http://ec.europa.eu/health/archive/ph_risk/committees/04_scenihr/docs/scenihr_o_013.pdf

Secker-Walker, R., Gnichn W., Platt, S., & Lancaster, T. (2002). Community interventions for reducing smoking among adults. *Cochrane Database of Systematic Reviews, 2*, CD001745. doi: 10.1002/14651858.CD001745

Sponsiello-Wang, Z., Weitkunat, R., & Lee, P. (2008). Systematic review of the relation between smokeless tobacco and cancer of the pancreas in Europe and North America. *BMC Cancer, 8*, 356.

Substance Abuse and Mental Health Services Administration. (2011). *Results from the 2010 national survey on drug use and health: National findings.* Retrieved from www.samhsa.gov/data/NSDUH/2k11Results/NSDUHresults2011.pdf

Substance Abuse and Mental Health Services Administration. (2012). *Results from the 2010 national survey on drug use and health: Detailed tables.* Retrieved from www.samhsa.gov/data/NSDUH/2k10ResultsTables/NSDUHTables2010R/PDF/Cover.pdf

Thomas, R., & Perera, R. (2006). School-based programmes for preventing smoking. *Cochrane Database of Systematic Reviews, 3*, CD001293. doi: 10.1002/14651858.CD001293.pub2

Thrasher, J., Carpenter, M., Andrews, J., Gray, K., Alberg, A., Navarro, A., Friedman, D., & Cummings, K. (2012). Cigarette warning label policy alternatives and smoking-related health disparities. *American Journal of Preventive Medicine, 43*(6), 590–600.

Tobacco Use and Dependence Guideline Panel. (2008). *Treating tobacco use and dependence: 2008 update.* Rockville, MD: US Department of Health and Human Services. Retrieved from www.ncbi.nlm.nih.gov/books/NBK63952

US Food and Drug Administration. (2012, August 29). *Overview of the Family Smoking Prevention and Tobacco Control Act.* Retrieved from www.fda.gov/tobaccoproducts/guidancecomplianceregulatoryinformation/ucm246129.htm

US Department of Health and Human Services. (2004). *The health consequences of smoking: A report of the surgeon general.* Atlanta: US Department of Health and Human Services, Centers for Disease Control and Prevention, National Center for Chronic Disease Prevention and Health Promotion, Office on Smoking and Health.

US Department of Health and Human Services. (2006). *The health consequences of involuntary exposure to tobacco smoke: A report of the surgeon general—Executive summary.* Atlanta: US Department of Health and Human Services, Centers for

Disease Control and Prevention, Coordinating Center for Health Promotion, National Center for Chronic Disease Prevention and Health Promotion, Office on Smoking and Health.

US Department of Health and Human Services. (2007). *Best practices for comprehensive tobacco control programs—2007.* Atlanta: US Department of Health and Human Services, Centers for Disease Control and Prevention, National Center for Chronic Disease Prevention and Health Promotion, Office on Smoking and Health.

US Department of Health and Human Services. (2008). *Treating tobacco use and dependence: 2008 update—clinical practice guidelines.* Rockville, MD: US Department of Health and Human Services, Public Health Service, Agency for Healthcare Research and Quality.

US Department of Health and Human Services. (2010). *How tobacco smoke causes disease: The biology and behavioral basis for smoking-attributable disease; a report of the surgeon general.* Atlanta: US Department of Health and Human Services, Centers for Disease Control and Prevention, National Center for Chronic Disease Prevention and Health Promotion, Office on Smoking and Health.

US Department of Health and Human Services. (2012). *Preventing tobacco use among youth and young adults: A report of the surgeon general.* Atlanta: US Department of Health and Human Services, Centers for Disease Control and Prevention, National Center for Chronic Disease Prevention and Health Promotion, Office on Smoking and Health.

US Department of Health and Human Services (2014). *The health consequences of smoking – 50 years of progress: A report of the surgeon general.* Atlanta: US Department of Health and Human Services, Centers for Disease Control and Prevention, National Center for Chronic Disease Prevention and Health Promotion, Office on Smoking and Health.

US Office of Personnel Management. (2013). *Section II: Guidelines for the development of effective agency tobacco cessation programs.* Retrieved from www.opm .gov/policy-data-oversight/worklife/reference-materials/tobacco-cessation -guidance-on-establishing-programs-designed-to-help-employees-stop-using -tobacco/#Program

Vallone, D., Duke, J., Cullen, J., McCausland K., et al. (2011). Evaluation of EX: A national mass media smoking cessation campaign. *American Journal of Public Health, 101,* 302–309.

Wilson, D. (2011, August 16). Cigarette companies file 2nd suit over warnings. *New York Times.* Retrieved from http://prescriptions.blogs.nytimes.com/2011/08/16 /cigarette-companies-file-2nd-suit-over-warnings

World Health Organization. (2012, May). *Tobacco: Fact sheet no. 339.* Retrieved from www.who.int/mediacentre/factsheets/fs339/en/index.html

CHAPTER 5

EATING BEHAVIORS

Food Choices, Trends, Programs, and Policies

Maya Maroto

Nutrition and food have taken center stage in many discussions related to promoting public health, and for good reason. The World Health Organization (2009) estimates that nutrition-related risk factors including high blood pressure, high blood glucose, overweight, obesity, and high blood cholesterol are responsible for more than sixteen million deaths per year globally (28% of global deaths). The vast majority of Americans fall far short of meeting the nutrition goals set out by the **Dietary Guidelines for Americans**, a national healthy-eating guide developed jointly by the US Departments of Health and Human Services and Agriculture. Health promotion professionals have an excellent opportunity to successfully change people's dietary habits if an ecological approach is adopted to increase personal responsibility and motivation while creating environments and policies that make the healthier choices the easier choices.

Eating Behaviors

Why did you eat that? People make around two hundred personal decisions related to food every day and report a multitude of drivers for their eating habits, many of which lay outside of health and nutrition (Scheibehenne, Miesler, & Todd, 2007; Wansink, 2007). As an entrant into the field of health promotion, it is important to understand the range of potential drivers of food choices in order to approach

LEARNING OBJECTIVES

After reading this chapter, the student will be able to:

- **Define the factors that influence people's eating patterns.**

- **Identify the relationship between eating patterns and health.**

- **Identify the benefits to healthy eating.**

- **Discuss the history of eating patterns.**

- **Explain historical changes to the food environment in America.**

- **Restate educational programs that assist people in making healthy food choices.**

- **Discuss local, state, and national policies that encourage healthy eating.**

- **Summarize nutrition programs at the community, work site, school, and individual levels.**

An ecological approach is one that involves change through different spheres to influence behavior modification. This involves individual behavior, along with family, school, workplace, community, and policy change. By targeting each level, improved health changes are more likely to be practiced.

the notion of dietary change from a realistic and informed viewpoint. Steptoe, Pollard, and Wardle (1995) reported "health is clearly not the only factor people take into account when choosing their food, and a focus on health may lead to exclusive emphasis on a set of motives that are of limited significance for many people" (p. 268).

> Our diet has changed more in the last 100 years than in the last 10,000, probably with the result that it is affecting our health.
>
> —Michael Pollan, food author; journalist; and University of California, Berkeley, professor

Dietary Guidelines for Americans
nutrition guidelines jointly issued and updated every five years by the Departments of Health and Human Services and Agriculture; provide authoritative advice for Americans ages two and older about consuming fewer calories, making informed food choices, and being physically active to attain and maintain a healthy weight, reduce risk of chronic disease, and promote overall health

Taste

Perhaps not surprisingly, taste is Americans' number one consideration when they make food purchasing decisions (International Food Information Council, 2011; Scheibehenne, Miesler, & Todd, 2007). The flavor of food is highly related to a person's preference. Research indicates that humans have biological preferences toward foods that are sweet, salty, and fatty. These characteristics may have been helpful for survival during early history because humans focused on foods that were calorically dense, physiologically beneficial, and safe to eat. Today's world offers an abundance of technologically created and heavily marketed processed foods that are high in sugar, salt, and fat, and low in nature's healthiest elements, such as vitamins, minerals, fiber, and phytochemicals (plant chemicals). This has resulted in an increasing number of people who are overweight or obese, domestically and internationally (Popkin, Adair, & Ng, 2012). Furthermore, studies suggest that for certain individuals, fat, sugar, and salt induce changes to the brain structure that are similar to those induced by addictive narcotics (Kessler, 2009).

Emotions

In addition to taste, food also delivers a sense of enjoyment often described as satisfaction, happiness, and comfort, depending on the situation. For example, a person may feel a sense of happiness in eating a healthy meal of fish, broccoli, and rice after a workout and that same person may derive happiness from eating pizza after a night out with friends or eating "comfort" foods when stressed (Antin & Hunt, 2012). There is no denying the important role of emotions and feelings in driving food choice. Numerous studies have linked increased stress levels with craving and consuming foods high in calories, sugar, and fat (Laran & Salerno, 2013; Tryon, Carter, DeCant, & Laugero, 2013; Zellner et al., 2006). Other studies have shown that individuals with lower socioeconomic status in the United States have the highest levels of chronic stress as measured by stress hormone levels (Cohen, Doyle, & Baum, 2006; Suglia, Staudenmayer, Cohen, Enlow, Rich-Edwards, & Wright, 2010). The links among stress, income, race, body weight, and eating habits are hot topics among nutrition and neuroscience researchers, who wish to explain the pathways between life circumstances and food choice.

Price

Cost is an important consideration for many people when selecting foods. Recent data indicate that in 2011, price was an important factor in food choices for almost 80% of consumers—up from 65% of consumers in 2006 (International Food Information Council, 2011). This trend aligns with the economic downturn beginning in 2008, illustrating that economic struggles drive people to seek foods that are less expensive. Although there is controversy within the world of economists about which foods are least expensive, much evidence suggests that the foods delivering the most calories for the least cost include refined grains (grains largely stripped of their fiber, vitamins, and minerals) and processed foods high in added sugar, fats, and salt. These foods tend to be tasty, highly convenient, and readily available (Drewnowski & Darmon, 2005). Other researchers contend that when foods are compared by weight or portion, healthy foods such as fruits, vegetables, and whole grains are actually less expensive than less-healthy "processed" foods (Carlson & Frazão, 2012). However, people on limited budgets generally perceive that healthy foods are more expensive than unhealthy foods (Antin & Hunt, 2012).

Convenience

Americans are in a rush—to do everything. Today's economy increasingly requires adult family members to work outside of the home, leaving less time and energy for food preparation. Research indicates that even in the twenty-first century, women continue to do the majority of household food preparation. The amount of time Americans spend cooking varies based on employment. For example, women who do not work outside of the home spend an average of seventy minutes per day on food preparation whereas women employed full-time spend about forty minutes per day on food preparation (Mancino & Newman, 2007). This creates a demand for accessible, affordable, quick, and easy-to-prepare meals including "ingredients" such as canned soups or "heat and eat" meals. Unfortunately, the less time people spend cooking, the more likely they are to be overweight or obese (Hamrick, Andrews, Guthrie, Hopkins, & McClelland, 2011).

The convenience food market is built on a shifting culture in which everyone seems to have a shortage of time. Consumer habits have drastically changed and many people are spending additional cash in exchange for already prepared meals. The focus of the convenience food industry is on products that can easily be divided into helpings, are resealable, and are easily prepared in a microwave oven. Fast food is not just left to restaurants with drive-through windows. Grocery stores have picked up on the convenience food trend and are now offering entrees and side dishes ready for the oven, microwave, and dinner plate. The demand for processed, convenience meals is on the rise and is especially in demand in households with children (Lee & Lin, 2012).

Health and Nutrition

Health and nutrition are also factors influencing food selection. Many consumers are interested in foods that will help them improve well-being and physical health, lose weight, and manage health conditions. Although health concerns play a role in food selection for some people, personal appearance is a distinct factor reported as well. Beyond selecting foods to avoid chronic disease such as type 2 diabetes and heart disease, consumers also report making "healthy" choices in order to achieve a certain body size, beautiful hair, and glowing skin (Antin & Hunt, 2012; Steptoe, Pollard, & Wardle, 1995).

According to a large study, the leading source of food information is the media, cited as the primary source of nutrition information by 70% of respondents. The media in this case included Internet articles, cooking shows, TV and radio news, magazines, newspapers, talk shows, and blogs and social networks, including Twitter and Facebook. Also, 59% of consumers reported the nutrition facts panel provided on food labels to be a major source of nutrition information (International Food Information Council, 2011).

When consumers read nutrition facts panels, they report they are most likely to focus on the information regarding calories, fat, sodium, sugar, and saturated fat (International Food Information Council, 2011). Food manu-facturers have responded to consumers' desire for healthier products with an array of lower fat-, sugar-, and sodium-processed food options. However, questions remain regarding how these products affect rates of obesity and other diet-related diseases. Furthermore, health professionals should be aware of the growing practice termed *leanwashing*, which refers to food manufacturers making exaggerated or misleading health claims through advertising, marketing, or packaging in order to convince consumers to purchase products that are less healthy than they appear (EnviroMedia Social Marketing, 2012).

Culture and Familiarity

Food selection is also influenced by culture and familiarity. Think back to a food you loved as a child and how it made you feel to consume that food. You may be flooded with powerful memories. Many people have strong connections to the foods native to their culture and upbringing. Foods are attached to a sense of identity and are a central feature of people's social lives, cultural identities, and holiday celebrations. Food is a powerful cultural identifier, reflecting unique values and beliefs related to food cultivation, production, preparation, and consumption (Montanari, 2006).

Environment

Foods readily available to consumers affect food selection. What types of food are near consumers' homes, schools, or workplaces? Consumers purchase food in a variety of venues, influenced by what is nearby and accessible, including grocery stores, farmer's markets, corner stores, liquor stores, fast food outlets, and coffee shops. Food availability affects food selection. The term *food desert* has been widely used to describe low-income areas that lack access to the array of foods carried in grocery stores. *Food swamp* may be a more appropriate term to describe the multitude of geographic areas with access to numerous corner stores, fast food outlets, and grocery stores. In a US Department of Agriculture report regarding food access, findings indicated that "easy access to all food, rather than lack of access to specific healthy foods, may be a more important factor in explaining increases in BMI and obesity" (Ploeg et al., 2009).

Marketing

Finally, food marketing influences food selection. Cohen (2008) contends that the "omnipresence of food advertising is artificially stimulating people to feel hungry and overconsume. Given the increasing availability of food over time, this stimulation follows suit, potentially explaining the continuing rises in obesity" (p. S138). Advances in food marketing research have identified the most effective methods to persuade and entice consumers to consume the foods being marketed. Food marketing research enables companies to design advertisements and packaging that immediately capture and hold consumer attention. Companies have also mastered the art of "branding," which creates an automatic and powerful connection between a product and consumer emotions (Cohen, 2008). Much controversy also exists regarding food marketing to children and whether the practice is healthy or ethical (Scully et al., 2012).

Nutrition, Eating Habits, and Health

Americans are eating poorly and suffering from high rates of numerous chronic diseases, including heart disease, cancer, stroke, and diabetes. Poor dietary choices, along with inadequate physical activity, smoking, and alcohol use, are linked to the nation's leading chronic diseases (Roberts & Barnard, 2005).

As identified in table 5.1, in 2010, of the top ten leading causes of death in the United States, five were chronic diseases that are nutrition related. The following section covers the links between various foods and nutrients and heart disease, cancer, stroke, diabetes, and kidney disease. It is notable that the nutrients that decrease the risk of these diseases are usually only protective when consumed from foods—studies of nutrients from dietary supplements have generally not shown the same powerful positive effects as nutrient-rich diets.

Table 5.1   Leading Causes of Death: Number of Deaths (United States, 2010)

- Heart disease: 597,689
- Cancer: 574,74
- Chronic lower respiratory diseases: 138,080
- Stroke (cerebrovascular diseases): 129,476
- Accidents (unintentional injuries): 120,859
- Alzheimer's disease: 83,494
- Diabetes: 69,071
- Nephritis, nephrotic syndrome, and nephrosis (kidney disease): 50,476
- Influenza and pneumonia: 50,097
- Intentional self-harm (suicide): 38,364

Note: Nutrition-related causes of death are highlighted.
Source: Centers for Disease Control and Prevention (2011a).

Heart Disease

Heart disease is the leading cause of death in developed countries for men and women (Centers for Disease Control and Prevention, 2011a). Diseases of the heart result from a buildup of plaque inside of artery walls, which may ultimately lead to a heart attack. Heart disease is most prevalent among populations with unhealthy diets, individuals who smoke, obese individuals, and among those who are not physically active.

The link between nutrition and heart disease has been researched for more than one hundred years; the first studies were conducted in the early 1900s (Roberts & Barnard, 2005). Several nutrients have been linked with increased risk of heart disease, including saturated fat, industrially produced trans fat, and sodium (salt). Studies have shown that people consuming diets rich in fiber, folate, and potassium have lower rates of heart disease and those who substitute monounsaturated fats, omega-3, and omega-6 poly-unsaturated fats in place of saturated fats also reduce their risk of heart disease.

Dietary patterns that are high in animal foods, refined carbohydrates, red meat, processed meat, high-sodium processed foods, sweets and desserts, high-fat dairy products, and sugar-sweetened beverages are most strongly linked to the development of heart disease. Those consuming diets high in fruits, vegetables, whole grains, fish (especially omega-3 fatty acid–containing varieties), chicken (when substituted for red meat), nuts, and legumes have a much lower risk of developing heart disease (Hankey, 2012; Roberts & Barnard, 2005; World Health Organization and Food and Agriculture Organization, 2003).

Following a healthy dietary pattern can decrease the risk of multiple chronic diseases. The dietary patterns that are protective against heart disease are also protective against hypertension (high blood pressure), which is a risk factor for heart disease (Roberts & Barnard, 2005). Hypertension is also a leading cause of kidney disease, which means these dietary patterns will also help decrease the risk of kidney disease, the fifth leading nutrition-related cause of death. Research shows that individuals who are obese can decrease their risk of heart disease by improving their diet and physical activity, even if weight loss is not achieved (Roberts & Barnard, 2005).

Cancer

Cancer is the second leading killer in the United States, accounting for 23% of all deaths in 2010 (Centers for Disease Control and Prevention, 2011a). Numerous studies suggest that lifestyle factors including smoking, physical

Heart disease
generally refers to conditions that involve narrowed or blocked blood vessels that can lead to a heart attack, chest pain (angina), or stroke

Cancer
term used for diseases in which abnormal cells divide without control and are able to invade other tissues

inactivity, and diet play a major role in the development of cancer. Although tobacco is the most important known avoidable cause of cancer, obesity is second (World Health Organization and Food and Agriculture Organization, 2003).

Specific nutrients have been studied for their possible relationship to cancer. Studies have shown that diets high in fat (saturated fat and omega-6 fats), calories, and alcohol are associated with an increased risk of cancer. Diets rich in omega-3 fats and fiber are protective against the risk of many cancers (Roberts & Barnard, 2005).

Diets associated with increased risk of cancer are high in red meat, charbroiled meat, fried meats, refined carbohydrates, sugar, and alcohol. Diets high in whole grains, fruits, vegetables, beans and legumes appear to protect against the development of several types of cancer (Roberts & Barnard, 2005).

Stroke

Stroke

occurs when the blood supply to part of the brain is interrupted or severely reduced, depriving brain tissue of oxygen and food; within minutes, brain cells begin to die

Stroke is the fourth leading cause of death in the United States and the leading cause of functional impairment of Americans, with up to 30% of stroke survivors suffering permanent disability (Apostolopoulou, Michalakis, Miras, Hatzitolios, & Savopoulos, 2012). Several lifestyle factors contribute to the risk of stroke, including dietary factors, excessive alcohol, and obesity. High blood pressure is a major contributor to stroke; following dietary guidance to reduce the risk of heart disease and high blood pressure will indirectly decrease the risk of stroke as well (Medeiros, Casanova, Fraulob, & Trindade, 2012).

Nutrients that have been found to increase the risk of stroke include trans fat, sodium, and saturated fat. Nutrients that appear to decrease the risk of stroke include antioxidants, folate, fiber, potassium, flavonoids (found in many fruits and vegetables as well as in red wine, tea, cocoa, and chocolate), and carotenoids, which are found in some yellow and red fruits and vegetables (Apostolopoulou, Michalakis, Miras, Hatzitolios, & Savopoulos, 2012; Hankey, 2012; Medeiros, Casanova, Fraulob, & Trindade, 2012).

Diets that increase the risk of stroke are high in animal protein, fried foods, butter, whole milk, and alcohol. Diets that lower the risk of stroke are rich in olive oil, omega-3–rich fish, fruits, vegetables (particularly cruciferous and green leafy vegetables such as cabbages, kale, and broccoli), low-fat dairy products, whole grains, coffee, tea, chocolate, and nuts (Apostolopoulou, Michalakis, Miras, Hatzitolios, & Savopoulos, 2012; Hankey, 2012; Medeiros, Casanova Mde, Fraulob, & Trindade, 2012).

Type 2 Diabetes

Type 2 diabetes develops when a person's body becomes resistant to the effects of insulin and the body is no longer able to produce sufficient insulin to overcome this resistance. These changes lead to elevated levels of glucose (a sugar) in the blood. Type 2 diabetes is increasing most rapidly in populations with unhealthy diets, among individuals who are overweight or obese, and among those who are not physically active.

Several nutrients have been found to either increase or decrease the risk of developing type 2 diabetes. Specific nutrients that have a possible effect on increasing the risk of type 2 diabetes include total fat, trans fats, and saturated fats. Consuming a high-calorie diet also increases the risk of type 2 diabetes (Roberts & Barnard, 2005; World Health Organization and Food and Agriculture Organization, 2003).

Populations consuming higher intakes of specific foods including processed and red meat, full-fat dairy products, refined grains (white bread, white rice, non-whole-grain pancakes, muffins, etc.), desserts, and sweets have a higher risk of developing type 2 diabetes. High intake of sugar-sweetened beverages is also associated with increased risk of diabetes (Hankey, 2012). Omega-3 fatty acids (from fish), fruits, vegetables, whole grains, and legumes have been found to protect against type 2 diabetes. Mothers who develop diabetes during pregnancy (known as gestational diabetes) give birth to children who are more likely to develop type 2 diabetes in the future. Children whose mothers do not breastfeed them exclusively for at least six months are also more likely to develop type 2 diabetes (Roberts & Barnard, 2005; World Health Organization and Food and Agriculture Organization, 2003).

Type 2 diabetes once known as adult-onset or noninsulin-dependent diabetes; is a chronic condition that affects the way the body metabolizes sugar (glucose), the body's main source of fuel; with type 2 diabetes, the body either resists the effects of insulin—a hormone that regulates the movement of sugar into the cells—or doesn't produce enough insulin to maintain a normal glucose level; untreated, can be life threatening

Obesity

Obesity is caused by consuming calories beyond one's daily needs and not being physically active enough. Researchers believe that the energy gap—calories consumed above and beyond what the body burns—that has led to today's obesity levels is in the range of one hundred to four hundred extra calories per day. The leading contributors of calories to the American diet are grain-based desserts, breads, chicken dishes, sugary drinks (soda, energy, and sports drinks), and pizza. Excessive calorie intake has led to very high levels of overweight and obesity in US children and adults (Dietary Guidelines Advisory Committee, 2010).

From 1976 until 2008, obesity prevalence has increased from 15% to 34% in adults and from 5% to 17% among children and adolescents (Centers for Disease and Prevention, 2011b). Obesity rates are generally higher among Hispanic and African Americans. Obesity is driven by biological,

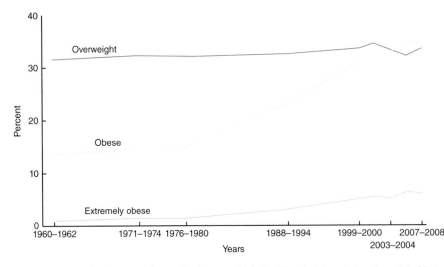

Figure 5.1   Trends in Overweight, Obesity, and Extreme Obesity among Adults Aged Twenty to Seventy-Four Years: United States, 1960–2008

Note: Age adjusted by the direct method to the year 2000 US Census Bureau estimates, using the age groups twenty to thirty-nine, forty to fifty-nine, and sixty to seventy-four years. Pregnant females were excluded. Overweight is defined as a body mass index (BMI) of twenty-five or greater but less than thirty; obesity is a BMI greater than or equal to thirty; extreme obesity is a BMI greater than or equal to forty.

Source: Centers for Disease Control and Prevention (2010).

cultural, and social factors contributing to limited opportunities for physical activity and an abundance of high-calorie foods. Obesity can be a serious health issue because it has been linked to increased risk for premature death, type 2 diabetes, hypertension (high blood pressure), dyslipidemia (abnormalities in blood such as high low-density lipoprotein cholesterol levels), heart disease (may lead to heart attack), stroke, gall bladder disease, sleep apnea, arthritis, and several kinds of cancer (Dietary Guidelines Advisory Committee, 2010) (see figure 5.1).

Benefits of Healthy Eating Habits

The previous section identified the links between dietary patterns and disease and illustrates that there are several dietary patterns that either increase or decrease the risk of most common chronic diseases. The 2010 Dietary Guidelines Advisory Committee, which is responsible for reviewing all published nutrition research to advise the government on dietary recommendations, summarized several of the most common global dietary patterns and the relationships of those diets to the risk of disease. Their research review shows that certain diets and dietary patterns are linked to reductions in risk for chronic disease and improved health outcomes. The typical American or Westernized diet, which is high in calories, processed foods, added sugars, solid fats, refined grains, and sodium, is associated with

Table 5.2   Different Dietary Patterns, Their Characteristics, and Disease Risk Impact

Dietary Pattern	Characteristics	Disease Risk Impact
Typical American or **Westernized diet**	High in calories, added sugars, solid fats, refined grains, sodium Low in whole grains, vegetables, fruits, and milk, dietary fiber, vitamin D, calcium, potassium, and omega-3 fatty acids (usually found in fish)	Increased risk for obesity, premature death, cardiovascular disease (CVD), type 2 diabetes, some cancers
DASH (dietary approaches to stop hypertension)-style eating pattern	High in vegetables, fruit, low-fat milk; includes whole grains, poultry, seafood, and nuts Low in red meat, sweets, sodium, and sugar-containing beverages	Lower blood pressure, improved blood lipids, and lower CVD risk
Mediterranean-style dietary pattern	High in plant foods, bread, vegetables, fruits, nuts, unrefined cereals, olive oil, fish, cheese, yogurt; includes red wine with meals Low in red meat, sweets, saturated fat, meat, and full-fat dairy products	Lower risk of coronary heart disease, lower risk of blood pressure, lower risk of stroke, lower risk of cardiovascular disease, lower risk of mortality
Vegetarian dietary pattern	High in carbohydrates and fiber Low in calories, saturated fat, animal products	Lower risk of high blood pressure
Traditional Southeast Asian diet	High in soybean products, fish, seaweeds, vegetables, fruit, green tea, rice Low in meat, milk and milk products	Increased longevity, lower rates of heart disease, lower blood pressure

Source: Dietary Guidelines Advisory Committee (2010).

increased risk for obesity and several major chronic diseases. Other dietary patterns (such as Mediterranean and Asian diets) that are higher in fruits, vegetables, seafood, and whole grains are associated with lower risk of disease. The impacts of nutrition (dietary patterns) on chronic diseases and health risk factors are identified in table 5.2.

Recommended Nutrition and Dietary Intake

Based on the research linking diet to chronic disease and other health outcomes, in 2010 the United States federal government released updated dietary guidance: the 2010 Dietary Guidelines for Americans. In 2011, the US Department of Agriculture (USDA) eliminated the food pyramid and introduced the MyPlate icon (see figure 5.2) as an interactive educational

Westernized diet
high in calories, processed foods, added sugars, solid fats, refined grains, and sodium; is associated with increased risk for obesity and several major chronic diseases

DASH (dietary approaches to stop hypertension)-style eating pattern
a low-sodium regimen for patients with hypertension that emphasizes fruits, vegetables, low-fat dairy foods, whole-grain products, fish, poultry, and nuts; low in saturated and total fat, cholesterol, red meat, sweets, and sugared beverages; high in magnesium, potassium, calcium, protein, and fiber

Mediterranean-style dietary pattern
emphasizes eating primarily plant-based foods, such as fruits and vegetables, whole grains, legumes, and nuts; replacing butter with healthy fats, such as olive oil; using herbs and spices instead of salt to flavor foods; limiting red meat to no more than a few times a month; eating fish and poultry at least twice a week; drinking red wine in moderation (optional)

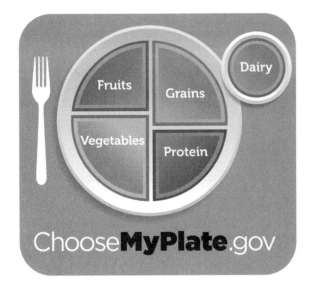

Figure 5.2   MyPlate Icon
Source: ChooseMyPlate.gov (nd).

tool to promote the healthy eating guidelines outlined in the 2010 Dietary Guidelines for Americans.

The 2010 Dietary Guidelines for Americans and MyPlate icon are intended to encourage Americans to increase their intake of certain foods while decreasing or limiting their intake of others. Americans are advised to eat more whole grains, vegetables, fruits, low-fat dairy products, seafood, fiber, potassium, vitamin D, and calcium and simultaneously decrease their intake of added sugars, refined grains, sodium, saturated fat, and trans fat.

Figure 5.3 compares the typical American diet to the dietary goals and limits set by the USDA and the Department of Health and Human Services in the 2010 Dietary Guidelines for Americans.

History of Nutrition and Dietary Patterns

Historical changes in civilization have dramatically affected the dietary patterns of our species and our country. Not too long ago, Americans' food consumption and physical activity were not out of balance on a large scale. It was only in the late 1980s and 1990s that obesity levels began to rise rapidly. However, obesity is not the only indicator of a lifestyle that is out of balance; the rates of cancer, heart disease, kidney disease, and type 2 diabetes are also rising among people of all weights, particularly affecting those who are carrying excess weight. This section provides information regarding how the human diet changed over thousands of years and more recently, in the

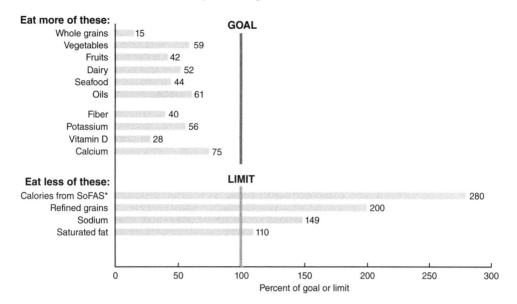

Figure 5.3 Comparison of Americans' Usual Dietary Intake to the 2010 Dietary Guidelines for Americans

Note: SoFAS = solid fats and added sugars.

Source: US Department of Agriculture and US Department of Health and Human Services (2010).

United States, with the advancement of technology and an increasing population.

What are the historic dietary patterns associated with the rise in chronic diseases (also called noncommunicable disease)? Dr. Barry Popkin, a prominent nutrition researcher at the University of North Carolina at Chapel Hill, describes five distinct dietary patterns that have emerged throughout human history.

Pattern 1: Paleolithic and Hunter-Gatherers

Foraging and food hunting and gathering have been the dominant forms of food acquisition sustaining the human race for the vast majority of human history. Preagricultural societies were largely omnivorous and consumed a variety of plant and animal species, including nuts, seeds, wild grasses, meat, and fish. Compared to the typical, current American diet, prehistoric diets were more than twice as rich in fiber, potassium, and calcium but contained very little sodium (Caballero & Popkin, 2002). Nutritional deficiencies were uncommon among hunter-gatherer populations (Popkin, 2006). The prehistoric diet was the dominant eating pattern for approximately the first 140,000 years of human history. Recent evidence suggests that many of our preagricultural ancestors had adult life spans of more than seventy years and were largely free of the chronic illnesses that are the leading causes of death in our culture today, including heart disease, cancer, and type 2 diabetes (Gurven & Kaplan, 2007).

Pattern 2: Advent of Agriculture

Approximately ten thousand years ago, with the advent of traditional agriculture, societies began shifting away from the hunter-gatherer diet. Human diets became heavily dominated by cereal grains (rice, wheat, corn), supplemented with legumes (beans), tubers (such as potatoes), and oil. Dietary variety was greatly decreased from prehistoric patterns and most diets in the early agricultural era were "highly monotonous and not very palatable" (Caballero & Popkin, 2002, p. 30). Archeological evidence suggests that average adult height during this period significantly decreased. Dependence on agriculture also subjected people to the harsh realities of famine, crop failure, and other natural disasters. However, farming enabled a tremendous increase in food calories per acre, which facilitated population growth and the formation of stratified civilizations (Caballero & Popkin, 2002). Early agriculture was based on processes such as crop rotation, cover crops, and the use of animals and human labor. All foods consumed during this era would be considered "organic" by today's standards because chemical pesticides and fertilizers had not yet been invented!

Pattern 3: Industrialization and Receding Famine

With the introduction of nonrenewable fossil fuels and electricity, farmers were able to transition to more modern farming methods. Modern farming relies on agricultural machinery for crop processing tasks and on synthetic fertilizers and pesticides to grow fruits, vegetables, and grains. Pharmaceuticals were also introduced to promote animal growth. The use of these technologies saw a marked rise in the 1960s during what was known as the "green revolution." In addition, crop varieties were developed that produced more reliable yields, and agricultural monoculture (growing of a single type of crop on a farm) began to replace agriculturally diverse farming. Modern farming methods significantly increased crop production, providing affordable food for a much larger number of people (Popkin & Gordon-Larsen, 2004). However, one of the major drawbacks of modern agriculture is the environmental damage caused by the use of synthetic pesticides, herbicides, and fertilizers. Additionally, concentrated animal feeding operations pose a threat to animal welfare and are a source of air and water pollution (Jacobson, 2006). This dietary pattern is characterized by increased consumption of fruits, vegetables, and animal protein and decreased consumption of starchy staple foods. However, diets continued to lack variety, similar to diets in pattern 2.

Pattern 4: Noncommunicable Disease

The noncommunicable disease dietary pattern is currently most dominant in the United States and is becoming the leading pattern globally as well. Barry Popkin writes that in the last two decades of the twentieth century "modern societies seem to be converging on a diet high in saturated fats, sugar, and refined foods but low in fiber often termed the 'Western diet' and on lifestyles characterized by lower levels of activity" (Popkin & Gordon-Larsen, 2004, p. S2). This dietary pattern emerged because of the convergence of many factors including modern food processing, marketing, and distribution; consumer demand for processed food, in part because of more women entering the workforce leaving less time for food preparation; global agricultural policies that have decreased the cost of grains and animal products; and global food advertising, among others (Popkin, 2006). In many countries, this dietary pattern is characterized by an increase in meals consumed away from home, larger portion sizes, rising consumption of animal foods, increased consumption of processed foods, and the replacement of water and milk by sugar sweetened beverages. This dietary pattern is associated with an increase in chronic diseases (cancer, heart disease, type 2 diabetes) and obesity (Popkin, 2006).

Pattern 5: Desired Societal and Behavior Change

In the United States, this pattern would be considered optimal adherence to the US federal government's dietary guidance, the Dietary Guidelines for Americans and MyPlate, as described in the previous section. It is not currently the dominant pattern in the United States, but it is the pattern that many health promotion professionals encourage to reduce chronic disease risk.

Changes to the American Food Environment

In the United States, since the 1980s, significant environmental changes have affected our diets and eating habits.

Food Supply and Consumption

Today's food environment presents people with a plethora of accessible, inexpensive food options. In 1970, there were 2,172 calories available in the food supply, per day, for every person in America; by 2009, that total had increased by more than 400 calories to 2,600 calories per person (Morrison,

Table 5.3   Food Availability in Pounds per Person

In Pounds per Person	Early 1900s	1970s	2005–2009
Grains	No data	133	197
Fruits and vegetables	No data	570	687[*]
Milk	36	32	21
Meat, eggs, nuts, beans	No data	225	242
Sweeteners	84	120	136
Fats and oils	36	56	87
Cheese	4	11	31
Total calories in food supply	No data	2,172	2,600

[*]Mostly potatoes, tomatoes, onions, and lettuce on sandwiches
Sources: Morrison, Buzby, and Wells (2010); US Department of Agriculture: Economic Research Service (2011).

Buzby, & Wells, 2010). In other words, there are more calories available and, as more calories have become available in the food supply, people have tended to eat them. Americans are consuming more calories than ever before in human history. But what are the sources of increased calories? In the following section, food availability and food consumption trends will be described. Table 5.3 summarizes the changes to the food supply in pounds of food available per person from the early 1900s until 2009.

grains
any food made from wheat, rice, oats, cornmeal, barley, or another cereal grain, such as bread, pasta, oatmeal, breakfast cereals, tortillas, and grits

Grains: A large part of the gain in calories available in the United States is a result of the increased production of flour and cereal products. These products rose from 133 pounds per person in 1970 to 197 pounds per person in 2008. Foods produced from these flours and cereals include grain-based snack foods and bakery items (e.g., crackers, cakes, cookies), as well as breads, buns, dough, and tortillas. These foods are frequently consumed away from home (Morrison, Buzby, & Wells, 2010). Americans are over-consuming refined grains and falling far short of recommended whole-grain intakes (US Department of Agriculture and US Department of Health and Human Services, 2010; Wells & Buzby, 2008).

fruits and vegetables
nutritionally speaking, similar to each other; generally lower in calories and fat than animal products; also contain health-enhancing plant compounds, such as fiber and antioxidants; loaded with vitamins and minerals

Fruits and vegetables: There are currently more fruits and vegetables available in the food supply than there were in 1970. In 2005, there were 687 pounds of fruits and vegetables (fresh and processed) available per person, up from 570 pounds per person in 1970. Although this may sound like good news, it is not so simple. Most of these vegetables typically come with a fast food meal: potatoes (mainly in the form of French fries), tomatoes, onions, and lettuce—the common accompaniments to fast food sandwiches

(Wells & Buzby, 2008). Americans are eating less than the recommended amounts and are also not eating the recommended pattern of vegetables, which should include ample amounts of dark green leafy vegetables, orange vegetables, and beans and peas. In order to meet the most current guidelines, intakes of all three of those categories would need to be consumed in quantities at least double the current intake patterns (US Department of Agriculture and US Department of Health and Human Services, 2010; Wells & Buzby, 2008).

Beverages: Americans are increasingly consuming soft drinks, juices and juice drinks, and bottled water, at the expense of milk. Milk availability declined from its peak of 44.7 gallons per person in 1945 to 21 gallons in 2008 (Morrison, Buzby, & Wells, 2010). The consumption of lower-fat milk began to increase in the 1990s as knowledge about cholesterol, saturated fat, and calories became more widely known by Americans (Putnam & Allshouse, 2003). Americans are currently not meeting the dietary guidelines of daily recommended milk intake, which is promoted for its contribution of nutrients (including calcium, vitamin D, and potassium); potential for improving bone health; and possible role in decreasing risk of type 2 diabetes and cardiovascular disease (US Department of Agriculture and US Department of Health and Human Services, 2010). However, it is also noteworthy that several leading health authorities, including Dr. Walter Willett of the Harvard School of Public Health, have publicly questioned the validity of the three-cup-of-milk-per-day recommendation of the federal government and instead urge people to maintain bone strength through adequate physical activity, vitamin D (from sunshine), and by consuming calcium from nondairy sources including collard greens, bok choy, fortified soy milk, and baked beans (Harvard School of Public Health, 2011).

Although milk consumption may be a controversial recommendation, it is universally agreed on that sugar-sweetened beverages are overconsumed by Americans. From 1977 to 2001, Americans tripled their daily caloric intake of soft drinks from 50 calories per day to 144 calories per day. The increase in soft drink consumption is primarily due to large increases in soda intake among children (aged two to eighteen) and young adults (aged nineteen to thirty-nine). Interestingly, humans do not compensate for consuming caloric beverages by reducing food intake as we do for consuming caloric foods; soft drinks are strongly associated with weight gain (Nielsen & Popkin, 2004; Popkin, 2011). For these reasons, soft drinks are a focus of many policy makers and health advocates who wish to improve dietary intake and decrease rising obesity rates.

Meat and other protein foods: The total amount of meat, eggs, and nuts available for consumption grew from 225 pounds per person in 1970 to

beverages include soft drinks, juices, and juice drinks, tap water and bottled water, coffee, tea, and milk (dairy and nondairy)

meat and other protein foods all foods made from meat, poultry, seafood, beans and peas, eggs, processed soy products, nuts, and seeds

242 pounds in 2005. A large portion of this increase is due to increasing production of chicken, which rose from 34 pounds per person in 1970 to almost 74 pounds in 2005 (Wells & Buzby, 2008). This increase was due to technological and pharmaceutical innovations facilitating the production of very large, meaty broiler chickens, and the development of boneless chicken breasts, chicken nuggets, and ready-to-eat products, such as precooked chicken strips. Although the consumption of chicken has been on the rise, red meat and egg consumption have steadily declined since the 1970s with increasing awareness of cholesterol and saturated fat. Consumption patterns suggest that Americans are overconsuming beef, pork, and chicken and underconsuming healthier protein foods including fish and seafood, beans, peas, nuts, and seeds.

added sweeteners, fats, and oils
found in a variety of processed foods, including soft drinks, breads, sauces, and desserts; added fats and oils found in processed foods such as French fries, baked goods, and snacks, and also used in food preparation and cooking

Added sweeteners, fats, and oils: Added sweeteners have also grown in availability. In 1909, there were 84 pounds of sweeteners available per person. In 2008, 136 pounds of sweeteners were available per person; almost 40% in the form of high fructose corn syrup (HFCS). HFCS is an inexpensive manufactured sweetener found in a wide array of processed foods ranging from soft drinks to spaghetti sauce to apple sauce and breakfast cereal (Morrison, Buzby, & Wells, 2010). Americans consumed 30 teaspoons per person per day of added sugars and sweeteners in 2005 (three times the recommended 8 teaspoons outlined in the dietary guidelines); the vast majority of this sugar comes from soft drinks. Thirty teaspoons of added sugars and sweeteners are equivalent to 477 calories per day, or about 24% of the total daily caloric intake for a person on a two-thousand-calorie-per-day diet (Wells & Buzby, 2008).

There is also more added fat in the food supply than ever before. Added fats and oils are found in a variety of processed foods, such as French fries, baked goods, and snacks, and are also used in food preparation and cooking. Added fats are consumed in addition to naturally occurring fats, such as fat in red meat and dairy products. There were 36 pounds of fats and oils per person in 1909; in 2008, there were 87 pounds per person. Americans consumed most of this fat in the form of cooking oil used in fried foods (Morrison, Buzby, & Wells, 2010; Wells & Buzby, 2008). The dietary guidelines recommend that fats and oils, both added and naturally occurring, contribute 20% to 35% of daily energy intake (in a two-thousand-calorie-per-day diet, that's 44 to 78 grams). Americans consumed 71.6 grams of added fats and oils per person per day in 2005 and this estimate does not include fats occurring naturally in foods such as meat and dairy products (Wells & Buzby, 2008). This high level of added fat consumption suggests that Americans may be eating too much fat.

Cheese: Cheese availability rose from 11 pounds per person in 1970 to 31 pounds in 2008. The proliferation of cheese in the food supply is attributed to the rise and spread of Italian and Mexican restaurants as well as innovative, convenient cheese packaging—such as string cheese (Morrison, Buzby, & Wells, 2010) and resealable bags of shredded cheese (Putnam & Allshouse, 2003). Convenience food is a major component of the growth in cheese consumption; more than half of our cheese comes from commercially manufactured and prepared foods such as fast food sandwiches and packaged snacks (Putnam & Allshouse, 2003).

Table 5.4 compares the 2010 Dietary Guidelines for Americans with the most recent dietary consumption data with regards to grains; fruits and vegetables; milk, meats, and protein; added sweets; and fats and oils.

Where Americans Eat

Harried Americans are increasingly consuming meals away from home, which tend to be higher in fat, sugar, and salt than home-prepared meals. From 1970 to 1995, the percentage of food dollars spent on meals away from home increased from 25% to 40%. Over that same time period, foods eaten

Table 5.4 A Comparison of the 2010 Dietary Guidelines and the Average American Diet

	Dietary Guidelines Recommendations (2010)*	Average American Consumption (2005)	Overconsumption of	Foods to Increase
Grains	6 ounces, half of which should be whole grains	6.4 ounces • 5.8 were refined grains • 0.6 were whole grains	Grain-based snack foods and bakery items (such as crackers, cakes, cookies) as well as breads, buns, dough, and tortillas	Brown rice, whole grain breads, whole wheat pastas, oatmeal, and other whole grain foods
Fruits and vegetables	2 cups of fruit 2.5 cups of vegetables	1 cup of fruit 1.6 cups of vegetables	Potatoes (mainly in the form of French fries), tomatoes, onions, and lettuce	Leafy green vegetables, orange vegetables, and beans
Milk	3 cups	1.5 cups	Whole-milk products	Reduced-fat milk products
Meats and proteins	5.5 ounces	6.5 ounces	Beef and pork	Fish and seafood, beans, peas, nuts, and seeds
Added sweets	8 teaspoons	30 teaspoons	Soft drinks, high fructose corn syrup, and sugar	N/A
Fats and oils	25%–35% of daily intake (44 g to 78 g)	33% of daily intake (72 g per day from added fats)	Processed foods such as French fries, baked goods, and snacks	Avocado, olive oil, nuts

*All recommendations are based on a two-thousand-calorie-per-day diet.

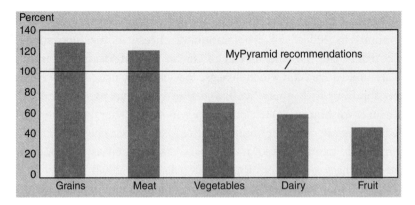

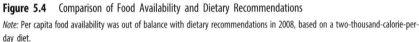

Figure 5.4   Comparison of Food Availability and Dietary Recommendations

Note: Per capita food availability was out of balance with dietary recommendations in 2008, based on a two-thousand-calorie-per-day diet.

Source: US Department of Agriculture: Economic Research Service (2011).

at fast food restaurants increased by 200% (Drewnowski & Darmon, 2005). More recent data indicate that Americans have somewhat cut back spending on restaurant meals due to the economic recession of 2007–2009 and are preparing slightly more meals at home (Kumcu & Kaufman, 2011).

Figure 5.4 compares food available in the United States with government recommendations on what people should consume (MyPlate, which was formerly MyPyramid). It is clear from this graphic that the food supply is not aligned with the dietary recommendations.

The Food Industry: Friend, Foe, or Both?

The food industry spends over $11 billion marketing its products to American consumers each year (Consumers Union, 2005). Marketing is a powerful driver of increased caloric intake from high-calorie foods and beverages. High calorie–low nutrient foods are highly available and heavily marketed, creating a perfect combination for people to eat them (Institute of Medicine, 2012). Many of the foods marketed to consumers are the very foods people should cut back on, according to the dietary guidelines. Furthermore, research indicates that African-American children are being exposed to even higher rates of food advertising, which is especially disconcerting given the documented high levels of childhood obesity in this population (Harris, Weinberg, Schwartz, Ross, Ostroffa, & Brownell, 2010).

Recently, there has been increased interest in foods marketed to children. The foods most heavily marketed to children typically contain high amounts of calories and do not often include whole foods, such as fruits, vegetables, and whole grains. The Interagency Working Group on Food Marketed to

Children (Interagency Working Group), composed of representatives from the Federal Trade Commission (FTC), the Centers for Disease Control and Prevention (CDC), the Food and Drug Administration (FDA), and the USDA, was directed by Congress to craft a set of voluntary standards that the food industry could use to guide their marketing efforts aimed at children. The Interagency Working Group proposed that foods marketed to children ages two to seventeen would include significant amounts of fruits, vegetables, whole grains, fat-free or low-fat milk, fish, extra lean meat or poultry, eggs, nuts and seeds or beans, and contain low amounts of sodium, saturated fat, trans fat, and added sugars (Interagency Working Group on Food Marketed to Children, 2011). These voluntary regulations were rejected by the trade associations representing the food industry on the basis of being too stringent and potentially devastating to their profits and were effectively abandoned by the FTC in 2011 (Nestle, 2011).

The food industry is certainly attempting to take an active role in nutrition and investing heavily in nutrition and health-related ventures. For example, Coca-Cola sponsors playgrounds and Walmart and Target sponsor anti-hunger programs and events. Many large companies have committed to lowering the sodium and fat in all products sold in their stores and Disney has enacted strict guidelines for future marketing of food products on their cable channel and in affiliation with their characters. However, food industry groups have been successful in derailing any attempt to tax soft drinks and effectively lobbied Congress to continue to classify pizza as a vegetable (due to the tomato paste content) in the National School Lunch Program in 2011. The role of the food industry in the movement toward healthier eating is a subject of heated debate; some advocate the inclusion of the food industry as a partner and others argue that "when the history of the world's attempt to address obesity is written, the greatest failure may be collaboration with and appeasement of the food industry" (Brownell, 2012, p. 1).

Farm Subsidies: The Culprit?

Farm subsidies are also a popular topic of discussion among nutrition-minded health professionals (see figure 5.5). Some argue that the billions of federal dollars paid to producers of corn and soybeans—often used in HFCS and other processed foods, oils, or cheap animal feed—are artificially lowering the price of less healthy food. Subsidies may also enable large food companies to spend more money marketing unhealthy foods to consumers. Others argue that farm subsidies do not contribute to the low prices of less healthy foods. Some suggest shifting subsidies and federal support to foods that Americans need to eat more of, such as fruits and

farm subsidies
paid to farmers and agribusinesses to supplement their income, manage the supply of agricultural commodities, and influence the cost and supply of such commodities; examples include wheat, feed grains (grain used as fodder, such as maize or corn, sorghum, barley, and oats), cotton, milk, rice, peanuts, sugar, tobacco, oilseeds such as soybeans, and meat products such as beef, pork, and lamb and mutton

Where the Money Goes: The Foods That Subsidies Support

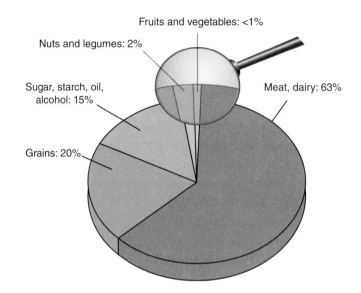

Fruits and vegetables: <1%

Nuts and legumes: 2%

Sugar, starch, oil, alcohol: 15%

Meat, dairy: 63%

Grains: 20%

Figure 5.5   Food Subsidies
Source: Physicians Committee for Responsible Medicine (2011).

vegetables—which currently receive less than 1% of federal subsidies (Fields, 2004). The Institute of Medicine (2012) recommended that the federal government "evaluate the evidence on the relationship between agriculture policies and the American diet" and examine the impact of farm subsidies on food prices, access, affordability, and consumption. The US Farm Bill governs agricultural subsidy policy and is reauthorized by the Congress approximately every five years.

Portion Sizes: Bigger but Not Better

The foods that Americans eat the most are generally tasty (by many people's standards), easy to get, cheap to buy, heavily marketed, and served in gigantic portions. Since the 1970s, portions have expanded at restaurants, grocery stores, and in prepackaged foods. Many studies suggest that when people are presented with larger portions of food, they tend to eat more. Restaurant meals are extremely large, often offering enough calories for an entire family in a single dish. Studies find that since the 1970s, people are eating larger portions of salty snacks, soft drinks, hamburgers, French fries, Mexican dishes, grains and cereals, and many beverages, such as orange juice, juice drinks, soft drinks, and alcohol (beer and wine) (Division of Nutrition and Physical Activity, 2006).

Recent Efforts to Promote Healthy Eating

Despite the numerous negative trends described in this chapter, there are also many positive developments in the world of health and nutrition that may enable the country to create future progress in improving eating habits. Nutrition promotion initiatives are most likely to be successful when they work on multiple levels of the ecological model, affecting public policy (national, state, and local), communities, organizations, interpersonal relationships, and the individual. Examples of nutrition-related efforts operating on several levels of the ecological model are explained in chapter 3 under the program planning models.

National Policy Actions

Nutrition is being addressed at the national level through various government initiatives. The landmark Patient Protection and Affordable Care Act (ACA) ushered in many changes to the American approach to health and health care and includes mandatory changes to the nutrition information available to consumers at restaurants. Under the law, all restaurants with twenty or more locations are required to list the calorie content for menu items directly on the restaurant menu. The restaurant also has to make other nutrient information available in writing upon request, including total calories, fat, saturated fat, cholesterol, sodium, total carbohydrates, sugars, fiber, and total protein. Furthermore, vending machine operators who operate more than twenty machines will also have to disclose calorie information in a manner that permits consumers to see how many calories are in an item before purchasing the item (Food and Drug Administration, 2010).

The United States government operates several programs aimed at improving the nutrition of Americans. One of those programs is the **Women, Infants, and Children (WIC) program** that provides supplemental food for low-income pregnant women and mothers with children up to the age of five. Currently, 53% of all infants in the United States are served by the WIC program, making it one of the most important federal nutrition programs. In 2007, the WIC food package was updated to align with the Dietary Guidelines for Americans; WIC began providing increased amounts of vegetables and low-fat dairy as well as fruit, whole grains, tofu, and soy milk for the first time. The new packages cut the amount of juice, cheese, and whole milk provided to participants (US Department of Agriculture: Food and Nutrition Service, 2009). Some believe that SNAP (the Supplemental Nutrition Assistance Program; commonly referred to as "food stamps") should also change to align with the dietary guidelines because the program currently allows participants to purchase almost any food or

Women, Infants, and Children (WIC) program provides supplemental food for low-income pregnant women and mothers with children up to the age of five

beverage with this government benefit (besides hot food and alcoholic beverages). Others argue that such changes to SNAP are paternalistic and that restrictions are unnecessary.

Finally, the federal government remains involved in providing dietary guidance to encourage Americans to make healthy food choices and to serve as a guide for nutrition policy. The 2010 Dietary Guidelines for Americans, released jointly by the Department of Health and Human Services and the USDA every five years, serve as the nation's nutrition guidance. The MyPlate icon and website (www.choosemyplate.gov) can serve as an eating guide for individuals. The National Weight Control Registry (www.nwcr.ws) was established to create successful long-term weight management habits among individuals. It is making a contribution to the obesity epidemic by tracking more than ten thousand individuals who have lost significant weight and maintained the weight loss.

State Policy Actions

California provides an example of a state that has enacted legislation to attempt to improve the nutrition of its residents. In 2008, a bill banning the use of trans fats in all food facilities in the state was signed into law. The law took effect in 2010 and prohibits California restaurants from using trans fat–containing oils in food preparation. The law does not ban the sale of packaged foods containing trans fats because, unlike restaurant foods, packaged foods have nutrition labels detailing the trans fat content and ingredients of the food product. Restaurants found to be in violation of the law are fined (California Directors of Environmental Health, 2010). Trans fats have been identified as a major dietary cause of heart disease, and legislation, such as that enacted in California, may have an effect on reducing future heart disease morbidity and mortality among the state's residents.

Local Policy Actions

Many local areas are using policy in attempts to improve the nutrition and health of their populations. New York City is an example of such an area; under former mayor Michael Bloomberg the city has undertaken a number of bold and sometimes controversial approaches to improving the diets of New York City residents. The New York City Department of Health required calorie listings on chain restaurant menus well before federal regulations mandated the practice. The city also has a policy establishing nutrition standards for foods served in hospitals, nursing homes, homeless shelters, and all city vending machines. A city program called *Health Bucks* extends the buying power of SNAP recipients to purchase fresh fruits and vegetables at participating farmers' markets (New York City Obesity Task Force, 2012). Perhaps most controversially, the New York City Health Department passed an ordinance restricting the sale of soft drinks in sizes exceeding sixteen ounces; however, the New York appeals court struck down the ruling, stating that the Department of Health exceeded its legal authority by limiting the size of a soda (Grynbaum, 2012; New York City Obesity Task Force, 2012).

Community Nutrition Efforts

Numerous communities are working together to promote healthy eating. Local and community efforts range from attracting more supermarkets to food deserts, to encouraging corner stores in urban areas to offer healthier food choices, to promoting farmers' markets, to providing nutrition education directly to consumers in grocery stores.

Many community organizations are actively engaged in nutrition outreach. The Philadelphia-based Food Trust is an organization that aims to increase healthy food access for all members of the community. The organization operates the Healthy Food Financing Initiative to bring supermarkets to underserved areas by providing loans and grants to interested entrepreneurs. Their Healthy Corner Store Initiative has increased nutritious offerings in corner stores and provides children with education about healthy snacking (The Food Trust, 2012). Shopping Matters, offered by local organizations nationwide, uses grocery stores as classrooms to teach participants how to purchase fruits and vegetables on a budget, compare unit prices, read food labels, and identify whole grains (Share Our Strength, 2012).

Since the 1990s there has been a dramatic rise in the number of farmers' markets in communities throughout the country. In 1994, there were 1,755 farmers' markets nationwide; by 2011 that number had more than quadrupled to 7,175 (USDA: Agricultural Research Service, 2012a). In 2006, a mere 444 farmers' markets nationwide accepted SNAP benefits; in 2010, that number had more than tripled to 1,607. In 2010, $64 billion total SNAP dollars were redeemed and $7.5 million of those dollars were redeemed at farmers' markets. Although this is a small percentage of total SNAP expenditures, it is certainly a dramatic increase from past years and indicates that over time more SNAP participants are choosing to spend their dollars at farmers' markets (Love, 2011). Programs to promote farmers' markets include the Wholesome Wave Double Value Coupon program and the USDA Know Your Farmer, Know Your Food program, launched to strengthen local and regional food systems by promoting farmers' markets, community-supported agriculture, and farm-to-school initiatives.

Work Site Wellness

Work site environments significantly influence health behaviors (Stokols, Pelletier, & Fielding, 1996). Millions of people consume meals and snacks at work every day; applying nutrition standards to foods offered in workplace cafeterias and vending machines can promote employee health and well-being. Additionally, providing nutrition education to employees while they are at work may also have a positive impact on their productivity and overall health—ultimately benefiting the employer's bottom line.

The US government is promoting a healthier workplace with the adoption of a set of health guidelines for foods sold in vending machines, in cafeterias, and at select conferences and events in federal government facilities. The goal of these guidelines is to increase healthy food and beverage offerings while eliminating trans fats, lowering sodium content, and increasing consumer information through menu and vending nutrition labeling. Under these guidelines, which were based on the Dietary Guidelines for Americans, cafeteria options include more whole grains, organic selections, low-fat milk, high-fiber cereals, and vegetarian choices. All cafeteria foods and vending options feature menu labeling, informing consumers of the calorie content of each item (US Department of Health and Human Services and General Services Administration, 2010).

The CDC considers nutrition a key component of work site wellness programs. Well-rounded programs also incorporate physical activity and clinical services. Educational programs addressing topics such as meal planning, food label reading, safe dietary supplement use, and food safety are encouraged by the CDC as a part of comprehensive work site wellness initiatives (Centers for Disease Control and Prevention, nd). Kaiser Permanente is a company with an award-winning work site wellness program entitled Live Well Be Well at their Northern California location. Live Well Be Well provides more than 250 services ranging from cooking classes to weight loss support groups to blood pressure and cholesterol screenings. Kaiser reports having successfully documented outcomes from their program in terms of healthy weight reduction and other positive health results (Brown, 2012).

Healthy Hunger-Free Kids Act of 2010
act that requires all school meals in the United States to include more fruits, vegetables, whole grains, and low-fat milk and less sodium and saturated fat; also calls for an update of nutrition standards for "competitive foods" (foods sold in addition to the school meals, such as a la carte and vending options)

School Food Environments

Most children spend a substantial amount of time at school during their impressionable developmental years. Children who participate in the National School Lunch Program and School Breakfast Program obtain nearly half of their calories at school (Gleason & Dodd, 2009). School meals are often identified as a contributor to childhood obesity and other health issues. The **Healthy Hunger-Free Kids Act of 2010** made inroads toward ensuring that school lunches and a la carte options are aligned with current health standards. Beginning in 2012, all school meals in the United States were required to include more fruits, vegetables, whole grains, and low-fat milk and less sodium and saturated fat (US Department of Agriculture: Food and Nutrition Service, 2012b). The Healthy Hunger-Free Kids Act also calls for an update of nutrition standards for "competitive foods" (foods sold in addition to the school meals, such as a la carte and vending options), which is important because improving the nutritional profile of those foods has been shown to significantly decrease children's intake of calories, total fat, and saturated fat (Snelling & Yezek, 2012).

Not only can schools promote health by improving nutritious food offerings, but they can also provide nutrition education to students. The USDA has developed a variety of resources through their Team Nutrition initiative, including the HealthierUS school challenge, recipe books, sample curriculum, and best practices documents (US Department of Agriculture: Food and Nutrition Service, 2012c).

Programs for the Individual

Recent studies affirm the effectiveness of one-on-one nutrition programs to improve food selection and promote positive health outcomes. Nutrition education programs implemented in supermarkets to assist shoppers with making healthy choices have been shown to positively affect people's purchasing of fruits and vegetables (Milliron, Woolf, & Appelhans, 2012). Many people receive nutrition counseling from registered dietitians or other qualified health professionals; researchers have found that one-on-one counseling can have a lasting effect on weight loss, lowering the risk of type 2 diabetes, hypertension (high blood pressure), and high cholesterol (Dansinger, Tatsioni, Wong, Chung, & Balk, 2007).

Summary

The importance of nutrition for maintaining good health is without question. Many of the leading causes of death and disability worldwide can be traced, at least in part, to poor dietary quality. Changes in dietary habits have occurred very recently in human history, with dramatic effects on the health of our species and our planet. The US food supply provides ample opportunities for individuals to consume foods that are low in nutrients and high in calories in the form of inexpensive processed foods and large restaurant meals and portions. Health promotion professionals must be able to make changes to the food environment as well as encourage individual behavior change through education and coaching in order to create successful and lasting dietary change.

KEY TERMS

1. **Dietary Guidelines for Americans:** nutrition guidelines jointly issued and updated every five years by the Departments of Health and Human Services and Agriculture; provide authoritative advice for Americans ages two and older about consuming fewer calories, making informed food choices, and being physically active to attain and maintain a healthy weight, reduce risk of chronic disease, and promote overall health

2. **Heart disease:** generally refers to conditions that involve narrowed or blocked blood vessels that can lead to a heart attack, chest pain (angina), or stroke

3. **Cancer:** term used for diseases in which abnormal cells divide without control and are able to invade other tissues

4. **Stroke:** occurs when the blood supply to part of the brain is interrupted or severely reduced, depriving brain tissue of oxygen and food; within minutes, brain cells begin to die

5. **Type 2 diabetes:** once known as adult-onset or noninsulin-dependent diabetes; is a chronic condition that affects the way the body metabolizes sugar (glucose), the body's main source of fuel; with type 2 diabetes, the body either resists the effects of insulin—a hormone that regulates the movement of sugar into the cells—or doesn't produce enough insulin to maintain a normal glucose level; untreated, can be life threatening

6. **Westernized diet:** high in calories, processed foods, added sugars, solid fats, refined grains, and sodium; is associated with increased risk for obesity and several major chronic diseases

7. **DASH (dietary approaches to stop hypertension)-style eating pattern:** a low-sodium regimen for patients with hypertension that emphasizes fruits, vegetables, low-fat dairy foods, whole-grain products, fish, poultry, and nuts; low in saturated and total fat, cholesterol, red meat, sweets, and sugared beverages; high in magnesium, potassium, calcium, protein, and fiber

8. **Mediterranean-style dietary pattern:** emphasizes eating primarily plant-based foods, such as fruits and vegetables, whole grains, legumes, and nuts; replacing butter with healthy fats, such as olive oil; using herbs and spices instead of salt to flavor foods; limiting red meat to no more than a few times a month; eating fish and poultry at least twice a week; drinking red wine in moderation (optional)

9. **Grains:** any food made from wheat, rice, oats, cornmeal, barley, or another cereal grain, such as bread, pasta, oatmeal, breakfast cereals, tortillas, and grits

10. **Fruits and vegetables:** nutritionally speaking, similar to each other; generally lower in calories and fat than animal products; also contain health-enhancing plant compounds, such as fiber and antioxidants; loaded with vitamins and minerals

11. **Beverages:** include soft drinks, juices, and juice drinks, tap water and bottled water, coffee, tea, and milk (dairy and nondairy)

12. **Meat and other protein foods:** all foods made from meat, poultry, seafood, beans and peas, eggs, processed soy products, nuts, and seeds

13. **Added sweeteners, fats, and oils:** found in a variety of processed foods, including soft drinks, breads, sauces, and desserts; added fats and oils found in processed foods such as French fries, baked goods, and snacks, and also used in food preparation and cooking

14. **Farm subsidies:** paid to farmers and agribusinesses to supplement their income, manage the supply of agricultural commodities, and influence the cost and supply of such commodities; examples include wheat, feed grains (grain used as fodder, such as maize or corn, sorghum, barley, and oats), cotton, milk, rice, peanuts, sugar, tobacco, oilseeds such as soybeans, and meat products such as beef, pork, and lamb and mutton

15. **Women, Infant, and Children (WIC) program:** provides supplemental food for low-income pregnant women and mothers with children up to the age of five

16. **Healthy Hunger-Free Kids Act of 2010:** act that requires all school meals in the United States to include more fruits, vegetables, whole grains, and low-fat milk and less sodium and saturated fat; also calls for an update of nutrition standards for "competitive foods" (foods sold in addition to the school meals, such as a la carte and vending options)

REVIEW QUESTIONS

1. What are the factors that influence people's eating patterns?

2. How have these factors changed over the decades?

3. What are the trends of overweight and obesity for children and adults in the United States?

4. What are the benefits of healthy eating?

5. What education tools are available to guide healthy eating?

6. What are the five historic dietary patterns of eating?

7. What has been the availability of food over the past one hundred years?

8. How does the food industry influence eating patterns?

9. What are some national and state policies to promote healthful eating?

10. What is the school food environment doing to promote healthful eating?

STUDENT ACTIVITIES

1.   Review the following quote from Cohen (2008, p. S141):

> A more accurate conceptualization of the obesity epidemic is that people are responding to the forces in their environment, rather than lacking in will power and self-control. A metaphor that more truly captures the phenomenon is the tsunami. The environmental tsunami of cues and stimuli artificially make people hungry and lead them to unintentionally overconsume and to remain excessively sedentary. The societal response to the tsunami has been to provide swimming lessons and cheerleaders. The response has clearly not been proportional to the threat. People cannot change their responses to cues they do not perceive. Unless we focus on a more appropriate response, the obesity epidemic will continue. The real solution would be to control and reduce those forces that are causing the tsunami, change the cues we are exposed to on a daily basis or make explicit the cues we cannot change. Only then will people be able to make good use of the swimming lessons they receive, and bring themselves into energy balance according to their individual preferences.

  a.   What do you think this quote means when it refers to "swimming lessons and cheerleaders"?

  b.   Do you believe the forces identified in the first question are substantial enough to change the public's eating habits and begin to reduce obesity? If so, why? If not, why not?

  c.   What do you think Cohen means when referring to the "forces that are causing the tsunami"? How do you think those forces play into nutrition choices?

  d.   Do you agree with Cohen's quote? Please explain why or why not.

2.   Several examples of nutrition programs on various levels of the ecological model were provided in the chapter. Find three additional examples of nutrition programs operating on various levels of the ecological model. Write a brief description of the program and outline your opinions on the strengths and weaknesses of each program.

3.   Take a tour of the food supply (www.cspinet.org/EatingGreen/tour.html) and use the Eating Green Calculator (www.cspinet.org/EatingGreen/calculator.html) to learn more about the environmental impacts of various dietary choices. What were three surprising or interesting facts you learned from completing these activities?

4.   Draw a schematic of leading causes of death and the nutrition factors.

References

Antin, T.M.J., & Hunt, G. (2012). Food choice as a multidimensional experience. A qualitative study with young African American women. *Appetite, 58*(3), 856–863

Apostolopoulou, M., Michalakis, K., Miras, A., Hatzitolios, A., & Savopoulos, C. (2012). Nutrition in the primary and secondary prevention of stroke. *Maturitas, 72*(1), 29–34. doi: 10.1016/j.maturitas.2012.02.006

Brown, M. (2012). *Kaiser Permanente's workplace wellness programs receive top honor from national business group on health.* Retrieved from http://share .kaiserpermanente.org/article/kaiser-permanentes-workplace-wellness-programs -receive-top-honor-from-national-business-group-on-health

Brownell, K. D. (2012). Thinking forward: The quicksand of appeasing the food industry. *PLoS Med, 9*(7), e1001254. doi: 10.1371/journal.pmed.1001254

Caballero, B., & Popkin, B. M. (2002). *The nutrition transition: Diet and disease in the developing world.* Amsterdam: Academic Press.

California Directors of Environmental Health. (2010). *California trans fat ban guidelines.* Retrieved from www.acgov.org/aceh/documents/TransFatBanGuide lines2010–01–07.pdf

Carlson, A., & Frazão, E. (2012). Are healthy foods really more expensive? It depends on how you measure the price. *Economic Information Bulletin, 96*, pp. 1–50.

Centers for Disease Control and Prevention. (2010). *Prevalence of overweight, obesity, and extreme obesity among adults: United States, trends 1960–1962 through 2007–2008.* Retrieved from www.cdc.gov/nchs/data/hestat/obesity _adult_07_08/obesity_adult_07_08.htm#figure2

Centers for Disease Control and Prevention. (2011a). Leading causes of death. Retrieved from www.cdc.gov/nchs/fastats/lcod.htm

Centers for Disease Control and Prevention. (2011b). CDC health disparities and inequalities report, United States. *Morbidity and Mortality Weekly Report, 60*, 1–116.

Centers for Disease Control and Prevention. (nd). *Workplace health promotion: Nutrition.* Retrieved from www.cdc.gov/workplacehealthpromotion/implementation /topics/nutrition.html

ChooseMyPlate.gov. (nd). *MyPlate graphic resources.* Retrieved from www.choose myplate.gov/print-materials-ordering/graphic-resources.html

Cohen, D. A. (2008). Obesity and the built environment: Changes in environmental cues cause energy imbalances. *International Journal of Obesity, 32*(Suppl. 7), S137–S142.

Cohen, S., Doyle, W. J., & Baum, A. (2006). Socioeconomic status is associated with stress hormones. *Psychosomatic Medicine, 68*(3), 414–420.

Consumers Union. (2005). *Out of balance: Marketing of soda, candy, snacks and fast foods drowns out healthful messages.* Retrieved from http://consumersunion .org/wp-content/uploads/2005/09/OutofBalance.pdf

Dansinger, M. L., Tatsioni, A., Wong, J. B., Chung, M., & Balk, E. M. (2007). Meta-analysis: The effect of dietary counseling for weight loss. *Annals of Internal Medicine, 147*(1), 41–50.

Dietary Guidelines Advisory Committee. (2010). *Report of the Dietary Guidelines Advisory Committee on the dietary guidelines for Americans, 2010: To the Secretary of Agriculture and the Secretary of Health and Human Services.* Washington, DC: US Department of Agriculture, US Department of Health and Human Services.

Division of Nutrition and Physical Activity. (2006). *Research to practice series no. 2: Portion size.* Atlanta: Centers for Disease Control and Prevention.

Drewnowski, A., & Darmon, N. (2005). The economics of obesity: Dietary energy density and energy cost. *American Journal of Clinical Nutrition, 82*(1 Suppl.) 265S–273S.

EnviroMedia Social Marketing. (2012). *Leanwashing index: Help keep advertising honest.* Retrieved from www.leanwashingindex.com

Fields, S. (2004). The fat of the land: Do agricultural subsidies foster poor health? *Environmental Health Perspectives, 112*(14), A820–A823.

Food and Drug Administration. (2010). *Menu and vending machines labeling requirements.* Retrieved from www.fda.gov/Food/IngredientsPackagingLabeling /LabelingNutrition/ucm217762.htm

The Food Trust. (2012). *What we do: In corner stores.* Retrieved from http:// thefoodtrust.org/what-we-do/corner-store

Gleason, P. M., & Dodd, A. H. (2009). School breakfast program but not school lunch program participation is associated with lower body mass index. *Journal of the American Dietetic Association, 109*(2 Suppl.) S118–S128. doi: 10.1016/j .jada.2008.10.058

Grynbaum, M. (2012). Health panel approves restriction on sale of large sugary drinks. *New York Times.* Retrieved from www.nytimes.com/2012/09/14 /nyregion/health-board-approves-bloombergs-soda-ban.html

Gurven, M., & Kaplan, H. (2007). Longevity among hunter-gatherers: A cross-cultural examination. *Population and Development Review, 33*(2), 321–365.

Hamrick, K. S., Andrews, M., Guthrie, J., Hopkins, D., & McClelland, K. (2011). How much time do Americans spend on food? *Economic Information Bulletin, 64* (EIB-86).

Hankey, G. J. (2012). Nutrition and the risk of stroke. *Lancet Neurology, 11*(1), 66–81. doi: 10.1016/s1474–4422(11)70265–4

Harris, J. L., Weinberg, M. E., Schwartz, M. B., Ross, C., Ostroffa, J., & Brownell, K. D. (2010). *Trends in television food advertising progress in reducing unhealthy marketing to young people?* New Haven, CT: Rudd Center for Food Policy and Obesity.

Harvard School of Public Health. (2011). *The bottom line: Calcium is important; but milk isn't the only, or even best, source.* Retrieved from www.hsph.harvard.edu /nutritionsource/what-should-you-eat/calcium-and-milk/index.html

Institute of Medicine. (2012). *Accelerating progress in obesity prevention: Solving the weight of the nation*. Washington, DC: National Academies Press.

Interagency Working Group on Food Marketed to Children. (2011). *Preliminary proposed nutrition principles to guide industry self-regulatory efforts: Federal Trade Commission (FTC), the Centers for Disease Control and Prevention (CDC), the Food and Drug Administration (FDA), and the United States Department of Agriculture (USDA)*. Retrieved from http://cspinet.org/new/pdf/IWG_food _marketing_proposed_guidelines_4.11.pdf

International Food Information Council. (2011). *2011 Food and health survey: Consumer attitudes toward food safety, nutrition & health*. Retrieved from www .foodinsight.org/Content/3840/2011%20IFIC%20FDTN%20Food%20and% 20Health%20Survey.pdf

Jacobson, M. (2006). *Six arguments for a greener diet*. Washington, DC: Center for Science in the Public Interest.

Kessler, D. A. (2009). *The end of overeating: Taking control of the insatiable American appetite*. New York: Rodale.

Kumcu, A., & Kaufman, P. (2011). Food spending adjustments during recessionary times. *Amber Waves*. Retrieved from www.ers.usda.gov/amber-waves/2011 -september/food-spending.aspx#.UvAMCbRn1Ns

Laran, J., & Salerno, A. (2013). Life-history strategy, food choice, and caloric consumption. *Psychological Science, 24*(2), 167–173.

Lee, J.-Y., & Lin, B.-H. (2012). A study of the demand for convenience food. *Journal of Food Products Marketing, 19*(1), 1–14. doi: 10.1080/10454446.2013.739120

Love, D. (2011). Farmers market SNAP sales soar in 2010. Retrieved from http:// farmersmarketcoalition.org/snap-sales-soar-2010

Mancino, L., & Newman, C. (2007). *Who has time to cook? How family resources influence food preparation* (No. 55961). Washington, DC: US Department of Agriculture, Economic Research Service.

Medeiros, F., Casanova, M., Fraulob, J. C., & Trindade, M. (2012). How can diet influence the risk of stroke? *International Journal of Hypertension, 763507*. doi: 10.1155/2012/763507

Milliron, B.-J., Woolf, K., & Appelhans, B. M. (2012). A point-of-purchase inter-vention featuring in-person supermarket education affects healthful food pur-chases. *Journal of Nutrition Education and Behavior, 44*(3), 225–232.

Montanari, M. (2006). *Food is culture*. New York: Columbia University Press.

Morrison, R. M., Buzby, J. C., & Wells, H. F. (2010). Guess who's turning 100? Tracking a century of American eating. *Amber Waves*. www.purl.umn.edu/122141

Nestle, M. (2011). *Congress caves in again: Delays IWG recommendations*. Retrieved from www.foodpolitics.com/2011/12/congress-caves-in-again-delays-iwg -recommendations

New York City Obesity Task Force. (2012). *Reversing the epidemic: The New York City Obesity Task force plan to prevent and control obesity*. Retrieved from www.nyc.gov/html/om/pdf/2012/otf_report.pdf

Nielsen, S. J., & Popkin, B. M. (2004). Changes in beverage intake between 1977 and 2001. *American Journal of Preventive Medicine, 27*(3), 205–210. doi: 10.1016 /j.amepre.2004.05.005

Physicians Committee for Responsible Medicine. (2011). *USDA's new MyPlate icon at odds with federal subsidies for meat, dairy.* Retrieved from www.pcrm.org /media/news/usdas-new-myplate-icon-at-odds-with-federal

Ploeg, M. V., Breneman, V., Farrigan, T., Hamrick, K., Hopkins, D., Kaufman, P. . . . Kim, S. (2009). Access to affordable and nutritious food measuring and understanding food deserts and their consequences. *Administrative Publication, 160* (AP-036).

Popkin, B. M. (2006). Global nutrition dynamics: The world is shifting rapidly toward a diet linked with noncommunicable diseases. *American Journal of Clinical Nutrition, 84*(2), 289–298.

Popkin, B. M. (2011). Agricultural policies, food and public health. *EMBO Reports, 12*(1), 11–18. doi: 10.1038/embor.2010.200

Popkin, B. M., Adair, L. S., & Ng, S. W. (2012). Global nutrition transition and the pandemic of obesity in developing countries. *Nutrition Reviews, 70*(1), 3–21. doi: 10.1111/j.1753-4887.2011.00456.x

Popkin, B., & Gordon-Larsen, P. (2004). The nutrition transition: Worldwide obesity dynamics and their determinants. *International Journal of Obesity, 28*, S2–S9. doi: 10.1038/sj.ijo.0802804

Putnam, J., & Allshouse, J. (2003, June). Trends in U.S. per capita consumption of dairy products, 1909 to 2001. *Amber Waves: The Economics of Food, Farming, Natural Resources, and Rural America.*

Roberts, C. K., & Barnard, R. J. (2005). Effects of exercise and diet on chronic disease. *Journal of Applied Physiology, 98*(1), 3–30. doi: 10.1152/japplphysiol.00852.2004

Scheibehenne, B., Miesler, L., & Todd, P. M. (2007). Fast and frugal food choices: Uncovering individual decision heuristics. *Appetite, 49*(3), 578–589. doi: 10.1016/j.appet.2007.03.224

Scully, M., Wakefield, M., Niven, P., Chapman, K., Crawford, D., Pratt, I. S., . . . Na, S.S.T. (2012). Association between food marketing exposure and adolescents' food choices and eating behaviors. *Appetite, 58*(1), 1–5.

Share Our Strength. (2012). *Shopping matters.* Retrieved from http://join.strength .org/site/PageNavigator/SOS/SOS_ofl_shoppingmatters_home

Snelling, A. M., & Yezek, J. (2012). The effect of nutrient-based standards on competitive foods in 3 schools: Potential savings in kilocalories and grams of fat. *Journal of School Health, 82*(2), 91–96. doi: 10.1111/j.1746–1561.2011.00671.x

Steptoe, A., Pollard, T. M., & Wardle, J. (1995). Development of a measure of the motives underlying the selection of food: The food choice questionnaire. *Appetite, 25*(3), 267–284. doi: 10.1006/appe.1995.0061

Stokols, D., Pelletier, K. R., & Fielding, J. E. (1996). The ecology of work and health: Research and policy directions for the promotion of employee health. *Health Education Quarterly, 23*(2), 137–158. doi: 10.1177/109019819602300202

Suglia, S. F., Staudenmayer, J., Cohen, S., Enlow, M. B., Rich-Edwards, J. W., & Wright, R. J. (2010). Cumulative stress and cortisol disruption among black and Hispanic pregnant women in an urban cohort. *Psychological Trauma: Theory, Research, Practice, and Policy*, 2(4), 326.

Tryon, M. S., Carter, C. S., DeCant, R., & Laugero, K. D. (2013). Chronic stress exposure may affect the brain's response to high calorie food cues and predispose to obesogenic eating habit. *Physiology & Behavior*, *120*, 233–242.

US Department of Agriculture: Economic Research Service. (2011). *Food availability spreadsheets*. Retrieved from www.ers.usda.gov/data-products/food-avail ability-%28per-capita%29-data-system.aspx#.UzrqU4VgHl8

US Department of Agriculture: Food and Nutrition Service. (2009). *Special supplemental nutrition program for women, infants and children (WIC): Revisions in the WIC food packages—Interim rule*. Retrieved from www.fns.usda.gov/wic /interim-rule-revisions-wic-food-packages

US Department of Agriculture: Agricultural Research Service. (2012a). Monitoring America's Nutritional Health. Retrieved from www.ars.usda.gov/is/AR/archive /mar12/March2012.pdf

US Department of Agriculture: Food and Nutrition Service. (2012b). *Nutrition standards for school meals*. Retrieved from www.fns.usda.gov/cnd/governance /legislation/nutritionstandards.htm

US Department of Agriculture: Food and Nutrition Service. (2012c). *Team nutrition*. Retrieved from www.fns.usda.gov/tn/team-nutrition

US Department of Agriculture and US Department of Health and Human Services. (2010). *2010 Dietary Guidelines for Americans*. Washington, DC: Government Printing Office. Retrieved from http://health.gov/dietaryguidelines/dga2010 /DietaryGuidelines2010.pdf

US Department of Health and Human Services and General Services Administration. (2010). *Health and sustainability guidelines for federal concessions and vending operations*. Retrieved from www.cdc.gov/chronicdisease/pdf/guide lines_for_federal_concessions_and_vending_operations.pdf

Wansink, B. (2007). *Mindless eating: Why we eat more than we think*. New York: Bantam-Dell.

Wells, H. F., & Buzby, J. C. (2008). *Dietary assessment of major trends in U.S. food consumption, 1970–2005* (EIB-33). Washington, DC: US Department of Agriculture Economic Research Service. Retrieved from www.ers.usda.gov /publications/eib-economic-information-bulletin/eib33.aspx#.UzrtG4VgHl8

World Health Organization. (2009). *Global health risks*. Geneva: World Health Organization.

World Health Organization and Food and Agriculture Organization. (2003). *Diet, nutrition and the prevention of chronic diseases*. Geneva: World Health Organization.

Zellner, D. A., Loaiza, S., Gonzalez, Z., Pita, J., Morales, J., Pecora, D., & Wolf, A. (2006). Food selection changes under stress. *Physiology & Behavior*, *87*(4), 789–793.

CHAPTER 6

PHYSICAL ACTIVITY BEHAVIORS

Benefits, Trends, Programs, and Policies

Jennifer Childress

People do not stop moving because they grow old; they grow old because they stop moving. Humans are designed to be physically active. Yet, with an increasing number of barriers, including personal, social, physical, and environmental factors, such as lack of time, limited access to walking paths and safe sidewalks, longer commutes, sedentary jobs, weather, and lower levels of health, people move less on a daily basis.

More than 80% of adults do not meet government-recommended physical activity guidelines for aerobic and muscle-strengthening activities. Similarly, more than 80% of adolescents do not participate in enough aerobic physical activity to meet the guidelines (US Department of Health and Human Services, 2012a). To address these behaviors, the Healthy People 2020 goals were established with the intention of increasing physical activity through a multidisciplinary approach, reaching people where they live, work, and play and promoting active daily living.

As a nation, we have many opportunities to engage and encourage people to be more physically active, from building healthier environments, to increasing motivation and personal responsibility, to developing policies that support these goals. As health promotion professionals, increasing physical activity among the population is a simple yet complex issue to address. Health promoters can learn from current efforts that have been proven effective and strive to build on them and innovate.

Just move!

LEARNING OBJECTIVES

After reading this chapter, the student will be able to:

- Define four different types of physical activity.

- Explain the benefits from being physically active.

- Identify the amount of physical activity recommended for individuals.

- Explain societal trends that have influenced physical activity patterns.

- Discuss the barriers to regular physical activity.

- Identify recent educational efforts to promote physical activity behavior.

- Summarize local, state, and national policies that are designed to promote physical activity.

Physical Activity

physical activity
any bodily movement produced by skeletal muscles that requires energy expenditure

Physical activity and exercise are often used interchangeably; however, there is a difference between the two terms. **physical activity** is defined as any bodily movement produced by skeletal muscles that requires energy expenditure (World Health Organization, 2012a). Any movement during the day is physical activity, including walking, climbing stairs, and housework. **exercise** is a subset of physical activity that is planned, structured, and repetitive and has as a final or an intermediate objective to improve or maintain physical fitness level (Caspersen, Powell, & Christenson, 1985). The US government, in aiming to reduce sedentary behavior, typically focuses on "lifestyle activity," the incorporation of physical activity into everyday life, such as taking the stairs, doing yard work or housework, brisk walking, and recreational activities.

exercise
a subset of physical activity that is planned, structured, and repetitive and has a final or an intermediate objective to improve or maintain physical fitness level

There are four primary types of physical activity: aerobic, muscle-strengthening, bone-strengthening, and stretching (National Heart, Lung, and Blood Institute, 2011).

aerobic (endurance) activity
any activity that uses the large muscle groups in the body to increase heart rate and benefit the strength of the cardiovascular system

aerobic (endurance) activity is most beneficial for the strength of the cardiovascular system (heart and lungs) and includes activities that move the large muscle groups in the body (arms and legs). Examples include running, jumping, bicycling, dancing, and walking.

muscle-strengthening activities
any activity that improves muscular strength, power, and endurance

muscle-strengthening activities involve improving muscular strength, power, and endurance. Examples include lifting weights, climbing stairs, and doing push-ups.

bone-strengthening activities improve bone density by causing impact on the musculoskeletal system. Examples include jumping rope, running, walking, and resistance training.

bone-strengthening activities
any activity that improves bone density by causing impact on the musculoskeletal system

stretching activities improve flexibility and joint mobility. Examples include general stretching and yoga.

Muscle and bone-strengthening activities can be aerobic if heart rate increases (e.g., running, jumping jacks, speed walking).

stretching activities
any activity in which a specific muscle or tendon is lengthened in an effort to improve flexibility and joint mobility

Recommended Physical Activity Levels

Physical inactivity is the fourth leading risk factor for global mortality, causing an estimated 3.2 million deaths each year (World Health Organization, 2012b). It is a significant, unnecessary health threat in the United States. Only 20% of Americans participate in recommended levels of daily physical activity (aerobic and muscle strengthening). In 2008, in response to these behaviors and health risks, the US Department of Health and Human Services developed the first ever national guidelines for physical activity, the **2008 Physical Activity Guidelines for Americans (PAG)** (US Department of Health and Human Services, 2012b), recommending specific physical activity levels by age group. Although the guidelines recommend minimum activity levels based on frequency and intensity, the underlying premise is that some activity is better than none. Table 6.1 identifies the 2008 PAG and table 6.2 provides examples of moderate and vigorous activity.

2008 Physical Activity Guidelines for Americans (PAG) a report released by the US Department of Health and Human Services recommending specific physical activity levels by age group

Table 6.1 The 2008 Physical Activity Guidelines for Americans Recommendations

	Children and Adolescents (Ages Six to Seventeen)	Adults (Ages Eighteen to Sixty-Four)	Older Adults (Ages Sixty-Five and Older)	Pregnant and Postpartum Women
Time	At least 1 hour daily	2.5 hours (150 minutes) weekly (at moderate intensity) *or* mixing it up (see following) In at least 10-minute bursts preferably spread throughout the week	Follow adult guidelines; if not possible due to limitations, be as physically active as possible	If not already doing vigorous activity, 2.5 hours (150 minutes) weekly at moderate intensity spread through the week
Level	Most of the hour should be either moderate or vigorous	2.5 hours (150 minutes) of moderate intensity weekly *or* 1 hour and 15 minutes (75 minutes) vigorous intensity *or* equivalent combination of moderate and vigorous intensity aerobic physical activity	Follow adult guidelines; if not possible due to limitations, be as physically active as possible	If already regularly engaged in vigorous-intensity aerobic activity or high activity, may continue as long as conditions don't change
Notes	Vigorous intensity at least 3 days per week	Additional health benefits when activity is increased to 5 hours (300 minutes) weekly of moderate intensity *or* 2 hours 30 minutes weekly of vigorous intensity or combination of both	Do activities that maintain balance	Check with your physician
Muscle and bone strengthening	Muscle and bone strengthening 3 days per week	Do muscle-strengthening activities involving all major muscle groups 2 or more days weekly	Do muscle-strengthening activities involving all major muscle groups 2 or more days weekly	Check with your physician

Table 6.2   Examples of Activities at Various Levels of Intensity

Moderate Activities (Ability to Talk; But Not Sing while You're Doing Them)	Vigorous Activities (Ability to Say a Few Words without Stopping to Catch Breath)
• Ballroom and line dancing	• Aerobic dance
• Biking on level ground or with a few hills	• Biking faster than ten miles per hour
• Canoeing	• Fast dancing
• General gardening (raking, trimming shrubs)	• Heavy gardening (digging, hoeing)
• Catch and throw sports (baseball, softball, volleyball)	• Hiking uphill
• Tennis (doubles)	• Jumping rope
• Using a manual wheelchair	• Martial arts (e.g., karate)
• Using hand cyclers (ergometers)	• Race walking, jogging, or running
• Walking briskly	• Sports with a lot of running (basketball, hockey, soccer)
• Water aerobics	• Swimming fast or swimming laps
	• Tennis (singles)

Source: US Department of Health and Human Services (2008).

Benefits of Physical Activity

The benefits of physical activity are numerous and include lowered risk of heart disease, stroke, high blood pressure, and type 2 diabetes. Additional benefits include reduced risk of developing osteoporosis, reduced risk of depression, and improved quality of life. Through physical activity, people increase their energy expenditure, helping to maintain energy balance and maintaining a desirable body weight. Being physically active helps improve self-esteem, mental activity, and energy levels. In addition, it improves learning, memory, and mood.

Based on a review of the scientific evidence, the health benefits identified in table 6.3 are associated with regular physical activity (www.health .gov/PAGuidelines/factsheetprof.aspx).

Sedentary Behavior

A review of studies on sedentary behaviors and outcomes in adults from 1996 to 2011 (Thorp, Owen, Neuhaus, & Dunstan, 2011) indicated that there is a consistent relationship between sedentary behavior and mortality and weight gain from childhood to adulthood. Time spent being sedentary was linked to an increased risk for site-specific cancers and diabetes, as well as an increased risk of cardiovascular disease, symptomatic gallstone disease, mental disorders, and hypertension.

Table 6.3 Benefits of Physical Activity

	Strong Evidence	Moderate to Strong Evidence	Moderate

Adults	• Lower risk of
	  • Early death
	  • Heart disease
	  • Stroke
	  • Type 2 diabetes
	  • High blood pressure
	  • Adverse blood lipid profile
	  • Metabolic syndrome
	  • Colon and breast cancers
	• Prevention of weight gain
	• Weight loss when combined with diet
	• Improve cardiorespiratory and muscular fitness
	• Prevention of falls
	• Reduced depression
	• Better cognitive function (older adults)
		• Better functional health (older adults)
		• Reduced abdominal obesity
			• Weight maintenance after weight loss
			• Lower risk of hip fracture
			• Increased bone density
			• Improved sleep quality
			• Lower risk of lung and endometrial cancers

Children and adolescents	• Improved cardiorespiratory endurance and muscular fitness • Favorable body composition • Improved bone health • Improved cardiovascular and metabolic health biomarkers	• Reduced symptoms of anxiety and depression	

Sedentary time is not simply time spent in front of the television. Although television viewing is the most common adult sedentary behavior, it may only occupy a small part of the day. The average amount of adult sedentary behavior per day is seven to ten hours, with workplace sitting occupying the majority of this time. Similarly, youths spend two to four hours each day in sedentary screen-based behaviors and a total of five to ten hours each day sedentary (Salmon, Tremblay, Marshall, & Hume, 2011). Data suggest that time spent in sedentary behavior may lead to poor health outcomes in adults, independent of physical activity. Yet, when adjusting for body mass index and the limitations of self-report measures, the evidence becomes less conclusive that sedentary behavior is a distinct risk factor for poor health outcomes (Thorp, Owen, Neuhaus, & Dunstan, 2011).

To address sedentary behaviors, the 2008 Physical Activity Guidelines for Americans promotes limiting the amount of sedentary time for children and adults. Healthy People 2020 (US Department of Health and Human Services, 2012b) sets objectives specifically addressing sedentary and screen time for children and adolescents as follows:

* No television or videos on an average weekday for children ages zero to two

* No more than two hours daily of television, videos, or video games for children ages two years to twelfth grade

* No more than two hours daily of computer use or computer game playing outside of school (for nonschool work) for children ages two years to twelfth grade

The Healthy People 2020 adult objectives aim to increase daily physical activity but do not set any specific guidelines regarding sedentary behavior other than to limit it and strive to meet the minimum guidelines.

Identifying ways to reduce sedentary time for children and adults remains an important focus area for health promoters and public health professionals. Additional research is needed to examine the evidence of associations between overall sedentary time and health determinants of sedentary behaviors, including identifying behavioral, social, and environmental factors that support antisedentary behavior interventions (Rhodes, Mark, & Temmel, 2012).

Physical Activity Patterns

This section examines the trends in physical activity levels in the United States with information provided for adolescents, adults, and older adults.

Historical Patterns

Changes in occupational patterns, advances in transportation and technology, and suburban growth have affected our nation's levels of physical activity over the past century. An examination of occupational trends since the 1960s (Church et al., 2011) suggests that almost half the jobs in private industry in the United States fifty years ago required at least moderate intensity physical activity, compared to now, where less than 20% demand that intensity. Since 1969, with the popularity of the automobile and the growth of the suburbs, there has been a steady decline in the proportion of trips to work by public transportation or walking. Between 1977 and 1995, the proportion of trips by walking decreased by 2.1% every ten years. These trends result in an overall trend of declining total physical activity. Thus, without good long-term data, it appears that a combination of changes to the built environment and more people engaging in sedentary behavior has resulted in a decrease in the amount of physical activity.

1990s to Present

An examination of physical activity from 1990 to 2008 suggests slight but significant increases in activity levels. In looking at data and trends over a ten-year period, from 1990 to 2000, there was a 1.9% increase, from about 24% in 1990 to about 26% in 2000, among adult men and women meeting the recommended physical activity levels described in table 6.2. (Brownson & Boehmer, 2005). Table 6.4 suggests that this trend continued through 2008. However, less than half of the adult population meets these recommendations and national obesity levels continue to rise. There is significant opportunity for improvement, especially among adult populations that are relatively inactive, including females, older adults, non-Hispanic blacks, adults with lower levels of education, and individuals with higher body mass indexes (Carlson, Fulton, Schoenborn, & Loustalot, 2010; Evenson, Buchner, Morland, 2012).

It is important for us to also look at physical activity among youth because participation in physical activity drops as children age (Centers for Disease Control and Prevention, 2010a). In a nationally representative survey, 77% of children ages nine to thirteen years reported participating in free-time physical activity during the previous seven days. At the high school level, only 29% percent of students had participated in at least sixty minutes per day of physical activity on each of the seven days before the survey and 14% did not meet recommendations on any of the 7 days before the survey (Centers for Disease Control and Prevention, 2011a). Instilling the importance of and benefits from daily physical activity daily over the course of one's lifetime is important in improving the health of our nation.

Physical Activity Behaviors and Barriers

There are multiple variables affecting a person's decision to be physically active, such as individual factors (e.g., physical capacity, attitudes,

Table 6.4   Comparison of Healthy People 2020 Activity Criteria and 2008 Physical Activity Guidelines for Americans

Healthy People 2020 Physical Activity Criteria (President's Council on Physical Fitness and Sports, 2001)	2008 Physical Activity Guidelines for Americans (US Department of Health and Human Services, 2012b)
Regular, preferably daily, moderate physical activity for at least 30 minutes per day	150 minutes of moderate intensity weekly *or* 75 minutes vigorous intensity weekly *or* equivalent combination of moderate and vigorous intensity aerobic physical activity weekly
Vigorous physical activity 3 or more days per week for 20 or more minutes per occasion	
Activities that enhance and maintain muscular strength and endurance 2 or more days per week	Muscle-strengthening activities involving all major muscle groups 2 or more days weekly
Percentage of adults aerobically active at the recommended levels according to this criteria:	Percentage of adults aerobically active at the recommended levels according to this criteria:

1998	2008
29.7	32.9

1998	2008
40.1	43.4

Evidence showing that more adults were aerobically active according to the 2008 guidelines was higher than the Healthy People 2010 criteria because the 2008 guidelines didn't include any activity frequency requirement (e.g., minutes per day per week) and moderate and vigorous intensity activity could be combined (Carlson, Fulton, Schoenborn, & Loustalot, 2010).

Healthy People 2020 Physical Activity Criteria (Same as the 2008 Physical Activity Guidelines for Americans)
Selected Targets

* 47.9% of adults engaged in aerobic physical activity of at least moderate intensity for at least 150 minutes per week, or 75 minutes per week of vigorous intensity, or an equivalent combination.

* 31.3% of adults engaged in aerobic physical activity of at least moderate intensity for more than 300 minutes per week, or more than 150 minutes per week of vigorous intensity, or an equivalent combination.

* 20.1% of adults meet the objectives for aerobic physical activity and for muscle-strengthening activity.

preferences, time demands), the built environment (e.g., land use patterns), and the social context (e.g., social norms or public policies) (Committee on Physical Activity, Health, Transportation, and Land Use, 2005). Similar to eating habits and smoking, promoting physical activity follows an ecological approach. This section examines the factors influencing an individual's physical activity behaviors using an ecological framework or construct, as presented in figure 6.1. A historical context is also provided when applicable.

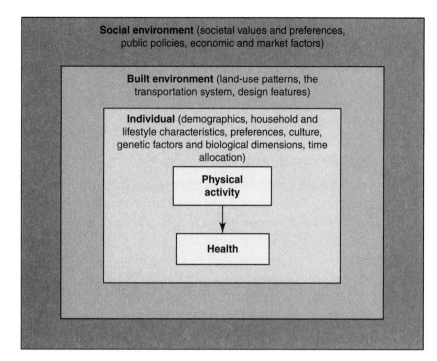

Figure 6.1   Ecological Approach to Physical Activity
Source: Committee on Physical Activity, Health, Transportation, and Land Use (2005).

Individual

Individual factors include demographics, household and lifestyle characteristics, preferences, culture, genetic factors and biological dimensions, and time allocation. For example, if the norm within the home is to spend the evenings and weekends watching TV instead of playing or being active, family members are more likely to be sedentary. A person's attitude regarding physical activity is also relevant. If people do not feel they have the time or that physical activity is not important or fun, they will be less likely to be physically active. Therefore, increasing people's physical activity level also hinges on finding internal significance or reasons why the person would be more likely to engage in physical activity and continue to be physically active.

Recreation

In 2005, 98% of all households had a television, compared to only 10% in 1950. The average hours of television viewed per day has doubled since that time; average household TV watching has increased by thirty-six minutes every ten years. A 2003 Harris Poll indicated a decline in the percentage of adults whose favorite pastime involved exercise (gardening, walking, housework, yard work), from 38% in 1995 to 29% in 2003 (Committee on Physical Activity, Health, Transportation, and Land Use, 2005).

According to the CDC, beginning 1988, 31% of the US population reported participating in no leisure-time physical activities; that percentage decreased to about 28% in 2000 and then to 25% in 2008 (Moore, Harris, Carlson, Kruger, & Fulton, 2012).

Built Environment

built environment

human-made surroundings that provide the setting for human activity; the human-made space in which people live, work, and recreate on a day-to-day basis

The **built environment** refers to human-made surroundings that provide the setting for human activity; the human-made space in which people live, work, and recreate on a day-to-day basis (Roof & Oleru, 2008). The role of the built environment as it relates to physical activity is a fast-growing area of scientific inquiry. Urban sprawl, suburbs, and the "freeway era" have affected the way people travel. City engineering and design are critical components in developing areas that are conducive to promoting physical activity in the spaces where people live and work. The decline of physically active occupations, increases in labor-saving devices, housing choices, and increases in automobile use have broadly affected physical activity levels.

Occupation

A study identifying patterns and long-term trends related to structural changes in society and the economy (Committee on Physical Activity, Health, Transportation, and Land Use, 2005) found that the percentage of the labor force in high activity occupations has declined from 16.4% in 1990 to 14.3% in 2000. Changes in employment types discussed previously in this chapter resulted in expending one hundred calories less each day on the job than earlier in the twentieth century. Researchers conclude that this one hundred calories could be adequately compensated for if adults met the 2008 Physical Activity Guidelines for Americans.

Commuting and Transportation Choices

The Committee on Physical Activity, Health, Transportation, and Land Use (2005) study also examined travel behavior using National Household Transportation Survey data. Data suggest that all adults spend an average of fifty-five minutes per day driving. People living in larger urban areas (over one million) with rail transit systems are much more likely to walk to work or for pleasure than people living in other areas. With increases in expendable income over the past few decades, however, the number of cars per household has increased, often to more cars than drivers per household.

Neighborhoods

Studies show that people walk and cycle more when their neighborhoods are more densely populated, there is mixed land-use (e.g., shops and homes), and connected streets. However, since 1945, the development of freeways and suburbs has resulted in people increasing their dependence on automobiles for work and socializing (Committee on Physical Activity, Health, Transportation, and Land Use, 2005). Proximity to safe play areas has been shown to increase physical activity in kids (Tappe, Glanz, Sallis, Zhou, & Saelens, 2013). Perceptions of safer neighborhoods are positively associated with transport walking, and perceived lower violence is associated with more leisure walking among adults (Frank et al., 2010). Therefore, to increase physical activity, health promoters must identify and work to increase levels of walking, promote access to public transportation, promote safety, and encourage the redesign of neighborhoods to facilitate increasing safe and accessible physical education activities and opportunities, including walking, cycling, and parks in which to engage in these activities.

Social Environment

According to the **social learning theory**, "human behavior is explained in terms of a three-way, dynamic, reciprocal theory in which personal factors, environmental influences, and behavior continually interact. And, that people learn through their own experiences and by observing actions of others and the results of those actions" (National Cancer Institute, 2012). Formal and informal policies and cultures affect the way people behave. For example, in an office where the expectation is that people work through their lunch breaks at their desks, employees might participate in less physical activity than in an office where the expectation is that people leave the building during the lunch hour. Or, if there's a corporate policy requiring that participation in health promotion activities (including being physically active) occur off the clock, employees might be less inclined to participate. A school policy preventing students from walking or riding their bikes to school would likely discourage physical activity. These types of situations create a culture or environment that does not promote physical activity.

social learning theory a theory of behavior that posits personal, environmental, and behavioral factors continuously interact to influence a person's behavior, along with past experiences and actions of others

In contrast, if a workplace has groups of people who informally get together to walk or participate in recreational physical activity during breaks, or if teachers incorporate physical activity into learning activities, or if families play or go out for walks together, then these activities help build social environments that support being physically active.

Efforts and Initiatives to Increase Physical Activity

As the nation's working and living landscapes continue to evolve, there has been a cultural change in how people are physically active. The fitness and recreation industries recognize that people will be physically active if there are opportunities that are convenient, appealing, and social. In the last ten years, the benefits of physical activity and its links to reducing chronic disease have been more formally promoted by government and the private sector through a variety of methods.

Technology

Social support is a critical element in successful behavior change. As society becomes increasingly technologically savvy, people are using smartphones, the Internet, and online applications to manage their health and fitness, locate and participate in group physical activities, and join virtual health or fitness-focused groups to stay accountable (Deutsche Telegroup Deteon Consulting, 2011). The private sector is continually exploring ways to tap into this market and find out what interests these individuals and what keeps them motivated. New and yet-to-be-developed technological tools will likely continue to support increased physical activity among our nation's children and adults.

Tracking Activity

Many people build accountability into their physical activity through virtual or online tracking, whether using GPS devices, applications (RunKeeper, MapMyWalk/Bike/Run, Spark People), or devices such as the FitBit or Body Bug. These tools enable people to monitor, track, and share their physical activities. New applications, such as Plus3 Network, are being released that not only track physical activity and nutrition to measure well-being but also examine health in a more holistic sense, giving people credit for community-focused activities such as carpooling and participating in volunteer activities, in some cases linking those activities, along with physical activity, to a charitable cause.

Virtual Social Support

In addition to being able to track activities, many sites offer members the opportunity to network with one another, access information and resources, ask questions, and post comments and questions in online forums. Jenny Craig, Spark People, and Weight Watchers are some examples of companies that offer websites that provide members with a virtual social community and support in reaching physical activity or health goals. The CDC has developed and promoted social media tools to support overweight and obesity prevention activities, including e-cards, badges, podcasts, and online videos, all of which are free.

Education Programs in Work Sites, Schools, and Communities

There are many opportunities to connect people with opportunities for physical activity where they live, work, and play. The key is to minimize barriers and provide a variety of activities while promoting what is available. Because adults spend most of their waking hours at their jobs, and children at school, work site and school settings provide opportunities for captive audiences. Additional community sites, such as faith-based organizations, also provide opportunities for physical activity engagement.

Work Sites

Work sites are small communities well positioned to encourage participation and engagement in physical activity programming and education. Work site policies, such as allowing employees to participate in physical activity while on the job, offering flexible work hours, and providing physical activity incentives (gym membership subsidies, gift cards, recognition, etc.) can significantly affect employee levels of physical activity (Partnership for Prevention, 2007). Increasingly, employers are modifying work environments to support physical activity, implementing walking workstations (treadmills with desks) and standing workstations, and encouraging walking meetings or huddles when team members don't require technology during a meeting. Larger employers may provide on-site fitness centers or walking and bike paths. Even smaller organizations can implement stretch breaks, post signs to encourage the use of the stairs, sponsor teams to participate in charity races (Sherwin, 2014), or provide "lunch 'n' learns" on health and fitness topics.

Education for employees at the workplace is useful in increasing physical activity. By providing follow-up consultation by health educators, coaches, or nurses after employees complete a health risk assessment, employees are able to set goals and better monitor their progress (Centers for Disease Control and Prevention, 2011b). Work site efforts build social support for behavior change and assist in the development of individualized strategies that empower employees to make lasting change.

A 2008 study (Linnan et al., 2008) examined 2004 National Worksite Health Promotion Survey data to assess to what degree work sites provide

GET ACTIVE!

The late Dr. Toni Yancey, a former professor at the UCLA School of Public Health, developed Instant Recess!, a program that invites workplaces to make time for ten minutes of physical activity into each workday through a practical, science-based, fun, friendly approach. In partnership with KEEN shoes, Instant Recess is a toolbox for employers designed to bring recess back through playful ways to get outside and get active, including videos and activities organized by areas of health in fun ways: Time to Roam, Short Escapes, High Energy, Taking a Breather, Kid Appropriate, and Good Balance (see http://recess.keenfootwear.com /recess-at-work).

environments supportive of physical activity. The study indicated that 27.6% of work sites offered on-site shower facilities, 14.6% had on-site fitness facilities, 13.5% offered fitness or walking trails, and 6.2% provided signage to encourage stair use. Data suggest that the higher number of employees at a work site increased the likelihood that the site offered supports conducive to physical activity.

Schools

Schools remain an important setting for delivering physical education programs and encouraging children to be physically active. Evidence indicates that children who are physically active tend to perform better academically. Active Living Research completed an examination of existing studies and determined that schools do not have to reduce physical activity to make gains in academic scoring. In the majority of studies reviewed, students who had higher levels of physical activity time during the school day did perform better academically. Studies also suggest that children who are physically fit have improved attendance patterns, are more focused, and better behaved in the classroom (Active Living Research, 2009). SHAPE America, formerly AAHPERD, establishes national standards and guidelines for physical education in grades K–12 (SHAPE America, nd). Table 6.5 displays the key points of a quality physical education program. Sadly, although evidence indicates that children who are physically active perform better academically, budget cuts and an increased focus on standardized testing has resulted in an astonishingly low percentage of elementary schools providing daily physical education: 3.8% (Active Living Research and San Diego State University, 2009).

Table 6.5   Key Points of Quality Physical Education

1. Opportunity to Learn:

- All students are required to take physical education
- Instructional periods totaling 150 minutes per week (elementary) and 225 minutes per week (middle and secondary school)
- Physical education class size consistent with that of other subject areas
- Qualified physical education specialist provides a developmentally appropriate program
- Adequate equipment and facilities

2. Meaningful Content:

- Written, sequential curriculum for grades P–12, based on state or national standards for physical education
- Instruction in a variety of motor skills designed to enhance the physical, mental, and social-emotional development of every child
- Fitness education and assessment to help children understand, improve and maintain physical well-being
- Development of cognitive concepts about motor skill and fitness
- Opportunities to improve emerging social and cooperative skills and gain a multicultural perspective
- Promotion of regular amounts of appropriate physical activity now and throughout life

3. Appropriate Instruction:

- Full inclusion of all students
- Maximum practice opportunities for class activities
- Well-designed lessons that facilitate student learning
- Out-of-school assignments that support learning and practice
- Physical activity not assigned as or withheld as punishment
- Regular assessment to monitor and reinforce student learning

4. Student and Program Assessment:

- Assessment is an ongoing, vital part of the physical education program
- Formative and summative assessment of student progress
- Student assessments aligned with state and national physical education standards and the written physical education curriculum
- Assessment of program elements that support quality physical education
- Stakeholders periodically evaluate the total physical education program effectiveness

Faith-Based Organizations

Religion and belief in a higher purpose are linked to a person's overall well-being. Nearly 37% of the US population reports attending religious services at least once a week (Lipka, 2013). Faith-based settings, therefore, are another important and effective environment for providing opportunities for and inspiring and engaging members in physical activity.

faith-based interventions
interventions offering some degree of spiritual or religious involvement, referencing the Bible or other religious text, institutionalized into the faith-based organization, and delivered by trained faith-based organization volunteers

faith-placed interventions
interventions that occur within the faith-based setting but do not have a spiritual or religious component; typically delivered by health promotion professionals

Faith-based interventions are defined as those offering some degree of spiritual or religious involvement, referencing the Bible or other religious text, institutionalized into the faith-based organization, and delivered by trained faith-based organization volunteers. **Faith-placed interventions** do not have a spiritual or religious component but are located on the site of a faith-based organization. Among faith-based interventions, those that ranged from six to eight months showed a significant increase in physical activity among participants immediately following the program and in the one-year follow-up.

There is further need to conduct research regarding physical activity interventions within faith-based organizations to help identify evidence-based best practices that can serve as models. The Let's Move! initiative has developed a toolkit (White House Office of Faith-Based and Neighborhood Partnerships, nd) to promote and assist faith-based and neighborhood organizations to transform neighborhoods, engage communities, and promote healthy choices. The toolkit provides step-by-step guides and examples to support faith-based efforts to improve community health.

Other Settings

The initiative of the American College of Sports Medicine (ACSM), Exercise is Medicine, encourages primary care physicians and other health care providers to include exercise in their patient treatment plans. It also advocates that doctors make physical activity a routinely assessed "vital sign" during every patient visit (www.exerciseismedicine.org). In addition to providing training and resources for medical students and doctors, ACSM also provides information, resources, and credentialing for health and fitness professionals in establishing partnerships with health care providers to promote and implement exercise as medicine.

Innovative interventions in a variety of community-based settings can be effective in planning, improving, and evaluating health promotion efforts. Researchers from the University of North Carolina Chapel Hill have been examining beauty salons as potential settings for reaching and promoting health among African American women. In a pilot study, cosmetologists were trained to deliver health messages regarding daily physical activity, weight management, and nutrition as part of an overall cancer prevention message. Researchers found that customers who spoke with their cosmetologists about health also reported higher percentages of increased readiness for and actual behavior changes after the seven-week study and twelve months postintervention (Linnan et al., 2005).

Policies That Promote Increasing Physical Activity

Policies at the national, state, and local levels have been implemented to support increasing opportunities for physical activity. These range from focusing on changing the built environment to organizing schools for successful and active kids to promoting financial and benefits polices within the workplace. The federal government has provided physical activity guidelines as well as funding to stimulate the design of programs to promote active lifestyles and to measure their impact.

National Policy

The federal government has the capability to affect levels of physical activity for adults and children across the country through legislation, resources, funding, research, and technical assistance. Among the most widely known, current legislation is the Patient Protection and Affordable Care Act (ACA). As part of the ACA, the Small Business Wellness Grant program was created, allocating $200 million in grant funding from 2011 through 2015. Dissemination of these grants will extend pieces of the Healthy Workforce Act, assisting small businesses to develop comprehensive work site health promotion programs in which physical activity is a component. Additionally, a regulation of the ACA is an allowance for employers to provide health plan premium differentials to employees who achieve health goals or participate in wellness programs (Health Promotion Advocates, 2012).

The National Coalition for Promoting Physical Activity (2011), an association that advocates for policies that encourage Americans of all ages to become more physically active (www.ncppa.org), tracks the status of legislation related to physical activity. During every Congress, a number of new pieces of legislation are introduced for review by committees; however, a very small percentage of these bills actually make it out of the committee and into law.

Federal legislation and budget resolutions support health and fitness by providing funding to federal agencies that are proponents of health and fitness, including the Department of Health and Human Services, the Department of Education, and the Department of Transportation. Each year, these departments fund projects and develop resources that support the promotion of physical activity, including state and community grants.

One of these efforts is the CDC's Community Transformation Grants (CTG) program. In 2011, this program awarded $103 million to sixty-one state and local government agencies, tribes, territories, and nonprofit

The term *Complete Streets* means much more than the physical changes to a community's streets. Complete Streets means changing transportation planning, design, maintenance, and funding decisions. A Complete Streets policy ensures that, from the start, projects are planned and designed to meet the needs of [all] community member[s], regardless of their age, ability, or how they travel. Doing so allows a community to save money, accommodate more people, and create an environment where every resident can travel safely and conveniently. (Seskin, 2012, p. 6)

organizations (see table 6.6). Two of the focus areas incorporated elements related to increasing opportunities for physical activity and making healthier and safer environments, including sidewalk improvement and expanding access to public transportation (Centers for Disease Control and Prevention, 2012a).

State Policy

States have the opportunity to encourage physical activity through various strategies. The CDC's *State Indicator Report for Physical Activity, 2010* (Centers for Disease Control and Prevention, 2010b) presents twelve policy and environmental indicators representing four different types of strategies to increase physical activity at the state and community levels (see table 6.7). States and communities are encouraged to act on or leverage as many of the strategies as possible. These guidelines

Table 6.6   Community Transformation Grants (CTG)

Physical activity and physical environment projects that received funding through the CTG program include the following:

* *Maryland:* Nineteen school districts (urban and rural) are implementing and monitoring USDA local wellness initiatives, including comprehensive physical activity strategies as well as strategies that involve other opportunities for physical activity (walking and biking-to-school programs, physical activity breaks, and intramural or physical activity clubs). The Maryland goal is that by the end of September 2016, 739,000 people (including school-age children and teens) will have access to physical activity opportunities throughout the state.

* *Broward County, Florida:* Broward County received funding to partner with experts and leaders to develop and implement Complete Streets standards and Smart Growth principles in at least 55% of its municipalities and increase opportunities for physical activity to improve overall health.

* *Oklahoma Counties:* Three counties in Oklahoma received funding to serve sixty thousand residents, focusing on low-income, racial and ethnic minority, and medically underserved communities and persons affected by mental illness or substance abuse. The funds will assist with implementing Project CORE (Community Outreach and Rural Education), with improving the quality of physical activity in schools, workplaces, and the community as one of its goals (Centers for Disease Control and Prevention, 2012b).

Table 6.7   Strategies for Increasing Physical Activity in the Community

Create or enhance access to places for physical activity	• Percentage of middle and high schools that allow community-sponsored use of physical activity facilities by youth outside of usual school hours
	• Percentage of youth with parks or playground areas, community centers, and sidewalks or walking paths available in their neighborhood
	• Percentage of census blocks that have at least one park located within the block or one-half mile from the block boundary
	• Percentage of census blocks that have at least one fitness or recreation center located within the block or one-half mile from the block boundary
Enhance physical education and activity in schools and physical activity in child care settings	• State requires or recommends regular elementary school recess minimum of twenty minutes
	• State policy requiring elementary, middle, and high schools or districts to teach physical education
	• Percentage of middle and high schools that support or promote walking or biking to and from school
	• State regulation specifying that children shall be engaged in moderate- or vigorous-intensity physical activity in licensed, regulated child care centers
Support urban design, land use, and transportation policies	• Existence of at least state-level-enacted community-scale urban design or land use policy (e.g., standards promoting destination walking and mixed-use zoning)
	• Existence of at least state-level-enacted street-scale, urban design or land use policy (e.g., improve street lighting, cross walks, enhance streetscape, and improve safety)
	• Existence of at least state-level-enacted transportation and travel policy (opportunities for biking and walking, e.g., bike racks, subsidies for or access to public transportation, incentives for car pools)
Develop and maintain a public health workforce competent in physical activity	• Number of state health department full-time equivalent personnel primarily focused on state physical activity (to develop, monitor, and support physical activity programming and partnerships throughout the state)

The Eat Smart, Move More initiative had significant success with policies passed during the 2009–2010 session, including the implementation of the following strategies:

- Fitness testing in schools—Develop guidelines for public schools to use evidence-based fitness testing for students statewide K–8 as recommended by the Legislative Taskforce on Childhood Obesity.

- Honors courses in healthful living classes—Develop or identify academically rigorous honors-level courses in healthful living education that can be offered at the high school level.

- Establish sustainable communities task forces.

- Counties and schools share PE equipment—State boards of education encourage local boards of education to enter into agreements with local governments and entities regarding joint use of physical activity facilities.

provide state and local officials with concrete steps for improving the physical and social environments to promote physical activity in their communities.

All fifty states are actively engaged in these types of strategies, to varying degrees. A couple of these efforts are described in the following: one in North Carolina and a second in New York.

North Carolina's Eat Smart, Move More Initiative

North Carolina's Eat Smart, Move More initiative is a good example of the types of state action that can influence physical activity. This initiative began with a policy strategy platform, which is a list of policy recommendations aimed at helping North Carolina meet the goals in its obesity prevention plan by influencing the environment to support healthy behavior change (Eat Smart, Move More North Carolina, 2012). For more information, see www.eatsmartmovemorenc.com.

Healthy Schools New York

The state of New York has focused attention on school-based efforts to improve student health. It received CDC funding to enhance school-based physical education, which includes strategies to increase the length of or activity level in school-based physical education classes. With only 14% of its school districts meeting state education department regulations for physical education, the state issued grants for organizations to work with school districts to develop and implement board of education–approved physical education policies. The physical activity goal is to increase the quantity or quality of physical education to meet or exceed 120 minutes per week for K–6 students. Ongoing training is provided for healthy school coordinators to assist school districts in developing and implementing physical education plans and classroom physical education instruction (Centers for Disease Control and Prevention, 2011c).

HEALTHY SCHOOLS NY

Working with a districtwide wellness committee to

* Assess current school wellness policies
* Identify priority areas based on need and realistic goal setting

We provide

- Technical assistance
- Professional development
- Evidence-based strategies and success stories
- Leadership institute
- Networking opportunities

The Healthy Schools NY Leadership Institute (HSNYLI) is funded by the NYS Department of Health and is designed to increase the number of schools that effectively implement policy, systems, and environmental changes that support tobacco-free norms, promote the consumption of healthy foods and beverages, comply with state physical education regulations, and expand opportunities to be physically active. HSNYLI aims to

- Establish a cohort of school health leaders with advanced skills to strengthen school health policy.
- Develop a network of mentors (school health leaders) [who] will transfer knowledge and skills gained through the HSNYLI to other schools within their catchment area.
- Expand the number of school health policy advocates who encourage action by other administrators and decision makers in their catchment area and statewide.

Source: Excerpted from New York State Center for School Safety (2011).

Local Policy

Government officials at the local level play a primary role within the community to enact policies supporting healthy community design. (See table 6.7.) Elected and appointed members of city councils and county commissions, zoning boards, and school boards, as well as government officials within transportation and planning departments, health departments, human services departments, parks and recreation departments, and school divisions, can develop and implement local policies and programs that directly affect the physical activity levels of local residents. Systemic change takes time; goals for the short term and long term should be set and continually measured to assess the community's performance and adjust goals as necessary (Khan et al., 2009).

Table 6.8 lists recommended strategies to prevent obesity that the CDC developed for local jurisdictions (Khan et al., 2009).

Table 6.8   Local Strategies to Prevent Obesity

Strategies to Encourage Physical Activity or Limit Sedentary Activity among Children and Youth	Strategies to Create Safe Communities That Support Physical Activity	Strategy to Encourage Communities to Organize for Change
• Require physical education in schools • Increase the amount of physical activity in PE programs and schools • Increase opportunities for extracurricular physical activity • Reduce screen time in public service venues	• Improve access to outdoor recreational facilities • Enhance infrastructure supporting bicycling • Enhance infrastructure supporting walking • Support locating schools in residential neighborhoods • Improve access to transportation • Zone for mixed-use development • Enhance personal safety where people are or could be physically active • Enhance traffic safety in areas where persons are or could be physically active	• Participate in community coalitions or partnerships to address obesity

Examples of successful local-level implementation of these strategies are listed in the following sections from West Palm Beach, Florida, and Corning, California.

West Palm Beach, Florida

In West Palm Beach, Florida, a project was implemented to improve the street environment for nonmotorized users to enhance aesthetics and to improve driving behavior (Lockwood & Stillings, 1998). The town enacted a downtown-wide traffic-calming policy. Prior to the project, the city had little street connectivity, many abandoned buildings, commercial rental rates were low, streets weren't suitable for physical activity, and vacancy rates were over 80%. The project resulted in enhanced traffic and personal safety, increased street connectivity, and mixed-use zoning. Changes included two-way traffic, wide shaded sidewalks, narrowed streets, raised intersections, on-street parking, and shortened crosswalks. Abandoned buildings were renovated into a mixed-use development. Other benefits included a doubling in property values, reduced vacancy rates, and increased rental property rates with the attraction of major retailers, restaurants, and bars.

City of Corning and Corning Union School District, California

In another project aimed at increasing community access to safe places for physical activity, the City of Corning and Corning Union School District in

California established a joint-use agreement to open school recreation facilities and resources for public use (Strategic Alliance ENACT, 2008). Through the agreement, the public could use the facilities when school was out of session, including evenings and weekends. The facilities that were available for use included gymnasiums, swimming pools, tennis courts, and athletic fields. The school and the city shared responsibility for facility maintenance and repairs.

Community Policy

Communities may be smaller areas within a local government jurisdiction or may bridge multiple local government jurisdictions. The Task Force on Community Preventive Services has identified four areas where there is sufficient evidence for increasing physical activity (Guide to Community Preventive Services, 2011). Embedded within the task force recommendations are research-tested intervention programs, which provide useful information on the practical application of the task force's recommendations. These programs are designed to help health promotion professionals identify how interventions could be incorporated into their communities (see table 6.9).

Community Partner Initiatives and Multisectorial Strategies

Multisectorial approaches are helpful for bringing together communities to leverage resources and address community member needs. Through partnerships, communities create environments that support active living. Using the multisectorial approach broadens access to opportunities for physical activity. Cost and location are barriers to some for participating in physical activity. For other communities, safety, sidewalks, and neighborhoods inadvertently cause access limitations. Therefore, public-private partnerships and community collaboration is essential in successfully implementing programming.

Recognizing that there are countless venues and collaborative opportunities available, the national government, in partnership with public and private entities, developed efforts aimed at increasing physical activity from a cross-sectorial approach.

The National Physical Activity Plan (NPAP)

The **National Physical Activity Plan (NPAP)** (www.physicalactivityplan .org) is a comprehensive set of policies, programs, and initiatives that aim

multisectorial approaches partnerships among multiple sectors to leverage resources and address community member needs

National Physical Activity Plan (NPAP) a comprehensive set of policies, programs, and initiatives that aim to increase physical activity in all segments of the American population

Table 6.9   Community Actions to Promote Physical Activity

Strategy	Community-scale urban design and land use policies	Creation of or enhanced access to places for physical activity combined with informational outreach activities	Street-scale urban design and land use policies	Point of decision prompts to encourage use of stairs
Description	Multifaceted efforts including urban planners, architects, engineers, developers, and public health professionals changing the physical environment of urban areas of several square miles with design elements such as the distance of residential areas to stores, jobs, school, and recreational areas; the connectivity and continuity of streets and sidewalks; and aesthetic and safety aspects of the environment	Efforts within communities at work sites, among coalitions, and agencies; creating walking trails, building exercise facilities, or providing access to existing nearby facilities	Efforts of urban planners, architects, engineers, developers, and public health professionals to change the physical environment of small geographic areas (a few blocks in size); includes building codes, roadway designs, environmental changes, improved lighting, and infrastructure for safe street crossing, traffic	Motivational signs or art or music near or in stairwells or at the bottom of elevators and escalators encouraging individuals to increase stair use
What the supporting studies show	Increases the number of walkers and cyclists; increases sense of community and choice of where to live; reductions in crime and stress; improvements in green space	Increases in aerobic capacity and energy expenditure; participants reporting some leisure-time physical activity and exercise scores; shown to be effective across age, gender, income, and environments	Overall median improvements in physical activity and green space; reductions in crime and stress	More people using stairs when prompts were involved; interventions shown to be effective in a variety of settings and among a wide population (age, weight, sex, and race)

to increase physical activity in all segments of the American population. The plan aims to transform American culture into one that supports more physically active lifestyles to improve health, prevent disease and disability, and enhance quality of life. The NPAP provides recommendations in eight sectors to support people being physically active where we live, work, and play:

- Business and industry
- Education

- Health care

- Mass media

- Parks, recreation, fitness, and sports

- Public health

- Transportation, land use, and community design

- Volunteer and nonprofit

The NPAP identifies policies and objectives for implementation and provides its multisectorial partners (coalitions, nonprofits, and businesses) with priorities, resources, and success stories from organizations who have achieved inspiring measurable change.

Let's Move!

The Let's Move! Campaign (www.letsmove.gov), launched by First Lady Michelle Obama, is dedicated to solving the problem of obesity within a generation. It is designed to promote healthier lifestyles, especially among communities with lower socioeconomic status. It's about eating healthier, being more active, and improving food labeling. The initiative provides parents helpful information for fostering healthier environments that support healthy choices and recognizes that a multisectorial approach is critical to improving the health of the nation. Let's Move! engages parents, caregivers, elected officials from all levels of government, schools, health care professionals, faith-based and community-based organizations, and private-sector companies.

Rails-to-Trails

The mission of Rails-to-Trails (www.railstotrails.org/index.html) is to create a nationwide network of trails from former rail lines and connecting corridors to build places for people to become healthier. To date, Rails-to-Trails has supported the development of more than 1,600 preserved pathways that form the foundation of a growing trail system spanning communities, regions, states, and the entire country. In addition to providing places for people to walk and bike, the trails can also be used for other physical activities including in-line skating and horseback riding. Other benefits include wildlife conservation, historical preservation, stimulation of local economies by increasing tourism and promoting local business, and providing safe and accessible routes for commuting.

Bike Shares

During the 2000s, urban public bike-sharing programs increased in popularity. Since 2008, there are now thirty bike-share programs in the United States (Gustafson, 2012). City governments often develop bike-sharing programs to alleviate traffic, diminish the economic impact of higher gas prices on residents, facilitate tourism and urban activities, encourage exercise and economic investments, reduce pollution, and better link people between locations and public transportation. Through bike-share programs, bikes are made available to people for free or at a low cost at strategic locations throughout the city. Customers can rent bikes using credit or debit cards or through memberships to the bike-share system for specified periods of time and return bikes to any sponsored parking racks or stations when done.

YMCA Initiatives

The YMCA of the USA (2009) promotes health of body, mind, and spirit. In addition to youth development programs, it focuses on healthy living in the broader context of healthier communities and social responsibility (see table 6.10).

Table 6.10   YMCA Physical Activity Community Initiatives

Pioneering Healthier Communities (PHC)	Activate America	Community Healthy Living Index (CHLI)
Focuses on collaborative engagement with community leaders, how environments influence health and well-being, and the role policy plays in sustaining change; with support from the CDC and other donors, 117 YMCAs across the country are reaching out to a broad adult population, in particular health seekers and socioeconomic groups that are most in need of health interventions to promote physical activity	Working with communities to support healthy living; currently, more than 160 YMCAs are collaborating with community leaders to make changes within their communities at the physical environment and policy levels; areas of focus include creating safer walking routes to school and increasing physical education and activity throughout the school day	Helps communities assess their support for healthy living and equips them with tools to help reverse the trend of unhealthy living while building community partnerships; includes six different assessments for key community settings (after-school child care, early childhood programs, neighborhoods, schools, work sites, and the community at large); respondents are asked questions about policies and practices supporting healthy lifestyles; each question identifies a best practice or idea for improvement on that topic; a guide and toolkit are provided to help facilitate discussion, identify barriers and opportunities, and incorporate community input (www.ymca.net /communityhealthylivingindex)

Blue Zones Project

The Blue Zones Project (www.bluezonesproject.com) is a community well-being improvement initiative designed to make healthy choices easier through permanent changes to environment, policy, and social networks. The Blue Zones Project is based on the idea of a social movement focused on encouraging positive healthy change. Communities can strive to earn Blue Zone certification through a concentrated effort among work sites, restaurants, grocery stores, and schools. Blue Zone certification includes achieving the following (www.bluezonesproject.com/communities/mason-city/certification_progress):

- 20% of citizens signing up with the Blue Zones Project and complete at least one action

- 25% of schools becoming Blue Zones schools

- 25% of locally owned or independent restaurants becoming Blue Zones restaurants

- 25% of grocery stores becoming Blue Zones grocery stores

- 50% of the top twenty community-identified work sites becoming Blue Zones work sites

- Implementing at least one policy from each section of the community policy action list

- Completing at least two changes to the built environment to help people adopt healthier behaviors

- Earning at least 50% of the total available points for community policy pledge actions

Summary

There are many opportunities to increase physical activity levels among the entire US population. People's decisions to be physically active are influenced not only by personal factors but also by social and environmental factors. The most successful efforts are those that are multifaceted addressing personal, social, and environmental factors. The more variety, access, and points of confluence that exist, the more likely it is to build and sustain environments that are conducive to active living. The important thing is to just move! Be more active and encourage others around you to be as active as they can be. Even small increases make a difference.

Additionally, health promotion professionals can advocate for health and well-being legislation by contacting local health departments, city councils, and representatives, voicing support for initiatives that promote health and physical activity.

KEY TERMS

1. **Physical activity:** any bodily movement produced by skeletal muscles that requires energy expenditure

2. **Exercise:** a subset of physical activity that is planned, structured, and repetitive and has a final or an intermediate objective to improve or maintain physical fitness level

3. **Aerobic (endurance) activity:** any activity that uses the large muscle groups in the body to increase heart rate and benefit the strength of the cardiovascular system

4. **Muscle-strengthening activities:** any activity that improves muscular strength, power, and endurance

5. **Bone-strengthening activities:** any activity that improves bone density by causing impact on the musculoskeletal system

6. **Stretching activities:** any activity in which a specific muscle or tendon is lengthened in an effort to improve flexibility and joint mobility

7. **2008 Physical Activity Guidelines for Americans (PAG):** a report released by the US Department of Health and Human Services recommending specific physical activity levels by age group

8. **Built environment:** human-made surroundings that provide the setting for human activity; the human-made space in which people live, work, and recreate on a day-to-day basis

9. **Social learning theory:** a theory of behavior that posits personal, environmental, and behavioral factors continuously interact to influence a person's behavior, along with past experiences and actions of others

10. **Faith-based interventions:** interventions offering some degree of spiritual or religious involvement, referencing the Bible or other religious text, institutionalized into the faith-based organization, and delivered by trained faith-based organization volunteers

11. **Faith-placed interventions:** interventions that occur within the faith-based setting but do not have a spiritual or religious component; typically delivered by health promotion professionals

12. **Multisectorial approaches:** partnerships among multiple sectors to leverage resources and address community member needs

13. **National Physical Activity Plan (NPAP):** a comprehensive set of policies, programs, and initiatives that aim to increase physical activity in all segments of the American population

REVIEW QUESTIONS

1. What are the benefits of physical activity?

2. What are the health risks associated with a sedentary lifestyle?

3. What percentage of adolescents, adults, and older adults are meeting physical activity recommendations?

4. What are the individual and social barriers to achieving physical activity?

5. How do you define the variables of social environment, built environment, and individual factors as they relate to physical activity?

6. What is a multisectorial approach to physical activity?

7. Why is a policy approach important to increasing physical activity?

8. How do you describe policy approaches at the national, state, and local levels?

9. What are four of the twelve policy and environmental indicators that the CDC recommends for states and communities?

STUDENT ACTIVITIES

1. Many physical activity advocates state that physical activity has been engineered out of daily living. What does that statement mean? What are the strategies being used to reengineer activity back into our lives? Identify the barriers and opportunities.

2. We live in a time when athletes are setting world records for sporting events. Yet, concurrently we also have a high percentage of children who are overweight and showing signs of chronic disease. What causes such disparities?

3. For the following target audiences, create and describe one creative physical activity program:

    a. Children two to four years old

    b. Adults at the work site

    c. Seniors seventy years and older

References

Active Living Research. (2009). *Active education physical education, physical activity and academic performance.* San Diego: Active Living Research.

Active Living Research and San Diego State University. (2009, September 25). *New evidence strengthens case for increasing school-based physical activity.* Retrieved from www.rwjf.org/en/research-publications/find-rwjf-research/2009/09/new-evidence-strengthens-case-for-increasing-school-based-physic.html

Brownson, R. C., & Boehmer, T. K. (2005). *Patterns and trends in physical activity, occupation, transportation, land use, and sedentary behavior.* Paper for Transportation Research Board Special Report 282. Retrieved from http://onlinepubs.trb.org/onlinepubs/archive/downloads/sr282papers/sr282Brownson.pdf

Carlson, S., Fulton, J. E., Schoenborn, C. A., & Loustalot, F. (2010). Trend and prevalence estimates based on the 2008 physical activity guidelines for Americans. *American Journal of Preventive Medicine, 39*(4), 305–313.

Caspersen, C. J., Powell, K. E., & Christenson, G. M. (1985). Physical activity, exercise, and physical fitness: Definitions and distinctions for health-related research. *Public Health Reports, 100*(2), 126–131.

Centers for Disease Control and Prevention. (2009). *Healthy communities: What local governments can do to reduce and prevent obesity.* Retrieved from www.cdc.gov/obesity/downloads/CDC_Healthy_Communities.pdf

Centers for Disease Control and Prevention. (2010a). *The association between school-based physical activity, including physical education, and academic performance.* Atlanta: US Department of Health and Human Services. Retrieved from www.cdc.gov/healthyyouth/physicalactivity/facts.htm

Centers for Disease Control and Prevention. (2010b). *State indicator report on physical activity, 2010.* Atlanta: US Department of Health and Human Services.

Centers for Disease Control and Prevention. (2011a). *Adolescent and school health, physical activity facts.* Retrieved www.cdc.gov/healthyyouth/physicalactivity/facts.htm

Centers for Disease Control and Prevention. (2011b, April 25). *Physical activity.* Retrieved from www.cdc.gov/workplacehealthpromotion/implementation/topics/physical-activity.html

Centers for Disease Control and Prevention. (2011c, July). *Program highlights enhanced school-based physical education.* Retrieved from www.cdc.gov/obesity/downloads/SchoolBasedPhysicalEducation.pdf

Centers for Disease Control and Prevention. (2012a, September 24). *Community transformation grants (CTG).* Retrieved from www.cdc.gov/communitytransformation/accomplishments/index.htm

Centers for Disease Control and Prevention. (2012b, October 12). *Community transformation grants—small community awards summary of proposed project activities.* Retrieved from www.cdc.gov/communitytransformation/smallcommunities/awardees.htm

Church T. S., Thomas, D. M., Tudor-Locke, C., Katzmarzyk, P. T., Earnest, C. P., et al. (2011). Trends over 5 decades in U.S. occupation-related physical activity and their associations with obesity. *PLoS ONE 6*(5), e19657. doi: 10.1371/journal .pone.0019657

Committee on Physical Activity, Health, Transportation, and Land Use. (2005). *Does the built environment influence physical activity? Examining the evidence.* Transportation Research Board Special Report 282. Retrieved from http:// onlinepubs.trb.org/onlinepubs/sr/sr282.pdf

Deutsche Telegroup Deteon Consulting. (2011, July). *Mobile health applications for low socio-economic communities.* Retrieved from www.slideshare.net/applica tionsforgood/mobile-health-apps-for-low-income-communities#btnNext

Eat Smart, Move More North Carolina. (2012, March). *Policy strategy platform: Summary of state legislation.* Retrieved from www.eatsmartmovemorenc.com /PolicyStrategy/Texts/ESMM%20NC%20PSP%20Summary%20of%20State% 20Legislation%20FINAL%202012%203-21.pdf

Evenson, K. R., Buchner, D. M., & Morland, K. B. (2012). Objective measurement of physical activity and sedentary behavior among US adults aged 60 years or older. *Preventing Chronic Disease, 9,* 110109. doi: http://dx.doi.org/10.5888/pcd9.110109

Frank, L. D., Sallis, J. F., Saelens, B. E., Leary, L., Cain, K., Conway, T. L., & Hess, P. M. (2010). The development of a walkability index: Application to the neighborhood quality of life study. *British Journal of Sports Medicine.* doi: 10.1136/bjsm .2009.058701

Guide to Community Preventive Services. (2011). *Increasing physical activity: Environmental and policy approaches.* Retrieved from www.thecommunity guide.org/pa/environmental-policy/index.html

Gustafson, E. (2012, August 19). *U.S. hits 30 bike shares in just four years.* Climate Progress. Retrieved from http://thinkprogress.org/climate/2012/08/19/708941 /us-hits-30-bike-shares-in-just-four-years/?mobile=nc

Health Promotion Advocates. (2012). *Health Promotion Advocates advocacy priorities.* Retrieved from http://healthpromotionadvocates.org/legislative-priorities

Khan, L. K., Sobush, K., Keener, D., Goodman, K., Lowry, A., Kakietek, J., & Zaro, S. (2009, July 24). Recommended community strategies and measurements to prevent obesity in the United States. *MMWR, 55*(7), 1–26. Retrieved from www.cdc.gov/mmwr/preview/mmwrhtml/rr5807a1.htm

Linnan, L. A., Bowling, M., Childress, J., Lindsay, G., Blakey, C., Pronk, S., Wieker, S., & Royall, P. (2008). Results of the 2004 National Worksite Health Promotion survey. *American Journal of Public Health, 98*(8), 1503–1509.

Linnan L. A., Ferguson, Y. A., Wasilewski, Y., Lee, A. M., Yang, J., Solomon, F., & Katz, M. (2005). Using community-based participatory research methods to reach women with health messages results from the North Carolina BEAUTY and Health Pilot Project. *Health Promotion Practice, 6*(2), 164–173.

Lipka, M. (2013, September 13). *What surveys say about worship attendance—and why some stay home.* Pew Research Center. Retrieved from www.pewresearch .org/fact-tank/2013/09/13/what-surveys-say-about-worship-attendance-and -why-some-stay-home

Lockwood, I., & Stillings, T. (1998). *Traffic calming for crime reduction & neighborhood revitilization.* West Palm Beach, FL: City of West Palm Beach.

Moore, L. V., Harris, C. D., Carlson, S. A., Kruger, J., & Fulton, J. E. (2012). Trends in no leisure-time physical activity—United States, 1988–2010. *Research Quarterly for Exercise and Sport, 83*(4), 587–591.

National Cancer Institute. (2012, June 8). *Theory at a glance: A guide for health promotion practice.* Retrieved from www.cancer.gov/cancertopics/cancerlibrary /theory.pdf

National Center for Safe Routes to School. (nd). *Safe routes.* Retrieved from http:// saferoutesinfo.org

National Coalition for Promoting Physical Activity. (2011, June 28). *Public policy— Current physical activity legislation.* Retrieved from www.ncppa.org/static /assets/Physical_Activity_Legislation-112th_Congress_Updated_6–28–11.pdf

National Heart, Lung, and Blood Institute. (2011). *Types of physical activity.* Retrieved from www.nhlbi.nih.gov/health/health-topics/topics/phys/types.html

New York State Center for School Safety. (2011). *Healthy Schools NY.* Retrieved from http://nyscenterforschoolsafety.org/what.cfm?subpage=508910

Partnership for Prevention. (2007). *Leading by example feature sheets.* Retrieved from www.prevent.org/data/files/initiatives/lbe_profile_sheets.pdf

President's Council on Physical Fitness and Sports. (2001, March). *Healthy People 2010: Physical activity and fitness.* Retrieved from www.presidentschallenge.org /informed/digest/docs/200103digest.pdf

Rhodes, R. E., Mark, R. S., & Temmel, C. P. (2012). Adult sedentary behavior: A systematic review. *American Journal of Preventive Medicine, 42*(3), e3–e28.

Roof, K., & Oleru, N. (2008). Public health: Seattle and King County's push for the built environment. *Journal of Environmental Health, 71*(1), 24–27. Retrieved from www.cdc.gov/nceh/ehs/Docs/JEH/2008/july-aug_w_case_studies/JEH_ Jul-Aug_08_Seattle.pdf

Salmon, J., Tremblay, M. S., Marshall, S. J., & Hume, C. (2011). Health risks, correlates, and interventions to reduce sedentary behavior in young people. *American Journal of Preventive Medicine, 41*(2), 197–206.

Seskin, S. (2012, August). *Complete Streets local policy workbook.* Smart Growth America and National Complete Streets Coalition. Retrieved from www.smart growthamerica.org/documents/cs-local-policy-workbook.pdf

SHAPE America. (nd). Key points of quality physical education. Retrieved from www.shapeamerica.org/publications/resources/teachingtools/qualitype/qpe _keypoints.cfm

Sherwin, J. (2014, January 29). *A look into MD Anderson Cancer Center's wellness program—An employer case.* Retrieved from www.corporatewellnessmagazine .com/article/a-look-into-md-anderson-cancer-center-s-wellness-program-an -employer-case-.html

Strategic Alliance ENACT. (2008). *Policy detail: Corning Union High School District facilities use agreement.* Retrieved from http://eatbettermovemore.org/sa/polic ies/policy_detail.php?s_Search=&issue=&env=&keyword=73&s_State=Califor nia&jurisdiction=3&year=&policyID=333

Tappe, K. A., Glanz, K., Sallis, J. F., Zhou, C., & Saelens, B. E. (2013). Children's physical activity: Parents' perception of the neighborhood environment; neigh-borhood impact on kids study. *International Journal of Behavioral Nutrition and Physical Activity.* doi: 10.1186/1479–5868–10–39

Thorp, A. A., Owen, N., Neuhaus, M., & Dunstan, D. W. (2011). Sedentary behaviors and subsequent health outcomes in adults. *American Journal of Preventive Medicine, 41*(2), 207–215

US Department of Health and Human Services. (2008, October 17). At-a-glance: A fact sheet for professionals. *Physical activity guidelines for Americans.* Retrieved from www.health.gov/PAGuidelines/factsheetprof.aspx

US Department of Health and Human Services. (2012a, September 6). *Physical activity.* HealthyPeople.gov. Retrieved from www.healthypeople.gov/2020/topics objectives2020/overview.aspx?topicid=33

US Department of Health and Human Services. (2012b, November 27). *Physical activity guidelines.* Retrieved from www.health.gov/paguidelines

White House Office of Faith-Based and Neighborhood Partnerships. (nd). *Let's move!* Retrieved from www.hhs.gov/partnerships/resources/Pubs/lets_move _toolkit.pdf

World Health Organization. (2012a). *Global strategy on diet, physical activity and health: What is moderate-intensity and vigorous-intensity physical activity?* Retrieved from www.who.int/dietphysicalactivity/physical_activity_intensity/en /index.html

World Health Organization. (2012b). *Health topics: Physical activity.* Retrieved from www.who.int/topics/physical_activity/en

YMCA of the USA. (2009). *Pioneering healthier communities lessons learned and leading practices.* Washington, DC: YMCA of the USA.

CHAPTER 7

STRESS, EMOTIONAL WELL-BEING, AND MENTAL HEALTH

Marty Loy

Sound mental and **emotional health** is linked to a wide range of positive outcomes, including better health status, educational achievement, productivity, higher earnings, improved interpersonal relationships, better parenting, closer social connections, greater resilience, and an overall improved quality of life (World Health Organization, 2010).

Conversely, poor mental health can impede our capacity to realize full potential, work productively, and make contributions to our families, work, and community. Consider the following statistics according to the National Alliance on Mental Illness (2013):

- One in four adults will experience a mental health disorder in any given year; one in seventeen lives with a serious mental illness such as schizophrenia, major depression, or bipolar disorder; and one in ten children suffer a mental or emotional disorder.

- Major depressive disorder affects 6.7% of adults, or about 14.8 million Americans, and it is the leading cause of disability in the United States between ages fifteen and forty-four.

- Anxiety disorders, including panic disorder, obsessive-compulsive disorder (OCD), posttraumatic stress disorder (PTSD), generalized anxiety disorder, and phobias, affect about 18.7% of adults, an estimated forty million.

LEARNING OBJECTIVES

After reading this chapter, the student will be able to:

- Define the elements of mental and emotional health.

- Describe the stress response or the fight-or-flight response.

- Identify statistics that support the rising levels of stress in our country.

- Describe how stress is linked to chronic disease and stress physiology.

- Explain the opportunities for managing stress.

- Identify strategies for managing individual and organizational stress.

- Describe mental health disparities.

- Summarize how stress affects children.

emotional health
our ability to attend to
our own emotional needs
and the skill with which
we are able to deal with
everyday life

- Suicide is the tenth leading cause of death in the United States and the third leading cause of death for people ages fifteen to twenty-four years.

- Less than one-third of adults and one-half of children with a diagnosable mental disorder receive mental health services in a given year and those rates are even lower among racial and ethnic minority groups.

- One in five children has some sort of mental, behavioral, or emotional problem. Of these only 30% receive any sort of intervention or treatment and the other 70% simply struggle through the pain of mental illness or emotional turmoil, doing their best to make it to adulthood.

The Origins of the Term *Stress*

Physician Hans Selye first introduced the term *stress* to the biologic science community in 1936. That does not mean that stress did not exist until then; it certainly did. Early humans probably struggled to find food and protect their young. Depression-era families certainly struggled to survive. Even so, recent research indicates that stress may be at an all-time high. Consider the following statistics according to the American Psychological Association (2009):

- More than 70% of Americans experience regular physical and psychological stress symptoms; over half rate their stress levels as moderate to high and a third of those report living with extreme stress. The American Academy of Family Physicians estimates that two-thirds of all office visits to family physicians are because of stress-related symptoms.

- At work, eight in ten employees report job-related stress and nearly half say they need help managing stress. The cost of job stress is estimated at more than $300 billion annually in the United States.

- Chronic stress is associated with a greater risk for many illnesses such as depression, cardiovascular disease, diabetes, autoimmune diseases, upper respiratory infections, and poorer wound healing.

Mental health and emotional well-being depends on our ability to deal with stress and maintain control of our emotions and behavior. The first step is to understand how the body handles stress.

The Fight-or-Flight Response

"Fight or flight" was a phrase first introduced to the literature by Walter Cannon in 1914. Cannon, a Harvard physiologist, used the term to describe

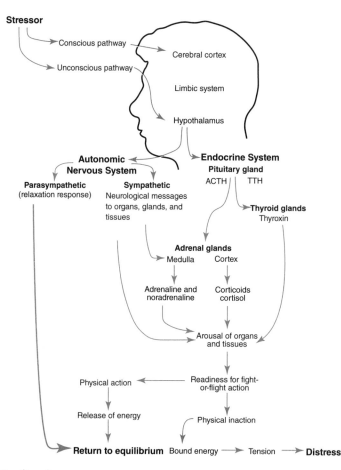

Figure 7.1   Stress Response
Source: Adapted from Seaward (2004 p. 38).

our body's physiologic response that produces the energy to either "fight" or "flee" when we are confronted with a stressor.

The **fight-or-flight response**, also known as the *stress response,* begins with the interpretation of an event (conscious or unconscious). Once recognized as a threat, a physiologic reaction occurs activating the nervous and endocrine systems, leading to the arousal of protective bodily functions. When the stressor is gone, the body returns to homeostasis (see figure 7.1).

The fight-or-flight response is often characterized by describing the two options cavemen had when confronted by a lion and the instinctive response to stay and fight the animal or to run away from it. Fight or flight is easily recognized when the stressor is physical in nature; however, the urge to fight or flee is also a reaction brought on by nonphysical stressors, such as pressure of an upcoming exam or a big project at work or a verbal encounter

fight-or-flight response
a human body's physiological response to stress; the response produces the energy needed to either fight back against a stressor or to flee from it

with someone. In some cases, even our imagination can elicit the stress response; consider the effects of a scary dream or the thought that a loved one who has not returned home on time may be lost.

Cannon identified physiologic reactions that occur to prepare for fighting or fleeing that have clear protective functions. For example, when under stress our heart rate increases carrying more oxygen to our muscles, arteries dilate in order to redirect blood flow to muscles and organs that need it, and we perspire more, using our body's innate cooling system (see figure 7.2).

Taylor, Klein, Lewis, Gruenewald, Gurung, and Updegraff (2000) coined the term *tend and befriend* to describe a behavioral response most often found in women, which is less confrontational and more nurturing. According to their research, the authors found that although men and women experience similar physiologic responses to a threat, women typically respond with an impulse to nurture and to befriend others. They theorized

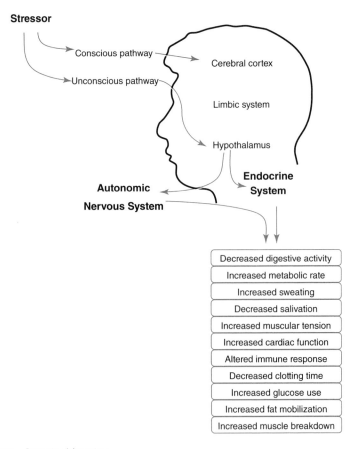

Figure 7.2   Protective Adaptations
Source: Adapted from Blonna (2005, p. 117).

that the tend-and-befriend behavior is the result of a combination of brain chemistry and gender-specific hormones released during the stress response, and there is no doubt that social mores also influence this gender-specific response.

Stress Physiology

The autonomic nervous system, endocrine system, and immune system are three physiologic pathways involved in the stress response and the stress-illness relationship (see figure 7.3).

The **autonomic nervous system (ANS)**, is the part of the peripheral nervous system (brain, spinal cord, and nerves) that regulates involuntary

autonomic nervous system (ANS)
the part of the peripheral nervous system that regulates involuntary bodily functions such as heart rate and respiration

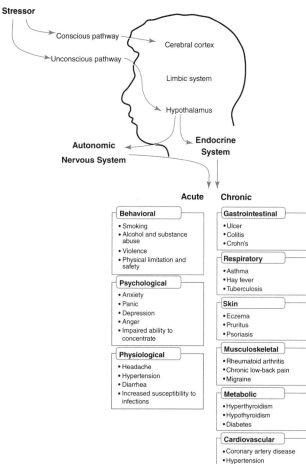

Figure 7.3   Effects of Stress on Health
Source: Adapted from Hesson (2010, p. 34).

body functions. Autonomic functions are automatic or reflexive, regulating many of our vital body functions, such as heart rate and respiration. This system has two parts: (1) the sympathetic nervous system, recognized as the stress system because it excites and speeds you up, and (2) the parasympathetic system, known for stimulating the relaxation response and helping the body return to a relaxed, normal state. Inciting the sympathetic system releases chemicals and hormones that initiate the stress response, increasing capabilities of essential organs of the body and constraining organs that are not essential.

endocrine system
a system of glands responsible for secreting hormones into the bloodstream

The **endocrine system** is made up of glands that secrete hormones into the bloodstream. Three major glands involved in the stress response are the pituitary, the thyroid, and the adrenal glands. The pituitary, a pea-sized gland located at the base of the skull, is often called the master gland because it controls all other glands. Pituitary hormones trigger hormone release in other organs. The thyroid gland, located in the front of the neck below the larynx, regulates metabolism, and in reaction to stress its hormones increase the rate with which the body can use energy. Adrenal glands, located on the top of each kidney, have two distinct parts: an outer part called the cortex, which produces steroid hormones such as cortisol, aldosterone, and testosterone, and an inner part called the medulla, which produces adrenaline and noradrenaline. The adrenal cortex produces a glucocorticoid called cortisol, which increases blood sugar and assists in metabolizing fat, protein, and carbohydrates. In recent years, there has been growing interest in using cortisol as an objective marker of stress because it is easy to trace in urine, saliva, and plasma. Cortisol has also been shown to affect immune function.

immune system
a system of biological structures responsible for protecting the human body from infectious external agents such as bacteria and viruses and against the body's own disease-causing agents

The **immune system** has as its primary role to protect the human body against infections such as bacteria, viruses, and cancerous cells. Stress has long been known to suppress immune function and increase susceptibility to infections and cancer; however, recent observations by Dhabhar (2009) suggest that stress may suppress immune function under some conditions and enhance it under others. Chronic or long-term stress seems to suppress immunity by decreasing immune cell numbers and function and increasing regulatory T cells; however, during acute stress, immune function can be enhanced (Dhabhar, 2009). The more that we learn about how stress affects immunity, the more we can see how our emotions influence illness and health.

eustress
"good" stress; stress that can be beneficial to the experiencer

distress
"bad" stress; stress that can be harmful to the experiencer, especially in excess amounts

Eustress and Distress

Not all stress is bad. The frequency, duration, and intensity each play a role in whether stress is good (**eustress**) or bad (**distress**). In his 1956 book titled

The Stress of Life, noted endocrinologist Hans Selye recognized stress as not only a demand but also commonly quite helpful. In the preface to his book he wrote,

> No one can live without experiencing some degree of stress all the time. You may think that only serious disease or intensive physical or mental injury can cause stress. This is false. Crossing a busy intersection, exposure to a draft, or even sheer joy are enough to activate the body's stress-mechanism to some extent. Stress is not even necessarily bad for you; it is also the spice of life, for any emotion, any activity causes stress. (Selye, 1956, p. vii)

It is important to remember that stress is most often good; after all, our body's physiologic response to a stressor is designed to help us achieve success and protect us from physical and psychological demands. Indeed, humans need stress to be healthy, happy, and productive. The Yerkes-Dodson law (Yerkes & Dodson, 1908) was conceptualized by two psychologists to show the interaction between arousal and performance. Applied more broadly, it demonstrates that having either too little or too much stress can create distress and harmful effects. People perform at peak levels when they are in the zone of optimal stress (see figure 7.4).

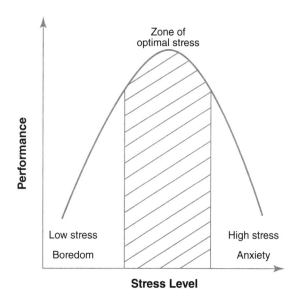

Figure 7.4   Optimal Stress Zone
Source: Adapted from Seward (2004, p. 8).

Hans Selye's research demonstrated that our bodies respond to stress in remarkably similar ways and that the physical response to a stressor goes through three predictable stages known as the **general adaptation syndrome (GAS)**: alarm, resistance, and exhaustion. The alarm stage, previously described as the fight-or-flight response, prepares our body for action. During the resistance stage, our body reduces arousal levels to more appropriate and manageable levels, which are necessary to continue to protect us for a longer duration. Our body's defenses against stress cannot go on forever, and once our protective resources are depleted we reach a state of exhaustion in which our body can no longer meet the demands placed on it and it fails to function properly. This is when chronic and serious illness can develop. Even if our stress is not particularly intense, if prolonged, it has been shown to lead to poor performance outcomes or poor mental health such as depression and illness (Cohen, Janicki-Deverts, & Miller, 2007).

general adaptation syndrome (GAS)
the physical response to a stressor involving three stages: alarm, resistance, and exhaustion

Life Stress and Illness

Two early researchers, Thomas Holmes and Richard Rahe (1967), studied the link between stress and illness. Holmes and Rahe found significant correlations between the severity of the life events (positive and negative) and medical histories of their study participants. Based on what they learned, they designed a Social Readjustment Rating Scale. Their scale assigned "life-change units" (LCUs) to each of forty-three stressful, yet common life events. According to Holmes and Rahe, a score of 150 LCUs or above indicated the potential for major health-related problems (see figure 7.5).

Coping: Stress Management Techniques

Most scholars agree that it is not the circumstance that is stressful, but the perception and interpretation of the circumstance (Seaward, 2011). How we

A basketball player is standing at the free throw line getting ready to take a shot that will determine the outcome of a championship game. The game is on the line. If she makes the shot her team wins; if she misses they will lose. It is the same shot she has easily made many times in practice: the rim is at the same height, she is standing the exact same distance from the hoop, and every ball is the same size and weight. The only difference is her perception. If she interprets the situation accurately she will maintain perspective and find herself in a state of eustress. Effectively having coped with the situation, she will in all likelihood make the shot to win the game.

INSTRUCTIONS: Mark down the point value of each of these life events that has happened to you during the previous year. Total these associated points.	
Life Event	**Mean Value**
1. Death of spouse	100
2. Divorce 3. Marital Separation from mate	73 65
4. Detention in jail or other institution	63
5. Death of a close family member 6. Major personal injury or illness	63 53
7. Marriage	50
8. Being fired at work 9. Marital reconciliation with mate	47 45
10. Retirement from work	45
11. Major change in the health or behavior of a family member 12. Pregnancy	44 40
13. Sexual difficulties	39
14. Gaining a new family member (i.e. birth, adoption, older adult moving in, etc.) 15. Major business readjustment	39 39
16. Major change in financial state (i.e. a lot worse or better off than usual)	38
17. Death of a close friend 18. Changing to a different line of work	37 36
19. Major change in the number of arguments w/ spouse (i.e. either a lot more or a lot less than usual)	35
20. Taking on a mortgage (for home, business, etc.) 21. Foreclosure on a mortgage or loan	31 30
22. Major change in responsibilities at work (i.e. promotion, demotion, etc.)	29
23. Son or daughter leaving home (marriage, attending college, joined mil.) 24. In-law troubles	29 29
25. Outstanding personal achievement	28
26. Spouse beginning or ceasing work outside the home 27. Beginning or ceasing formal schooling	26 26
28. Major change in living condition (new home, remodeling, deterioration of neighborhood or home etc.)	25
29. Revision of personal habits (dress manners, associations, quitting smoking) 30. Troubles with the boss	24 23
31. Major changes in working hours or conditions	20
32. Changes in residence 33. Changing to a new school	20 20
34. Major change in usual type and/or amount of recreation	19
35. Major change in church activity (i.e. a lot more or less than usual) 36. Major change in social activities (clubs, movies, visiting, etc.)	19 18
37. Taking on a loan (car, tv, freezer, etc.)	17
38. Major change in sleeping habits (a lot or a lot less than usual) 39. Major change in number of family get-togethers	16 15
40. Major change in eating habits (a lot more or less food intake, or very different meal hours or surroundings)	15
41. Vacation 42. Major holidays	13 12
43. Minor violations of the law (traffic tickets, jaywalking, disturbing the peace, etc.)	11
150pts or less means a relatively low amount of life change and a low susceptibility to stress-induced health breakdown	
150 to 300pts implies about a 50% chance of major health breakdown in the next 2 years	
300pts or more raises the odds to about 80%, according to the Holmes- Rahe statistical predication model	

Figure 7.5   Holmes and Rahe Stress Scale

Source: Adapted from Holmes and Rahe (1967).

interpret a situation or event will have a great deal to do with the stress that results and the outcome of the situation.

Some people may wrongly believe that the basketball player had little control over the stress of the moment, but this is not true. Processing of visual sensory information (interpretation) occurs quickly in the prefrontal cortex of the brain *before* being passed to the mid-brain, where the stress reaction begins. The prefrontal cortex, located in the part of the brain that we have conscious control of, makes it clear that we *can* consciously control our reaction to any given circumstance.

Four Coping Opportunities

One important moment in dealing with stress is at the very moment we encounter, perceive, and interpret a stressor; however, this is not the only moment that matters. Intervention in the stress-distress cycle is possible at any time and in many ways. The following sections describe four opportunities.

Opportunity 1

One of the first opportunities occurs at that very moment we encounter a stressor. This moment is key because shortly thereafter we interpret and act on what we perceive as a threat. This interpretation is what sets the physiologic stress response in motion. If we view a threat as being more or less than it really is, we risk being ineffective at dealing with it, and we will be harmed either by the stressor itself or by the stress hormones being produced. A few other stress management approaches that can help manage perceptions are mindfulness, spirituality, finding purpose and meaning, visualization and self-talk, gratitude, and managing our environment. Let's consider mindfulness as an example.

mindfulness
a way of paying attention, perceiving things as they truly are, and living in the moment

mindfulness, at its core, is a way of paying attention, perceiving things as they truly are, and living in the moment. Being mindful enables us to recognize habitual, often unconscious, emotional and physiological reactions to everyday events. Considering the role of perception on stress, it is easy to see how mindfulness can help accurately interpret and initiate an appropriate stress response.

Although mindfulness stems from Buddhist tradition, it is not a religious concept nor is it affiliated with any religious, cultural, or belief system. It is secular in nature; however, mindfulness practice has been shown to foster a sense of purpose and meaning and feelings of being grounded and connected with one's own spirituality. It is not uncommon for companies, hospitals, and community centers to provide mindfulness instruction to their employees, patients, or residents as a way of helping them succeed, reduce stress, cope with mental illness, or deal with chronic pain.

Mindfulness is a way of thinking and a skill that takes time and practice to learn. It can be practiced in a number of ways but is most often taught through meditation. One of the most frequently cited contemporary authorities on mindfulness is Jon Kabat-Zinn, professor of medicine at the University of Massachusetts Medical School. Kabat-Zinn developed an eight-week meditation-based training called the Mindfulness-Based Stress Reduction (MBSR). MBSR has demonstrated benefits for a wide range of emotional and physical issues, including stress, anxiety, depression (Goldin & Gross, 2010), and psychological distress in people with chronic somatic diseases (Bohlmeijer, Prenger, Taal, & Cuijpers, 2010). Mindfulness is a useful strategy to help react to stress appropriately, cope for the short and long term, and develop resiliency.

Opportunity 2

Shortly after the stress response occurs, we have a second opportunity to cope. The act of breathing is a simple yet powerful way to bring about a parasympathetic relaxation response that stops the flow of stress hormones, calms us, and returns our body to equilibrium. Deep breathing is a common technique used, but just about any type of breathing will work. All relaxation techniques as well as meditation have breathing as a core component. Imagery, progressive muscle relaxation, meditation, touch and massage, and anchoring are also effective ways to produce calm when under stress.

People who first try meditation or other stress management techniques often leave with the attitude that the relaxation exercise was quieting but they have a limited sense of its benefits. That is because starting a formal relaxation routine in many ways is similar to starting a formal exercise routine, and similar to exercise, it takes time for the benefits to become apparent. If you were asked to describe what it felt like after your first day of strength training, you would probably say "sore"; if asked again after six weeks, you would probably say that your muscles feel tighter and stronger; and if asked after six months, you would probably notice other people admiring your new look and say that strength training is a routine that you can't live without. The same is true with any formal relaxation routine; at first it may seem only vaguely helpful, but as you progress you will begin to experience its benefits and at some point you will begin to rely on them and it will become an activity that you can't live without.

There are many relaxation activities to choose from and all include or are enhanced by breathing; however, all relaxation techniques also have characteristics that are unique. Visualization and anchoring are two examples that illustrate how different techniques can be used to manage stress.

Visualization serves three purposes: (1) to bring calm to a stressful situation, (2) to support behavior change by enabling opportunities to experience the benefits of the desired change through imagining their benefits, and (3) to provide an opportunity to mentally rehearse and prepare for a potentially stressful situation. Visualization has been used extensively among athletes to help them practice desired standards of performance and think through potential stressful situations before they happen. In this way, visualization enables athletes to think through and rehearse their game plan and plan ahead of time for any stressful situation that might occur so they will be able to maintain perspective and keep stress at optimal levels when under the pressure of a big game. Considering its purposes, it is easy to see the many uses of visualization in day-to-day life.

Anchoring, which is different from visualization, is a tactic that helps prepare in advance for stress. An anchor is a physical or mental cue (e.g., touching our thumb and forefinger together, imagining our favorite beach) that stimulates a desirable conditioned response. For example, if we use a physical cue such as touching our thumb and forefinger whenever we are in a relaxed state, this conditions our body to associate the touching of our finger to our thumb with the state of relaxation. Practice this enough and it becomes a conditioned response that can be used to trigger relaxation whenever a stressful situation arises.

Opportunity 3

Exercise is one of *the* most helpful stress management techniques. To understand why, recall the stress physiology section of this chapter, and in particular the bottom of figure 7.1. Physical action, such as exercise, is one way of following through on the fight-or-flight response. By using major muscle groups during exercise, our body metabolizes excess blood sugar, fats, and stress hormones (adrenalin and cortisol), and with the hormones gone, our body can return to homeostasis. Not only does exercise help with the stress of the moment, but it is believed that regular exercise over time reduces the amount of adrenalin and cortisol released during other stressful times (Olpin & Hesson, 2010) and may weaken neural mechanisms involved in the stress response resulting in lower sympathetic nervous system activity in response to perceived stress (Kelley, 2009).

There is much evidence on the positive and lasting relationship between exercise and emotional health for the mentally healthy as well as psychiatric populations. For example, a number of studies have demonstrated a positive relationship between exercise and mental health in people with emotional and mental health issues that range from hostility and drug and alcohol abuse to clinical depression and schizophrenia (Daley, 2002).

Exercise has long been known to improve mood and reduce anxiety. It increases daily energy levels, boosts self-confidence, and creates a sense of accomplishment. Brain chemicals such as endorphins and serotonin are released during exercise and produce a feeling of euphoria sometimes called a "runners' high." These uplifting feelings can last for hours after the exercise is completed. All types of exercise can contribute to emotional and mental health, and activities such as yoga, tai chi, and qi gong can bring additional coping benefits, such as breathing work, being grounded, and maintaining perspective.

Opportunity 4

Music, art, and writing are each considered expressive coping strategies that are available to help manage stress and build resilience over time. Other examples of expressive therapies are drama, photography, dance, drumming, and play. These activities cater to a greater variety of communication styles, for example, verbal, visual, tactile, and so on, and provide supportive ways to communicate effectively and authentically. Expressive strategies help individuals quickly communicate relevant issues in ways that talk cannot accomplish. Expressive strategies can be particularly helpful for people with limited language skills, such as children, trauma victims, or older persons who may have suffered a stroke or are dealing with dementia. Each expressive strategy has its own unique properties and can play a variety of roles in sustaining emotional health and building resilience.

Music as a coping strategy can be as simple as a change in your emotional state by listening to uplifting music when feeling depressed. Music is routinely used by companies to achieve desired emotional effects or to sell products. Consider the use of "elevator music" as a way to calm clients who are waiting to be seen by a physician, rock and roll to excite players and fans at a professional sporting event, or jazz at a night club to portend romance. According to the American Music Therapy Association (2005), music can also effect positive changes in psychological, physical, cognitive, and social functioning, and it has the ability to break down strong emotional defenses and enable the expression of feelings. Not only is listening to music helpful, but also creating, singing, and moving to music can be therapeutic.

Art therapy, according to the American Art Therapy Association (2008), is the use of art media, the creative process, and the resulting artwork to help people explore and express feelings, deal with emotions, gain self-awareness, improve self-esteem, and reduce stress, fear, and anxiety. In some cases, such as with children, difficult emotions and information about stressful or traumatic events can be more easily expressed through drawings than through conversation. Art can also inspire a sense of freedom and personal well-being.

Writing is another expressive therapy that helps us understand and communicate perceptions, make reasoned interpretations, and consider appropriate responses. It can take many forms, such as journaling, poetry, letter writing, and blogging. Expressive writing provides opportunities to express and release emotions, make sense of stressful events, and process their meanings. If shared, writing can facilitate social support and enable opportunities to receive feedback and advice.

Only a few of the many available healthy coping strategies have been touched on here. Unfortunately, poor coping is all too common in response to stress. Overeating, using tobacco products, or consuming alcohol are unhealthy and counterproductive and can lead to a cycle of unresolved stress and a wide range of lifestyle illnesses. Thus, it is important to make healthy lifestyle choices and maintain a variety of healthy coping strategies.

Stress at Work

Stress is bad for business and it places workers at alarming levels of risk. A review of the literature completed by the American Psychological Association (2009) suggests an estimated fourteen million working days are lost to stress, depression, and anxiety in the United States each year at a cost to business and industry of more than $300 billion. Research shows that health care expenditures for employees with high stress are 47% higher than for those employees with low stress (Goetzel et al., 1998). Conversely, as organizations reduce stress they also reduce the associated costs; and as data suggests, their companies will also outperform their competitors (Brown, 2006), their workers will suffer fewer sick days, and they will become more productive and more engaged.

Demand and Control

The work of Karasek (1979) and later Karasek and Theorell (1990) has led to a deeper understanding of what factors play the greatest role in job stress.

Their work looked specifically at the relationships between psychological demands of any given job and the amount of control one has in his or her position. When looking at the demand-control relationship, it is somewhat surprising to learn that control is a greater predictor of job stress than demand is. As one might expect, the combination of high job demands coupled with low decision-making authority can place any job among the most stressful; however, because control is the variable that is most predictive of stress, the least stressful and often most satisfying jobs can be those that are among the most demanding (see figure 7.6).

When people have ownership in their work, they gain a sense of meaning, purpose, and control. Meaning and purpose will not only make a worker more productive and creative (Whyte, 1994) but also it will lower stress and provide greater personal satisfaction. Finding meaning in your work will increase control and confidence and will lead to a more creative, productive, and fulfilling work life (Loy, 2001).

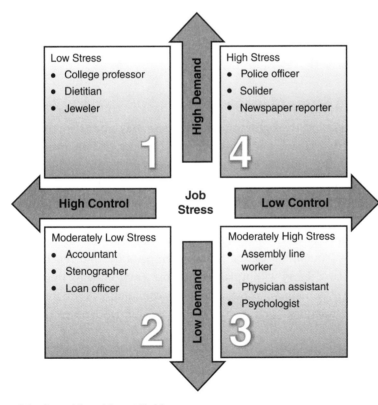

Figure 7.6 Demand-Control Support Model
Source: de Lange, Taris, Kompier, Houtman, and Bongers (2003, p. 282).

This concept is described in a story that is common among corporate culture experts.

A STORY ABOUT VISION, MEANING, AND LOW STRESS

A manager came upon three of his workers who were each busy breaking large pieces of granite, so he stopped to ask them, "What are you doing?" The first one sarcastically replied, "What does it look like I'm doing? I'm trying to break this granite." The second worker said, "I'm breaking granite so it can be chiseled to be sold as a corner stone." The third worker enthusiastically responded, "I'm part of a team of people who are building a beautiful cathedral."

This story illustrates the importance that having clear vision and purpose has on worker satisfaction and stress. Taking into account the importance of perceived control on stress, one could predict that stress levels became lower as the vision of their work became more meaningful.

Understanding the demand-control relationship provides insights that health promotion professionals can rely on when designing strategies that help workers see purpose and meaning in their jobs and when providing more decision-making authority, greater flexibility, and greater control at the work site.

Work Site Stress Management

work site stress management
a work site program designed to (1) create a healthier workplace and (2) build the capacity of employees to cope with stress through targeted stress management programs

The primary objectives of **work site stress management** are to (1) create a healthier workplace and (2) build the capacity of employees to cope with stress through targeted stress management programs (Girdano, Everly, & Dusek, 2001).Workplace stressors can come from the physical and social work environment, organizational policies, and from workers themselves.

The most obvious work environment stressors are noise, lighting, ergonomics (equipment design factors), temperature, and repetitive tasks. Other stressors found within particular work environments might include those caused by the psychosocial work environment or those found within specific job functions, such as the demands of shift work or excessive travel requirements.

There is broad recognition that the psychosocial environment at work can have profound emotional impact on people, individually and collectively. The National Institutes of Occupational Health and Safety (Howard, 2007) lists the following work environment factors that affect physical and mental health as well as organizational outcomes, such as work performance and effectiveness:

- Racism and racial and ethnic prejudice
- Sexism and sexual harassment
- Gender and racial discrimination
- Work-family integration and balance
- Support for diversity in the workplace and workforce

Organizational policies can also contribute to a stressful workplace (Greenberg, 2009). Wages, advancement opportunities, and career guidance will each play a role in job satisfaction and employee self-image and confidence levels. For example, employees who are in positions in which they are appropriately challenged and have opportunities to develop new skills and advance within their companies are far less stressed than those in companies with few advancement opportunities. Conversely, work that is above individual capacities through overspecialization, excessive time pressures, and job or decision-making complexity will cause stress. It is important to note that it is not only work that is too difficult that can be stressful. Low demand or meaningless work can also lead to boredom, low job satisfaction, and stress.

Employees who are better informed are more satisfied, feel more involved in the company, and ultimately contribute more to its success. In particular, communication that reveals shared values and reflects common commitments to organizational goals enables coworkers to forge and sustain productive relationships in organizations (Herriot, 2002).

Companies in which internal communication is a priority are more likely to have motivated employees who are focused on company goals, resolve conflicts, and improve employee productivity. The best workplace communication is open and honest and values ethics, transparency, and accountability (Proctor & Doukakis 2003). Among many functions of corporate communication are listening, information sharing, decision making, influencing, coordinating, and motivating (Cheney, Christensen, Zorn, & Ganesh, 2004). Job satisfaction is higher when supervisors are open and honest with their employees, share information, convey both good and bad news, evaluate job performance regularly, create a supportive climate, solicit input, and make appropriate disclosures.

Having clear policies, procedures, work objectives, job descriptions, and expectations are also essential characteristics of work site communication that affect employee stress. Too much bureaucracy, commonly called "red tape" because of its complex and seemingly arbitrary rules, can stifle employee creativity and lead to frustration, dissatisfaction, and stress.

Newer-generation employees tend to value flexible career paths more than past generations because their priority is work-life balance (Carless & Wintle, 2007). Furthermore, they tend to value relationships in the workplace, which can also be influenced by corporate and personal communication (Jablin & Krone, 1994). As self-managed work teams become commonplace in organizations, communication among and between employees becomes more important than ever before. New communication technologies (e.g., social networks, Twitter, blogs, photo sharing, and writing communities) show great promise for helping employers manage changing work environments and enhance internal communication.

Mental Health in Communities

Health statistics clearly show that mental health is one of our most pressing community health issues. For many healthy Americans, exposure to stressful lifestyles represents an increased risk of mental illness (McKenzie, Pinger, & Kotecki, 2005). Mental disorders are common throughout the United States and according to the National Institute of Mental Health (NIMH) affect tens of millions of people each year. What is most notable about NIMH data is that only a fraction of those affected by mental illness receive treatment.

The social costs of mental illness are staggering. The latest data available from the Centers for Disease Control and Prevention (2012) indicates a steady rise in US suicide deaths each year since 2000, with 38,364 suicide deaths reported in 2010. The 2010 figure, approximately 12.4 suicides per one hundred thousand people, places suicide as the tenth leading cause of death in the United States. A look at the most prescribed medications by drug class is another indicator of mental health in the United States. The Institute for Health Care Informatics reports antidepressants as the fastest growing class of prescription drugs in 2010, and second in overall sales behind lipid regulators with 253.6 million prescriptions filled. Perhaps the most disappointing observation that can be made about community mental health is that the United States still does not have an adequate mental health program.

Stress, as a contributor to mental health problems, is likely to remain important as life becomes increasingly complex. Even Americans who believe they have good mental health carry out their everyday activities under considerable stress (McKenzie, Pinger, & Kotecki, 2005). Although there will be opportunities for community health promotion professionals to affect stress and mental health in community populations through programming directly, much of the work will be directed toward referral and mental health policy change.

Patient Protection and Affordable Care Act (ACA)

Mental health policy has seen recent progress, especially in mental health parity laws that are part of the Patient Protection and Affordable Care Act (ACA) and are designed to stop insurers from arbitrarily limiting care for mental health disorders. Several other provisions of the act related to mental health are to (1) include mental health disorders in a set of health care service categories that must be covered by certain insurance plans as "essential services," including those offered through the exchanges and Medicaid; (2) allow people who are underinsured due to preexisting mental health conditions access to a new preexisting condition insurance plan; (3) prohibit insurers from denying coverage of mental illness as a preexisting condition or to use mental health conditions to raise premiums; and (4) require private plans to continue coverage for dependents until they turn twenty-six years old (Hyde, 2010).

Although care and support for people with mental illness have improved, the availability of such care and services is nowhere near complete. Significant challenges must be met before the goal of universally accessible, supportive services in the area of mental health can be met.

Meeting Community Mental Health Needs

Health promotion professionals play an important role in creating and advocating for community health policy at local, state, and national levels. When thoughtfully conceived, mental health policy improves the coordination of essential prevention and treatment services to ensure care is delivered to people in need while improving continuity and eliminating redundancies in the health system. Any community mental health plan must start with predetermined goals, objectives, and outcome measures and must be designed using evidence-based strategies. It should clarify the roles of multiple stakeholders in implementing the activities of the plan.

The World Health Organization (2010) section on mental health policy planning and service development suggests an optimal mix of mental health services and that most mental health care can be self-managed or managed informally through community mental health services; in doing so, health care costs could be greatly reduced (see figure 7.7).

Prevention is more cost effective and humane than treatment; thus, it must be the first goal of any community mental health promotion strategy.

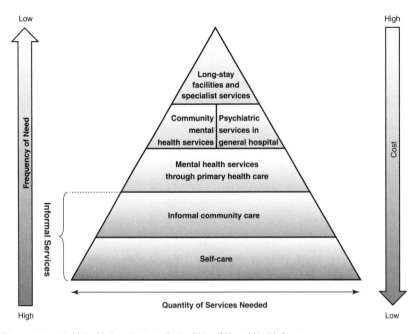

Figure 7.7   World Health Organization's Optimal Mix of Mental Health Services

Source: Department of Mental Health and Substance Abuse (2007).

There are many examples of preventive mental health programming in community settings (e.g., grief support groups, suicide prevention training, depression education) that are designed to address mental health issues before they manifest as mental health problems. For example, grief support groups are generally designed to normalize the grief experience and provide support and teach coping strategies that will protect participants from mental health issues, such as depression or prolonged grief disorder. Prevention programs for children that teach resilience are particularly beneficial, for example, art, music, poetry, martial arts, or dance focused on the expression of emotions, coping, healing, and community building (Mental Health Services Oversight and Accountability Commission, 2011).

Mental health treatment refers to the provision of systematic mental health intervention, support, and assistance for those already affected by a mental health issue. Treatment services provide appropriate medical, psychiatric, psychopharmacologic, and emotional support to those affected. Psychotherapy, cognitive behavioral therapy, assertive community treatment, supportive housing, self-help groups, support groups, and peer support services are all examples of treatment options for mental health issues. Assertive community treatment, for example, is an intense, integrated approach for community mental health service in which severely mentally ill recipients receive multidisciplinary round-the-clock staffing of a psychiatric team (e.g., psychiatry, social work, nursing, substance abuse, and vocational rehabilitation), but within the comfort of their own home and community.

It is important that any prevention- or treatment-based approach implement evidence-based practices. The term *evidence-based practice* refers to interventions for which there is consistent scientific evidence showing improved client outcomes. Standard guidelines, training materials, and toolkits can be designed using evidence-based practice to ensure consistent implementation practices and improve client outcomes (Drake et al., 2001). Guidelines are also available from organizations such as the American Psychiatric Association and other advocacy groups that are based on a mixture of scientific research and consensus of experts, and although not considered evidence-based in the strict sense, they are useful best practices to follow. Given that mental health resources are limited, people with mental health issues should be able to expect services with demonstrated effectiveness that are delivered competently and consistently.

Mental Health Disparities

Mental health disparities exist in many subpopulations. For example, homelessness and poverty are predictive of mental health, substance abuse, and physical health issues that add to the stress of this population and complicate prevention and treatment efforts. This is particularity problematic because homelessness and poverty are on the rise in the United States. According to a survey released by the US Conference of Mayors, 46.2 million Americans, or 15% of the population, are currently living in poverty, and on any given night, the number of homeless people is more than 633,000.

Older adults also have specific mental health issues, the most common being anxiety disorders (e.g., generalize anxiety and panic disorders), severe cognitive impairment (e.g., Alzheimer's disease), mood disorders (e.g., depression and bipolar disorder), and dementia. Nearly 60 percent of nursing home residents have Alzheimer's or another dementia (Alzheimer's Association, 2014).

According to the US Administration on Aging, the number of people sixty-five years or older is nearing forty million and is expected to grow to approximately seventy-two million by 2030, making up 20% of the population.

Lesbian, gay, bisexual, and transgender (LGBT) people experience mental illnesses. However, it is important to be aware of unique mental health risks that LGBT people may face. Research suggests that LGBT people are at higher risk for depression, anxiety, and substance use disorders

(Omoto & Kurtzman, 2006). The reason for these disparities is most likely related to societal stigma and resulting prejudice and discrimination that LGBT people often face.

Although each cultural group is unique in regards to mental health, in general, racial and ethnic minorities are shown to have equal or better mental health than white Americans, yet they suffer from disparities in mental health care (Jackson, Knight, & Rafferty, 2010). These disparities are the result of a general lack of attention to the mental health needs of minorities, cost of care, fragmented services, and insufficient cultural and language-appropriate mental health care in racial and ethnic minority communities (US Department of Health and Human Services, 2001).

Differences also exist in the types of stressors that various racial and ethnic groups experience. Considering the multitude of issues that still confront members of various racial and ethnic groups (hate crimes, fewer educational and employment opportunities, earning less pay for the same work, higher mortality and illness rates, lower access to health care, and feelings of isolation), it is clear that being of minority status can be a source of a great deal of stress (Payne, Hahn, & Lucas, 2009).

There are many examples of innovative approaches to mental health care that can help reach underserved groups, for example, stigma and discrimination programs, free transportation services, telemedicine, and at-home care, and outreach, transition centers, one-on-one support, and peer mentoring programs may be particularly helpful (Mental Health Services Oversight and Accountability Commission, 2011). Other innovative approaches to mental health must focus on increasing the quality and outcomes of services, promoting community collaboration, and reducing stigma and discrimination.

Health promotion professionals must understand mental health in a wide variety of subpopulations, consider the reasons that disparities exist, and develop strategies for addressing those disparities. Improved access, quality of care, better mental health education, and a more diverse mental health workforce would go a long way toward eliminating mental health disparities.

Stress Management with Children

Stress is often considered an adult-only issue. After all, what worries could a child possibly have? Children can be seen as happy, carefree, and worry free—and to a large extent, that perception is accurate. In most cases, children are loved, cared for, and protected from many of life's troubles. However, research tells us that children have their own set of day-to-day stressors that can have detrimental effects on their behaviors, moods, and overall health (Loy, 2010). In addition, many children can and do encounter changes or traumas that are extremely stressful, even by adult standards. Childhood stressors may be different from those encountered by adults, but they are no less detrimental. One reason that managing stress can be difficult for children is that the development of complex social and emotional understanding does not happen until about the age of ten, thus children often have difficulty putting stress into perspective, identifying and communicating emotions, and seeking appropriate support.

Effects of Stress on Children

A child's age, personality, and coping skills affect how he or she will deal with stress and react to it (Elkind, 2001). The type of stress, how long it lasts, and how intense it is will determine how taxing it is. Some research suggests that stress in children has a synergistic rather than a cumulative effect, multiplying the negative effects of stress by as much as four times with each added stressor present in a child's life (Brenner, 1997).

Among the first indicators of stress in children are changes in behavior such as fighting, teasing, or increased hostility toward siblings, family, or peers. Parents and teachers may notice communication problems, decreased concentration, compulsiveness, or sadness. Some children become easily tearful, whiny, anxious, demanding, fearful, and nervous. Physical symptoms may include complaints of upset stomach, headache, sore throat, or vomiting. Unusual physical behaviors such as fidgeting, stuttering, tremors, or shaking legs may arise from stress. When under stress, some older children revert to behaviors characteristic of younger children, such as baby talk, thumb-sucking, nose picking, or wetting themselves. Stressed children may bite their nails or bite, twirl, pull, or suck their hair.

There are also long-term physical and emotional consequences of mismanaged stress among children. Stress can impair a child's self-image, self-confidence, self-esteem, academic performance, and social skills. Childhood stress can increase long-term social anxiety and insecurity, and it can contribute to substance abuse, suicidal ideation, and suicide. Unidentified and untreated stress in children contributes to physical problems ranging from lowered immune function and migraine headaches to obesity, type 2 diabetes, respiratory tract illness, asthma, and several psychiatric disorders, including depression, anxiety, chronic posttraumatic stress disorder, and developmental physical and emotional delays (Loy, 2010). Some evidence suggests that many long-term consequences persist well into adulthood

(Middlebrooks & Audage, 2008) and can manifest in a range of adult emotional and physical problems such as insecurity, low self-confidence, social anxieties, substance abuse, and depression. Stress can influence everything from physical health and memory to social competence, marital success, and academic and socioeconomic attainment.

Children can appear outwardly resilient to the immediate effects of stress but, if the timing of the stress is during a critical period of personality development, they can carry the long-term effects with them for the rest of their lives. Many studies link trauma and chronic stress with poor physical and mental health over the long term (Brenner, 1997).

Stress Types among Children

In many cases, the same things that stress adults stress children; however, because levels of stress are influenced so strongly by one's perception, and because children often perceive circumstances differently than adults do, their stressors can be unique.

Childhood stressors can be placed along a continuum beginning with normal day-to-day situations, such as keeping up with an overloaded activity calendar; mid-range stressful situations, which are usually related to change and insecurity, such as a family move or a divorce; and those highly stressful, traumatic, and chronic stressors at the far end of the continuum that are difficult to handle, such as neglect or a death in the family.

Over half of all stressors described by children come from day-to-day occurrences at home or at school (Humphrey, 2004), such as time demands, parent or school expectations, social pressures, separation from parents, and punishments. Children who have siblings often report conflicts and rivalries with siblings as frequent stressors. Stressors related to change and insecurity, although somewhat common, rank higher on the severity of stress continuum. They include divorce or family discord, remarriage, moving, decline in family income, parent alcoholism, deployment, arrival of a new sibling, and hospitalization. Most children must deal with one or more of this type of stressor sometime during childhood.

Moderate change-related stressors can tax the individual resources of a child. At the pinnacle of the severity of the stress continuum lie traumatic and chronic stressors. They are serious, unexpected, and uncommon events, such as witnessing a death or experiencing the death of a family member. Emotional or sexual abuse, abandonment, natural disasters, and exploitation are examples of traumatic stress, as are neglect, poverty, or a major long-term illness (Courtois, 2008). All types of trauma pose serious risks to children in their youth and in later life; in most cases they require skillful, professional support.

During formative years, children must deal with a multitude of stressors. Most are common and short term, resulting in little more than short-lived poor behavior or a disagreeable mood and requiring only basic personal stress management skills and minimal support. Some stressors, especially when change and insecurity are involved, can be more taxing. If not dealt with properly, usually with the help of a skillful adult, these moderately stressful situations can lead to serious short- and long-term behavioral, emotional, or physical consequences. A few stressors involve traumas or chronic stressors that pose serious risks to children; in most cases, they just require skillful, professional support.

In any case, health promotion professionals and all adults who work with children should learn about childhood stress and be able to recognize the signs of stress in children, provide support to children when needed, and help children learn to manage stress for themselves.

Summary

The more we learn about mental health issues and stress, in particular, the more insight we will have into the factors that influence mental health. With this in mind, there are four areas that health promotion professionals must be able to address. Health promotion professionals must (1) understand the nature and origins of mental health-related issues and know how to respond appropriately; (2) empower individuals and communities, increasing personal control over decisions that affect mental health; (3) provide evidence-based best practices to ensure high-quality, consistent prevention, care, and treatment; and (4) assist in the coordination of services that enable individuals, families, groups, organizations, and communities to play active roles in achieving, protecting, and sustaining health.

KEY TERMS

1. **Emotional health:** our ability to attend to our own emotional needs and the skill with which we are able to deal with everyday life

2. **Fight-or-flight response:** a human body's physiological response to stress; the response produces the energy needed to either fight back against a stressor or to flee from it

3. **Autonomic nervous system (ANS):** the part of the peripheral nervous system that regulates involuntary bodily functions such as heart rate and respiration

4. **Endocrine system:** a system of glands responsible for secreting hormones into the bloodstream

5. **Immune system:** a system of biological structures responsible for protecting the human body from infectious external agents such as bacteria and viruses and against the body's own disease-causing agents

6. **Eustress:** "good" stress; stress that can be beneficial to the experiencer

7. **Distress:** "bad" stress; stress that can be harmful to the experiencer, especially in excess amounts

8. **General adaptation syndrome (GAS):** the physical response to a stressor involving three stages: alarm, resistance, and exhaustion

9. **Mindfulness:** a way of paying attention, perceiving things as they truly are, and living in the moment

10. **Work site stress management:** a work site program designed to (1) create a healthier workplace and (2) build the capacity of employees to cope with stress through targeted stress management programs

REVIEW QUESTIONS

1. How would you describe the stress response?

2. How is stress linked to chronic disease?

3. How would you describe stress physiology and the three systems it affects in the body?

4. What is the difference between eustress and distress?

5. What is a coping opportunity? Identify four opportunities.

6. How would you describe mental health disparities?

7. How would you describe what organizations are doing to help employees manage stress?

8. What are policies within the ACA that will improve mental health?

9. How would you describe the community mental health promotion strategy?

10. How would you describe the issues specifically affecting children's mental health?

STUDENT ACTIVITIES

1. Prepare a twenty-minute talk to consumers on the physiology of stress.

2. Using the PRECEDE-PROCEED model of program planning, outline a process for creating a stress management program for a department on a college campus.

3. Identify the different populations in a school. Identify potential stressors for each group and describe one stress management technique that could be used to address the stressors.

4. Identify statistics that support the rising levels of stress.

References

Alzheimer's Association. (2014). *Special care units.* Retrieved from http://www.alz .org

American Art Therapy Association. (2008). http://www.arttherapy.org/

American Music Therapy Association. (2005). *Definition and quotes about music therapy.* Retrieved from www.musictherapy.org/about/quotes

American Psychological Association. (2009). *Stress in America 2009.* Washington, DC: American Psychological Association.

Blonna, R. (2005). The physical basis of stress. *Coping with stress in a changing world* (3rd ed., p. 117). New York: McGraw-Hill.

Bohlmeijer, E., Prenger, R., Taal, E., & Cuijpers, P. (2010). The effects of mindfulness-based stress reduction therapy on mental health of adults with a chronic medical disease: A meta-analysis. *Journal of Psychosomatic Research, 68*(6), 539–544.

Brenner, A. (1997). *Helping children cope with stress.* San Francisco: Jossey-Bass.

Brown, P. B. (2006, September 2). Listen up. Know your audience. *New York Times.* Retrieved from http://www.nytimes.com/2006/09/02/business/02offline.html ?_r=1&

Carless, S. A., & Wintle, J. (2007). Applicant attraction: The role of recruiter function, work-life balance policies and career salience. *International Journal of Selection and Assessment, 15*, 394–404.

Centers for Disease Control and Prevention. (2012). *Suicide: Facts at a glance.* Atlanta: Centers for Disease Control and Prevention, National Center for Injury Prevention and Control, Division of Violence Prevention.

Cheney, G., Christensen, L. T., Zorn, T. E., & Ganesh Jr., S. (2004). *Organizational communication in an age of globalization: Issues, reflections and practices.* Prospect Heights, IL: Waveland Press.

Cohen, S., Janicki-Deverts, D., & Miller, G. E. (2007). Psychological stress and disease. *Journal of the American Medical Association, 298*(14), 1685–1687.

Courtois, C. A. (2008). Complex trauma, complex reactions: Assessment and treatment. *Psychological Trauma: Theory, Research, Practice, and Policy, 1* (S), 86–100.

Daley, A. J. (2002) Exercise therapy and mental health in clinical populations: Is exercise therapy a worthwhile intervention? *Advances in Psychiatric Treatment, 8*, 262–270.

de Lange, A. H., Taris, T. W., Kompier, M. A., Houtman, I. L., & Bongers, P. M. (2003). "The very best of the millennium": Longitudinal research and the demand-control-(support) model. *Journal of Occupational Health Psychology, 8*(4), 282–305.

Department of Mental Health and Substance Abuse. (2007). *The optimal mix of services for mental health.* Geneva: World Health Organization.

Dhabhar, F. S. (2009). Enhancing versus suppressive effects of stress on immune function: Implications for immunoprotection and immunopathology. *Neuroimmunomodulation, 16*(5), 300–317.

Drake, R. E., Goldman, H. H., Leff, S., Lehman, A. F., Dixon, L., Mueser, K. T., & Torrey, W. C. (2001). *Psychiatric Services.* doi: 10.1176/appi.ps.52.2.179

Elkind, D. (2001). *The hurried child growing up too fast too soon* (3rd ed.). Cambridge, MA: Perseus Publishing.

Girdano, D., Everly Jr., G. S., & Dusek, D. (2001). *Controlling stress and tension: A holistic approach* (6th ed.). Boston: Allyn & Bacon.

Goetzel, R. Z., Anderson, D. R., Whitmer, R. W., Ozminkowski, R. J., Dunn, R. L., Wasserman, J., & The Health Enhancement Research Organization (HERO) Research Committee. (1998). The relationship between modifiable health risks and health care expenditures: An analysis of the multi-employer HERO health risk and cost database. *Journal of Occupational and Environmental Medicine, 40* (10), 843–854.

Goldin, P. R., & Gross, J. J. (2010). Effects of mindfulness-based stress reduction (MBSR) on emotion regulation in social anxiety disorder. *Emotion, 10*, 83–91.

Greenberg, J. (2009). *Occupational stress comprehensive stress management* (11th ed., pp. 310–343). New York: McGraw-Hill.

Herriot, P. (2002). Selection and self: Selection as a social process. *European Journal of Work and Organizational Psychology, 11*, 385–402. doi: 10.1080/135943 20244000256

Hesson, O. (2010). The science of stress. *Stress management for life* (2nd ed., p. 34). Clifton Park, NY: Cengage Learning.

Holmes, T. H., & Rahe, R. H. (1967). The social readjustment rating scale. *Journal of Psychosomatic Research, 11*(2), 213–218.

Howard, J. (2007). Foreword. In M. A. Bond, A. Kalaja, P. Markkanen, D. Cazeca, S. Daniel, L. Tsurikova, & L. Punnett (Eds.), *Expanding our understanding of the psychosocial work environment: A compendium of measures, discrimination, harassment and work-family issues* (p. 3). Washington, DC: Department of Health and Human Services.

Humphrey, J. H. (2004). *Childhood stress in contemporary society* (11th ed.). Binghamton, NY: Haworth Press.

Hyde, P. S. (2010, August 19). *The Affordable Care Act & mental health: An update* [Blog]. Retrieved from www.healthcare.gov/blog/2010/08/mentalhealthupdate .html

Jablin, F. M., & Krone, K. J. (1994). Task/work relationships: A life-span perspective. In M. L. Knapp & G. R. Miller (Eds.), *Handbook of interpersonal communication*. Thousand Oaks, CA: Sage.

Jackson, J. S., Knight, K. M., & Rafferty, J. A. (2010). Race and unhealthy behaviors: Chronic stress, the HPA axis, and physical and mental health disparities over the life course. *American Journal of Public Health, 100*(5), 933–939.

Karasek, R. A. (1979). Job demands, job decisions latitude, and mental strain: Implications for job redesign. *Administrative Science Quarterly, 24*(2), 285–308.

Karasek, R. A., & Theorell, T. (1990). *Healthy work: Stress, productivity, and the reconstruction of working life*. New York: Basic Books.

Kelley, D. (2009). The effects of exercise and diet on stress. *Nutritional Perspectives: Journal of the Council on Nutrition, 32*(1), 37–39.

Loy, M. (2001). Combining heart and work: A prescription for a stress-free career. *The Communication Connection, 15*(3), 5–7.

Loy, M. (2010). *Children and stress: A handbook for parents, teachers, and therapists*. Duluth, MN: Whole Person Associates.

McKenzie, J. F., Pinger, R. R., & Kotecki, J. E. (2005). *An introduction to community health* (5th ed.). Sudbury, MA: Jones & Bartlett.

Mental Health Services Oversight and Accountability Commission. (2011). *Prevention and early intervention: Trends report 2011*. Sacramento, CA: Mental Health Services Oversight and Accountability Commission.

Middlebrooks, J. S., & Audage, N. C. (2008). *The effects of childhood stress on health across the lifespan*. Atlanta: Centers for Disease Control and Prevention, National Center for Injury Prevention and Control.

National Alliance on Mental Illness. (2013). *Mental illness: Facts and numbers*. Arlington, VA: National Alliance on Mental Illness.

Olpin, M., & Hesson, M. (2010). *Stress management for life: A research-based, experiential approach* (2nd ed.). Belmont, CA: Wadsworth, Cengage Learning.

Omoto, A. M., & Kurtzman, H. S. (2006). *Sexual orientation and mental health: Examining identity and development in lesbian, gay and bisexual people*. Washington, DC: APA Books.

Payne, W. A., Hahn, D. B., & Lucas, E. B. (2009). *Understanding your health* (9th ed.). Columbus, OH: McGraw-Hill.

Proctor, T., & Doukakis, I. (2003). Change management: The role of internal communication and employee development. *Corporate Communications, 8*(4), 268–277. doi: 10.1108/13563280310506430

Seaward, B. L. (2004). The physiology of stress. *Managing stress* (4th ed., p. 38). Sudbury, MA: Jones & Bartlett.

Seaward, B. L. (2011). *Managing stress: Principles and strategies for health and well-being.* Sudbury, MA: Jones & Bartlett.

Selye, H. (1956). *The stress of life* (Vol. 5). New York: McGraw-Hill.

Taylor, S. E., Klein, L. C., Lewis, B. P., Gruenewald, T. L., Gurung, R.A.R., & Updegraff, J. A. (2000). Biobehavioral responses to stress in females: Tend-and-befriend, not fight-or-flight. *Psychological Review, 107*(3), 411–429.

US, Department of Health and Human Services. (2001). *Mental health: Culture, race, and ethnicity.* Rockville, MD: US Department of Health and Human Services, Substance Abuse and Mental Health Services Administration, Center for Mental Health Services.

Whyte, D. (1994). *The heart aroused: Poetry and the preservation of the soul in corporate America.* New York: Currency and Doubleday.

World Health Organization. (2010). *Mental health and development: Targeting people with mental health conditions as a vulnerable group.* Geneva: WHO Press.

Yerkes, R. M., & Dodson, J. D. (1908). The relation of strength of stimulus to rapidity of habit-formation. *Journal of Comparative Neurology and Psychology, 18,* 459–482.

CHAPTER 8

CLINICAL PREVENTIVE SERVICES

Trends, Access, Promotion, and Guidelines

Casey Korba

It is empowering to realize that we have tremendous control over our health. What we eat; how often we exercise; our sleep habits, social habits, and coping mechanisms; and our use of preventive clinical services all influence our chances of developing certain illnesses and conditions. Although genetics plays a role, and not every health risk can be avoided, we can reduce our chances of developing many debilitating health conditions and contracting certain diseases while improving our overall health prognosis when we develop healthy habits and behaviors.

Through screening and other clinical preventive services that individuals receive at their primary care doctor's office, at their local pharmacy, or increasingly, at a work site or community-based health fair, individuals can detect certain conditions while they are asymptomatic, often leading to improved health outcomes (see table 8.1). Complications from chronic conditions and diseases such as cardiovascular disease and related risk factors, type 2 diabetes, certain types of cancer, and certain infectious diseases can be prevented by following evidence-based recommendations for specific preventive services based on age and gender.

Research demonstrates linkages between certain unhealthy behaviors, such as tobacco use, a sedentary lifestyle, and a high-fat, high-calorie diet, with chronic health conditions, which include heart disease, type 2 diabetes, and certain cancers. Changing or controlling these unhealthy behaviors can improve health outcomes.

LEARNING OBJECTIVES

After reading this chapter, the student will be able to:

- Define clinical preventive services.

- Describe how clinical preventive services are linked to promoting health.

- Identify aged-related clinical services to chronic disease.

- Describe the barriers and opportunities for accessing clinical preventive services.

- Identify what actions health care companies, communities, and work sites are doing to encourage preventive services.

- Describe how the Affordable Care Act incorporates clinical services into health care.

Table 8.1   Select Preventive Screenings Examinations

Screening Test	What the Test Is For	When It Should Be Conducted[*]

Blood pressure (BP)	High blood pressure
	Desirable blood
	  pressure is < 120/80
		Screening every two years with BP < 120/80
		Screening every year with systolic BP of 120–139 mmHg or diastolic BP
		  of 80–90 mmHg

Blood cholesterol
  level
	High blood cholesterol	For men who are not at increased risk for coronary artery disease, check every five years
		  after the age of thirty-five. For women who are at increased risk for coronary artery
		  disease, check every five years starting at age twenty.

Mammography	Breast cancer	Every two years between the ages of fifty and seventy-four
Colonoscopy	Colon cancer	Beginning at age fifty and continuing until age seventy-five
Height and weight	Overweight and obesity	Annually Clinicians should offer or refer patients with a body mass index (BMI) of 30 kg/m^2 or higher to intensive, multicomponent behavioral interventions.

[*]If no other risk factors are present, such as family history

For example, most risk factors for heart disease and stroke—specifically high blood pressure, high cholesterol, smoking, and obesity—are preventable and controllable. Yet heart disease is currently the number one cause of death in the United States, bringing about approximately six hundred thousand deaths each year in this country (Centers for Disease Control and Prevention, 2013). Controlling high blood pressure, high cholesterol, smoking, and obesity could reduce the risk of heart attack or stroke by more than 80% (US Department of Health and Human Services, 2013).

clinical preventive services

services provided at one's primary care physician's office, local pharmacy, or health fairs to detect and reduce the risk of specific health conditions from progressing; examples include screening tests, immunizations, counseling, and preventive medications

Benefits of Evidence-Based Clinical Preventive Services

Clinical preventive services include screening tests, immunizations, counseling, and preventive medications; many of these services are highly effective at extending and improving health and well-being. Screening tests, through the timely identification of reversible or treatable conditions, can reduce mortality from major chronic diseases by 15% to 30%. Immunization practices have eliminated many infectious diseases and dramatically reduced the rates of others. Effective health behavior counseling can reduce a significant percentage of deaths attributable to tobacco use, physical inactivity, unhealthy diet, and problem drinking (Krist, Rothemich, Kashiri, et al., 2012).

Recommended Levels of Preventive Services

Encouraging the use of certain clinical preventive services will save lives. In 2007, the Partnership for Prevention published a report concluding that one hundred thousand lives could be saved each year through the following actions related to six evidence-based preventive services:

* Increase the percentage of adults taking aspirin daily to prevent heart disease.

* Advise smokers to quit and provide assistance to facilitate quitting.

* Increase the percentage of adults age fifty referred for colorectal cancer screening.

* Increase the percentage of adults receiving the flu shot annually.

* Increase the percentage of adult women regularly screened for breast cancer.

* Increase the percentage of young women screened for chlamydial infection annually.

Patient Protection and Affordable Care Act

The Patient Protection and Affordable Care Act (ACA), otherwise known as the health care reform bill, was enacted in 2010. It includes many new policies and sets the stage for new regulations regarding clinical and community preventive health services that have recently gone into effect or will go into effect in the coming years (www.gpo.gov/fdsys/pkg/BILLS -111hr3590enr/pdf/BILLS-111hr3590enr.pdf).

The ACA included the creation of the National Prevention, Health Promotion, and Public Health Council (National Prevention Council), tasked with developing a national prevention strategy. The goal of the **National Prevention Strategy** is to move the nation from an emphasis on illness and disease to one based on prevention and wellness. The strategy's framework aims to guide the federal government and the nation on the most effective and achievable means for improving the health of the nation through prevention and health promotion policies and programs. The National Prevention Strategy has three cross-cutting priorities, which include a focus on healthy environments, prevention and public health capacity, and clinical preventive services. The National Prevention Strategy's 2011 framework states,

> Many clinical preventive services are effective in reducing death and disability and [are] cost-effective or even cost saving . . . Examples of

National Prevention Strategy guidelines developed as a result of the Affordable Care Act; provides guidance to the federal government and the nation regarding the most effective and achievable means for improving health through prevention and health promotion policies and programs

high impact, quality clinical preventive services recommended by the U.S. Preventive Services Task Force (USPSTF) include screening for tobacco use, high blood pressure, high cholesterol, HIV/AIDS and breast, cervical, and colon cancer and appropriate use of aspirin for the prevention of cardiovascular disease. As the USPSTF notes, screening services are only of value when followed up with high-quality, accessible education and treatment. Furthermore, the Advisory Committee on Immunization Practices recommends a range of vaccines, including childhood immunizations, annual influenza vaccines and vaccines for the prevention of infection with viral hepatitis. (Trust for America's Health, 2011)

History of Preventive Services

It is hard for many of us to believe that smoking in a hospital room used to be an accepted practice or that people drove in cars that did not have seat belts and that babies were held in laps rather than car seats. Through research, we have learned how to better keep people safe and healthy. Clinical preventive services have evolved over the years as growing evidence has demonstrated what works most effectively to improve the health and well-being of diverse populations. Science has guided public and private policies, as well as medical practices, influencing social norms.

Because clinical preventive services are typically addressed during a primary care office visit, clinicians have to make decisions about what services are feasibly covered in each office visit. As science evolves, these recommendations change over time. In the 1970s, pediatricians had fewer vaccines to provide, and childhood obesity was not as prevalent. In 2013, pediatricians are focused on the increase in developmental disorders such as autism and an increase in the number of vaccines available. It is likely that pediatricians do not spend time counseling parents of young children regarding motor vehicle safety, as they may have twenty years ago, considering that car seat use is addressed by state law, and social norms encourage parents to regularly use appropriate child safety restraints.

Health Resources and Services Administration (HRSA) the primary federal agency for improving access to health care services for people who are uninsured, isolated, or medically vulnerable

The **Health Resources and Services Administration (HRSA)**, the primary federal agency for improving access to health care services for people who are uninsured, isolated, or medically vulnerable, was formed in 1982. In 1984 the federal government formally established the US Preventive Services Task Force, which now serves as the gold standard in evidence-based clinical preventive services recommendations for physicians and clinicians, public health experts, government agencies, and health insurance plans.

The federal government's involvement in the public's health goes back to the earliest roots of our nation, with the passage of various bills to help the sick and disabled, and protect the public from the spread of infectious disease. In 1953, the Cabinet-level Department of Health, Education and Welfare was created under President Eisenhower. In 1979, the Department of Education Organization Act was signed into law, providing for a separate Department of Education. Health, Education, and Welfare became the Department of Health and Human Services in 1980. (US Department of Health and Human Services, 2014)

The US Preventive Services Task Force

Since it was first convened in 1984 by the US Public Health Service, the **US Preventive Services Task Force (USPSTF)** has worked to fulfill its mission of doing the following:

- Assessing the benefits and harms of preventive services in people asymptomatic for the target condition, based on age, gender, and risk factors for disease

- Making recommendations about which preventive services should be incorporated routinely into primary care practice

The Task Force makes recommendations based on rigorous reviews of the scientific evidence to help primary care professionals and patients decide together whether a preventive service is right for a patient's needs (US Preventive Services Task Force, 2013d). The Task Force does not conduct research studies but reviews and assesses the existing peer-reviewed evidence to make recommendations.

The Task Force chooses topics to review and makes recommendations based on the following criteria:

- Public health importance (i.e., burden of suffering and expected effectiveness of the preventive service to reduce that burden)

- Potential for the recommendation to have an impact on clinical practice

- New evidence that may change prior recommendations

- The need for a balanced portfolio of topics in clinical preventive services

US Preventive Services Task Force (USPSTF) an independent panel of national experts in prevention and evidence-based medicine composed of practicing doctors and nurses in the fields of family medicine, general internal medicine, gynecology-obstetrics, nursing, pediatrics, and preventive medicine, as well as health behavior specialists

Table 8.2   US Preventive Services Task Force (USPSTF) Grading System

Grade	Definition
A	The USPSTF recommends the service. There is high certainty that the net benefit is substantial.
B	The USPSTF recommends the service. There is high certainty that the net benefit is moderate or there is moderate certainty that the net benefit is moderate to substantial.
C	The USPSTF recommends selectively offering or providing this service to individual patients based on professional judgment and patient preferences. There is at least moderate certainty that the net benefit is small.
D	The USPSTF recommends against the service. There is moderate or high certainty that the service has no net benefit or that the harms outweigh the benefits.
I Statement	Evidence is lacking, of poor quality, or conflicting, and the balance of benefits and harms cannot be determined.

Although the primary audience of the Task Force recommendations is the primary care clinician, recommendations are also relevant to and widely used by policy makers, health insurance companies, public and private payers, quality improvement organizations, research institutions, and patients and consumers. Since 2010, the ACA requires that all new (non-grandfathered) health insurance plans cover USPSTF recommendations graded A or B, without cost sharing or copays. Services graded A or B are those services for which the Task Force has determined that the potential benefit of the preventive service outweighs its potential harms. The grading system of the USPSTF is presented in table 8.2.

Primary and Secondary Preventive Services

Task Force recommendations are intended to improve clinical practice and promote the public health. The Task Force's scope is to address primary and secondary preventive services targeting conditions that represent a substantial burden in the United States and that are provided in primary care settings or available through primary care referral. The USPSTF procedural manual provides the following definitions for primary, secondary, and tertiary prevention:

Primary preventive measures in a clinical setting are those provided to individuals to prevent the onset of a targeted condition (for example, the routine immunization of healthy children), whereas *secondary preventive measures* identify and treat *asymptomatic* persons who have already developed risk factors or preclinical disease but in whom the condition has not become clinically apparent (for example, screening for diabetes or colon cancer). Accordingly, most counseling topics and chemoprevention would today be categorized as primary prevention. Preventive measures that are part of the treatment and management of persons with clinical disease are usually considered *tertiary prevention* and are outside the scope of the USPSTF. (US Preventive Services Task Force, 2013b)

Although immunizations are considered primary prevention, the Task Force defers to another expert panel to make recommendations on immunizations. This group is called the Advisory Committee on Immunization Practices (ACIP) and is described later in this chapter.

Member Composition

Originally convened in 1984 by the US Public Health Service, since 1998, the Agency for Healthcare Research and Quality (AHRQ) has been authorized by the US Congress to convene the Task Force and to provide ongoing scientific, administrative, and dissemination support to the Task Force. AHRQ provides ongoing scientific, administrative, and dissemination support to the USPSTF. Currently the Task Force has sixteen members, appointed on a rolling basis for four years, with the possibility of a one- or two-year extension. Members are appointed by the director of AHRQ with assistance from the Task Force chairs and vice chair (US Preventive Services Task Force, 2014). Members serve on a voluntary basis and are national experts in prevention and evidence-based medicine. Task Force members are practicing doctors and nurses in the fields of family medicine, general internal medicine, gynecology-obstetrics, nursing, pediatrics, and preventive medicine, as well as health behavior specialists.

Identifying Evidence-Based Preventive Services

The USPSTF is widely recognized as having one of the most rigorous and consistent methodologies for choosing, reviewing, and rating the evidence. Its first step in undergoing a review of the evidence is to set a work plan and appropriately scope the topic, which means deciding what research questions are important to answer and what evidence (usually studies published in peer-reviewed journals) should be examined. Once the review is complete, the evidence is synthesized and the Task Force uses established rules to make a recommendation.

Grading System

Letter grades are assigned according to the strength of the evidence regarding the harms and benefits of a specific preventive service (US Preventive Services Task Force, 2008).

An "A" Recommendation   Blood pressure screening is an example of an A recommendation from the Task Force. In its review of the evidence, the Task Force weighed the benefits versus harms of this screening and determined that there was "good evidence that treatment of high blood pressure in adults substantially decreases the incidence of cardiovascular events" and "good evidence that screening and treatment for high blood pressure causes few major harms." In the final assessment, the USPSTF concluded "that there is high certainty that the net benefit of screening for high blood pressure in adults is substantial" (US Preventive Services Task Force, 2013c).

Other Recommendations   Services graded with a B are also recommended, but the evidence suggests the net benefit to be moderate rather than substantial. In general, the USPSTF states a C recommendation is when a service is offered or provided to individual patients based on professional judgment and patient preferences. There is at least moderate certainty that the net benefit is small. For example, the USPSTF recommendation for the prevention of falls in community-dwelling older adults contains both a B recommendation and a C recommendation. For community-dwelling individuals age sixty-five and older, who are at increased risks for falls, the Task Force recommends exercise or physical therapy and vitamin D supplementation. For adults sixty-five and older who do not reside in assisted-living facilities and are not at increased risk, there is not adequate evidence to recommend that clinicians routinely perform an in-depth assessment of risk of falling. The Task Force recommendation states that for this population, patients and clinicians should consider the balance of benefits and harms based on the circumstances of prior falls, comorbid medical conditions, and patient values (US Preventive Services Task Force, 2012a).

A D recommendation indicates evidence proves the risks outweigh the benefits and clinicians should not perform this intervention. An example of this would be screening for colorectal cancer in adults age eighty-five or older. The Task Force states that "for persons older than 85 years, competing causes of mortality preclude a mortality benefit that outweighs the harms" (US Preventive Services Task Force, 2008).

Benefits and Harms

The concept of benefits and harms is an important one for preventive services and one that is easily misunderstood by the public. It can sometimes be difficult for patients to understand that a screening may cause harm. Many times harm occurs after the screening, not during the screening itself. For example, some screening tests have a high rate of false positives, incorrectly identifying patients as having a risk for a condition they do not have. Or, the test may be so sensitive that it identifies a few cancerous cells that may not cause a problem in a person's lifetime. In these cases, patients may undergo a series of additional tests and procedures that can be harmful, either physically or psychologically. Psychological harms include the anxiety resulting from the uncertainty regarding a patient's condition or the anxiety caused by undergoing certain tests.

The Advisory Committee on Immunization Practices

Established under section 222 of the Public Health Service Act (42 USC § 2l7a), as amended and given a statutory role under section 13631 of the Omnibus Budget Reconciliation Act of 1993, the **Advisory Committee on Immunization Practices (ACIP)** consists of fifteen experts in fields associated with immunization who have been selected by the secretary of the US Department of Health and Human Services to provide advice and guidance to the secretary, the assistant secretary for health, and the CDC on the control of vaccine-preventable diseases. In addition to the fifteen voting members, the ACIP includes eight ex officio members who represent other federal agencies with responsibility for immunization programs in the United States and thirty nonvoting representatives of liaison organizations that bring related immunization expertise. The role of the ACIP is to provide advice that will lead to a reduction in the incidence of vaccine-preventable diseases in the United States and an increase in the safe use of vaccines and related biological products. The ACIP is responsible for determining the vaccine schedule for children and adults. It is recommended that children receive several vaccines before they turn two.

Advisory Committee on Immunization Practices (ACIP) consists of fifteen experts in fields associated with immunization who have been selected by the secretary of the US Department of Health and Human Services to provide advice and guidance to the secretary, the assistant secretary for health, and the CDC on the control of vaccine-preventable diseases

Vaccines: Myths and Misinformation

Vaccines are a major public health success story. Most children growing up today will rarely hear about the types of diseases that were common when their grandparents were growing up, including polio, measles, mumps, and many diseases. However, the viruses and bacteria that cause vaccine-preventable disease and death still exist and can be passed on to people who are not protected by vaccines.

Polio is a serious, life-threatening, and debilitating disease that can be prevented through vaccination; because the polio vaccination has been routine in the United States for many decades, it no longer occurs in the United States or anywhere in the western hemisphere. However, public health experts warn that because it is endemic in Afghanistan, India,

Nigeria, Pakistan, if US vaccinations were to stop, polio would return. According to the World Health Organization, widespread use of measles vaccine in the United States has led to a greater than 99% reduction in measles compared with the prevaccine era. Again, without immunization, measles eventually would increase to prevaccine levels.

The history of vaccinations and current issues surrounding vaccination policy are described in the following sidebar.

Unfortunately, in recent years, a small percentage of parents have opted to forego certain or all recommended vaccines for their children or to delay some vaccinations. The ACIP makes recommendations on the vaccination schedule to protect babies and children as early as possible from vaccine-preventable diseases. When parents opt to alter the recommended course of vaccines, they create their own schedule. They may receive guidance from their pediatricians, some of whom prefer the parents to space them out or delay them if the alternative would be forgoing the vaccines. However, most pediatricians do not have the expertise and have not reviewed the evidence as thoroughly as the ACIP; any schedule that modifies the CDC schedule is not based on the best available evidence.

Why do some parents delay or forgo all or selected vaccines, and why is this dangerous? Vaccines work because of herd immunity—when large numbers of people are vaccinated, it is more difficult for the chain of infection to continue (College of Physicians of Philadelphia, 2013a). There always will be people who cannot be vaccinated, such as people with compromised immune systems, very young infants, or people who are allergic to certain vaccine components. For most vaccine-preventable diseases, the disease can be kept at bay if between 80% and 95% of the population is vaccinated. When that percentage drops, the rates of disease will begin to increase.

MEASLES VACCINE CONTROVERSY

A few years after the measles vaccine was introduced in the late 1960s, measles cases in the United States dropped by 97% (College of Physicians of Philadelphia, 2013b). Measles is now given as part of the combined MMR (measles, mumps, and rubella) vaccine. In 1998, the *Lancet* published a now-discredited paper authored by a British physician, Andrew Wakefield, who claimed to have found evidence that the MMR vaccine was linked to autism. Wakefield's theory was that the vaccine inflamed the gut in a way that allowed toxins to cross into the bloodstream. The British media picked up the story and parental anecdotes began to circulate in support of the theory (College of Physicians of Philadelphia, 2013b). The paper was later formally withdrawn by the *Lancet* after several studies were not able to replicate the findings. In 2011, the *British Medical Journal* published a series of reports by an investigative journalist outlining evidence that Wakefield had falsified data and committed scientific fraud and that Wakefield stood to financially profit from his investigations in various ways (Baker & Clements,

2013). Dr. Wakefield's medical license was eventually revoked and he is no longer able to practice medicine in the United Kingdom. Unfortunately, however, the damage was done. Studies suggest that the discredited work of Dr. Wakefield was responsible for a decline in MMR vaccine rates in England and in the United States. As a result, rates of measles have increased (Baker & Clements, 2013).

Health Resources and Services Administration (HRSA)

In addition to requiring new health insurance plans to cover A and B recommendations of the USPSTF and routine recommendations of the ACIP, the ACA also included a requirement that new health insurance plans cover evidence-informed preventive care and screenings for infants, children, and adolescents identified in guidelines supported by the HRSA and evidence-informed preventive services for women identified in guidelines supported by HRSA. For children, these guidelines include well-baby and well-child visits, and for women, the services include well-woman visits, screening and counseling for sexually transmitted infections including HIV, screening for domestic violence, breastfeeding support and services, contraception counseling and services, and screening for gestational diabetes in pregnant women.

Promoting the Use of Preventive Services

In recent years the federal government has continued to support, promote, and encourage the use of clinical and community preventive services. In addition, new media outlets and advancements in science and medicine are successfully promoting and encouraging the use of preventive services. A few of these efforts are described in the following sections.

Health Care Coverage of Evidence-Based Preventive Services

The ACA has several sections related to prevention and wellness. Section 2713 of the act states that new (nongrandfathered) health plans offering coverage in the group and individual markets are required to cover certain services without cost sharing (e.g., a copayment, co-insurance, or deductible). These services include the following:

- Evidence-based services that have a graded A or B in the current recommendations of the USPSTF

- Routine immunizations for children, adolescents, and adults as recommended by the ACIP

- Evidence-informed preventive care and screenings for infants, children, and adolescents identified in guidelines supported by HRSA

- Evidence-informed preventive services for women identified in guidelines supported by HRSA

For the USPSTF, this provision means that recommendations once intended for primary care clinicians are now also required by law to be covered by health insurance plans (this applies only to the A and B recommendations). Increased attention and scrutiny of the Task Force has led to increased transparency and communication initiatives to ensure that the public understands and has input into Task Force processes. The Task Force invites public comment at all major steps of the recommendation process (see figure 8.1).

With the passage of the act, the Task Force is committed to making its work as transparent as possible so it can continue to serve as an open, credible, independent, and unbiased source of clinical recommendations. It has made substantial efforts to ensure that the public and the media have a clear understanding of its recommendations and processes. The public has the opportunity to comment on and help shape the research plan for each topic and comment on the evidence report that results from the research plan. The evidence report that results from the research plan and a draft recommendation statement are posted simultaneously for public comment. Typically comment periods of thirty days at both stages of the process are established for input. In addition, members of the public can also nominate new members to the Task Force and nominate new topics or request an update of an existing topic.

The Task Force produces plain language fact sheets for each of its final recommendations, designed to help the media and the public understand what the recommendation means for them. The plain language sheets provide information describing why the topic area is important for the public's health, providing specific information about the recommendation and what population(s) it applies to, explaining what the recommendation means, and listing resources for more information.

Medicare
federally funded health care services provided to individuals over the age of sixty-five years

Medicaid
federally funded health care services provided to individuals living below the poverty line or those who are disabled

Other Preventive Services Provisions

In addition to rules established for new group and individual plans in the private insurance market, there are specific preventive services provisions established for individuals enrolled in **Medicare** and **Medicaid**.

Create Research Plan

Draft Research Plan

The task force works with researchers from an evidence-based practice center (EPC) and creates a draft research plan that guides the review process.

Invite Public Comments

The draft research plan is posted on the USPSTF web site for public comment.

Finalize Research Plan

The task force and EPC review all comments and address them as appropriate, and the task force creates a final research plan.

Develop Evidence Report and Recommendation Statement

Draft Evidence Report

Using the final research plan, the EPC independently gathers and reviews the available published evidence and creates a draft evidence report.

then

Draft Recommendation Statement

The task force discusses the draft evidence report and the effectiveness of the service. Based on the discussion, the task force creates a draft recommendation statement.

Invite Public Comments

The draft evidence report and draft recommendation statement are posted simultaneously on the USPSTF web site for public comment.

Finalize Evidence Report

The EPC reviews all comments on the draft evidence report, addresses them as appropriate, and creates a final evidence report.

then

Finalize Recommendation Statement

The task force discusses the final evidence report and any new evidence. The task force then reviews all comments on the draft recommendation statement, addresses them as appropriate, and creates a final recommendation statement.

Disseminate Recommendation Statement

Publish and Disseminate Final Recommendation Statement

The final recommendation statement and supporting materials, including the final evidence report, are posted on the USPSTF web site at www.uspreventiveservicestaskforce.org. At the same time, the final evidence report and final recommendation statement are published together in a peer-reviewed journal. The final recommendation statement is also made available through electronic tools and a consumer guide.

Figure 8.1   USPSTF Recommendation Process
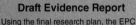

Source: US Preventive Services Task Force (2013d).

Section 4103 of the act requires that Medicare cover an annual wellness visit for individuals that results in a "personalized prevention plan" describing services recommended for that individual patient. Personalized prevention plan services include a health risk assessment and may include services such as updating family history, listing providers that regularly provide medical care to the individuals, measurement of BMI, and other screenings and services. Section 4104 of the ACA requires Medicare to waive co-insurance requirements for many preventive services, including those graded A or B by the USPSTF.

Section 4106 is a provision that incentivizes states to cover USPSTF graded A and B recommendations as well as ACIP-recommended immunizations with no cost sharing by providing them with an increased federal medical assistance percentage or one percentage point for these services. Under section 4107, states will be required to provide Medicaid coverage with no cost sharing for tobacco cessation services for pregnant women (Centers for Medicare and Medicaid Services, 2013).

Prevention and Public Health Fund

The ACA appropriated billions of dollars toward community preventive services through the Prevention and Public Health Fund. The goal of the fund is to support partnerships with states and communities to help control the obesity epidemic, fight health disparities, detect and quickly respond to health threats, reduce tobacco use, train the nation's public health workforce, modernize vaccine systems, prevent the spread of HIV/AIDS, increase public health program effectiveness and efficiency, and improve access to behavioral health services (Centers for Medicare and Medicaid Services, 2010).

Million Hearts Initiative

A major initiative to prevent heart disease through targeting risk factors is Million Hearts, launched in 2011 by the Department of Health and Human Services under the joint leadership of the CDC and the Centers for Medicare and Medicaid Services (CMS). This initiative is a public-private partnership with a goal to prevent one million heart attacks in five years. Million Hearts brings together communities, health systems, nonprofit organizations, federal agencies, and private-sector partners from across the country to fight heart disease and stroke (US Department of Health and Human Services, 2013).

Million Hearts promotes four interventions, called the ABCS, to prevent heart disease:

Aspirin therapy for recommended populations

Blood pressure control

Cholesterol management

Smoking cessation

The initiative includes strategies such as working with public and private partner stakeholders to promote programs, policies, and campaigns designed to make a positive impact across the spectrum of prevention and care. These efforts aim to promote the "ABCS" of clinical prevention, the use of health information technology and quality improvement initiatives to standardize and improve the delivery of care for high blood pressure and high cholesterol, and community efforts to encourage smoke-free air policies and reduce sodium in the food supply. Examples of Million Hearts programs and more information about the initiative can be found at www.millionhearts.hhs.gov.

Technology and the Media

Technology can be a significant tool to influence the use of preventive services. Most adults have access to e-mail and the Internet and many receive information every day on their mobile phones via applications and text messages. Initiatives using these technologies to educate the general public and target populations may successfully provide accurate information to patients and encourage the use of preventive services. It is unlikely that public health experts working to reach the public before the 1990s could have imagined the potential that technology has to reach people quickly with targeted information that can empower them to improve their health.

Text4baby

Text4baby is an example of a successful, evidence-based public-private partnership to advance public health and promote sound prenatal care and well-baby care. The program involves several mobile phone companies that waive text messaging charges for an educational service provided to pregnant women and new moms. Preventive health messages vetted by the CDC to promote healthy pregnancy and infants are texted to expectant mothers and new moms registered for the free service. Initiating the service is simple and involves sending a text message. Topics include recommended immunizations for pregnant women and infants, breastfeeding, oral health, nutrition, exercise, mental health, substance abuse, injury prevention and prevention of family violence, car seat safety, labor and delivery, and more. Partners include businesses, employers, health insurance plans, the media, advocacy organizations, elected officials, and health care providers (Text4baby, 2012).

Interactive Technology

Interactive voice technology is a platform many health plans use to remind people when they are due or overdue for recommended preventive screenings, based on their age, gender, and possible risk factors. More and more tech-savvy individuals are using mobile phone applications to upload results of their workouts or activity through information received from their pedometers or heart rate monitoring devices. Health plans and employers have web-based programs to reach out to members and employees to provide health information and offer interactive programs, such as health risk assessments and other tools, to connect individuals with programs and services aimed at improving health.

Nontraditional Sites of Care

Nontraditional sites of care that enable people to access clinical services outside the traditional primary care clinic are becoming more prevalent. Many employers host company-wide health fairs where employees can participate in a variety of screenings and gather information regarding a variety of important health topics. Some employers are building on-site clinics at the work site, encouraging employees to improve their health and making primary care services as convenient as possible for employees. Many health plans contract with retail clinics, such as drug stores, or are establishing their own retail clinics in underserved neighborhoods to expand access to care, preventive screenings, and other services.

Genetic Testing

Genome sequencing and genetic testing is a rapidly growing field that will continue to shape the prevention and early diagnosis of diseases. Genetic tests are tests on blood and other tissue to identify genetic disorders. Physicians use genetic tests to identify possible genetic diseases in unborn babies, determine if people carry a gene for a disease that may be genetically passed on, diagnose adults with genetic diseases prior to the appearance of symptoms, and to confirm a diagnosis of a disease in a person who is presenting symptoms (US National Library of Medicine, 2013).

Currently, the USPSTF has one recommendation for genetic risk assessment. The USPSTF recommends that women whose family history is associated with an increased risk for certain common mutations in breast cancer BRCA1 or BRCA2 genes be referred for genetic counseling and evaluation to test for these gene mutations. The USPSTF recommends against routine referral for genetic counseling or routine breast cancer susceptibility gene testing for women whose family history is not associated with an increased risk for these common mutations in breast cancer (US Preventive Services Task Force, 2013a).

As research evolves, whole-genome sequencing, a process that determines the complete DNA sequence of an organism's genome, will offer more information about what diseases individuals may be susceptible to and ideally help identify diseases early while providing information to best target treatment. However, not all results will be straightforward and there is the risk that ambiguous results will lead to increased worry, frequent screenings, and potentially unnecessary procedures—for diseases they might never develop or that we may not know how to treat. Dr. Francis Collins, a pioneer in the field for his work in discovering the gene that causes cystic fibrosis and the director of the National Institutes of Health, summarizes the challenge: "We are living in an awkward interval where our ability to capture the information often exceeds our ability to know what to do with it" (Kolata, 2012).

Advances in Behavioral Science

Behavioral science is another area that will continue to evolve and shape the evidence base for clinical and community preventive services. Although we have some information on what preventive services most benefit which individuals and research findings regarding what behaviors and habits can help keep us healthy, there is still more to learn about what motivates people to make decisions that influence their health-related behaviors. Advances in behavioral science can help us better understand how we can increase participation in recommended preventive services and what motivates people to make healthier eating choices or stop smoking. Research on how to engage consumers on health and health care will continue to inform program development, policies, and social norms.

Challenges to Increasing the Use of Evidence-Based Preventive Services

Although we have made great strides in building the evidence base for clinical and community preventive services, and promoting and encouraging the use of evidence-based preventive services, challenges remain. These challenges consist of educating the public and sharing accurate medical and health information with patients, medical research limitations, as well as health care barriers.

Educating the Public about Preventive Services

The media play a significant role in how scientific findings are shared with the public. Unfortunately, facts and accurate, consistent information often get lost in the message. Reporters do not always understand the science on which they report, and editors often condense stories to make them easier to read or to create controversy. News stories often present controversial topics as if there are two, equally relevant sides to the story. A good example is the case of the MMR vaccine, as described previously in the chapter.

In the age of social media, anyone can have a blog and frequently opinion gets passed on as fact. The discredited Wakefield measles study is a prime example of the power of media and the ways bad science and misinformation can be promoted and gain traction. One issue is that the media and bloggers do not always adequately capture the methodological difference between high-quality studies or the nuances between different kinds of studies that should not be compared or given equal weight. For example, laboratory studies and epidemiological studies serve different purposes. A vaccine laboratory study may involve studying the effects of a vaccine or vaccine component on a small group of animals or humans. Epidemiological studies show the effect of the vaccine on an entire population of people. An example of this is early studies examining the link between cigarette smoking and lung cancer. In 1939, a cancer surgeon was the first to propose the link between smoking and lung cancer, but results from laboratory studies on animals were inconclusive. A large epidemiological study in the 1950s clearly demonstrated the link and the dose response (the more people smoked, the greater their risk of lung cancer) (Doll & Hill, 1950). Similarly, several epidemiological studies have been helpful in demonstrating the safety of the US vaccine program.

Research Limitations

Sometimes, the USPSTF does a thorough review of the literature, only to find there is insufficient evidence to make a recommendation. The ACA requires the USPSTF to provide an annual report to Congress that outlines critical evidence gaps regarding clinical preventive services, as well as gaps in the evidence that exist for certain populations and age groups. Recent examples of USPSTF-identified high-priority topics with evidence gaps include screening for chronic kidney disease, screening for cervical cancer with human papillomavirus (HPV) tests, and screening for prostate cancer in African American men (US Preventive Services Task Force, 2012b).

Not all evidence reviews yield the same conclusions. Sometimes, recommendations from different groups may conflict or not completely align. For example, in its 2011 recommendation statement, the USPSTF concluded that the current evidence is insufficient to assess the balance of benefits and harms of screening for osteoporosis in men. The National Osteoporosis Foundation recommends bone-density testing for all men aged seventy years or older (US Preventive Services Task Force, 2012b).

Though there may be differences in clinical guidelines from various organizations, the USPSTF is widely recognized as gold standard because of its methodology and rigor. In 2011, the Institute of Medicine (IOM) published a report, commissioned by the US Congress, called *Clinical Practice Guidelines We Can Trust* (National Research Council, 2011). Because of the large number of clinical practice guidelines made by various organizations and expert panels, Congress called for the IOM to undertake a study on the best methods used in developing clinical practice guidelines to cut down on the confusion for practitioners and patients when determining which guidelines are of high quality. The aim of the IOM report was to provide a mechanism to immediately identify high-quality, trustworthy clinical practice guidelines and ultimately improve decision making—potentially improving health care quality and health outcomes. In the report, the IOM outlined eight standards for developing rigorous, trustworthy clinical practice guidelines. The standards are summarized as follows:

- Guideline issuers should have a transparent process (it should be clear who is making the recommendations and how the conclusions are made).

- Guideline issuers should appropriately manage conflicts of interest.

- The group issuing the guidelines should be balanced and multidisciplinary, and the public should be engaged on some level.

- The systematic reviews conducted should follow certain quality standards.

- The recommendations issued should be rated based on the strength of the evidence.

- Recommendations should be articulated in a standardized form.

- An external review process should be in place.

- There should be a plan in place for updating the recommendations. (National Research Council, 2011)

The methodology and processes of the USPSTF are supported by the IOM in this document because they incorporate many of these best practices.

Health Care Services Barriers

health care service barriers
any obstacle that prevents individuals from receiving the preventive services recommended for them including time, cost of travel, and lack of available services in their area

At the individual level, there are many **health care service barriers** that prevent patients from receiving the preventive services recommended for them. Some services are underused, meaning that not everyone in the appropriate population gets the recommended service. Some individuals may find it difficult to get to a doctor's office for a nonacute or non-emergency visit because of an inability to take time off work or find adequate child care (Office of the US Surgeon General, 2010). Individuals may be confused about what services they need and if they are up-to-date on these services. For example, they may hear a news report of a new study that recommends a particular service, but their physician may not have recommended the service to them. Or, they may not remember if they received a particular service.

Alternatively, some preventive services may be overused or misused, meaning some populations may get a service that is not recommended for them. In 2012, nine specialty societies partnered with the ABIM Foundation to launch the Choosing Wisely initiative (ABIM Foundation, 2013). Each specialty society convened to identify five tests or procedures commonly used in their field, whose necessity should be questioned and discussed. The resulting "Five Things Physicians and Patients Should Question" served to spark discussion about the need—or lack thereof—for many frequently ordered tests or treatments (ABIM Foundation, 2013). They were later joined by sixteen other specialty societies, and the initiative is ongoing. Examples of the forty-five services identified by the physician groups include the overuse of imaging for low back pain within the first six weeks and routine antibiotic prescribing for sinusitis.

Summary

Clinical preventive services are screenings, counseling, and related interventions including immunizations that individuals receive at their primary care doctor's office, at their local pharmacy, or a health fair that aim to detect certain conditions when they are asymptomatic, often leading to improved health outcomes. Recommended clinical preventive services are based on age and gender. The US Preventive Services Task Force, the Advisory Committee on Immunization Practices, and the Health Resource and Services Administration are the sources of recommended clinical preventive services authorized by the Affordable Care Act. Physicians, health insurance plans, employers, and communities promote recommended clinical preventive services with the goal of improving health outcomes. Promotion of preventive services includes educating individuals on what services they need, encouraging them to talk to their health care provider about these services, and increasing access to these services by offering them at work sites and retail clinics.

KEY TERMS

1. **Clinical preventive services:** services provided at one's primary care physician's office, local pharmacy, or health fairs to detect and reduce the risk of specific health conditions from progressing; examples include screening tests, immunizations, counseling, and preventive medications

2. **National Prevention Strategy:** guidelines developed as a result of the Affordable Care Act; provides guidance to the federal government and the nation regarding the most effective and achievable means for improving health through prevention and health promotion policies and programs

3. **Health Resources and Services Administration (HRSA):** the primary federal agency for improving access to health care services for people who are uninsured, isolated, or medically vulnerable

4. **US Preventive Services Task Force (USPSTF):** an independent panel of nonfederal experts in prevention and evidence-based medicine composed of primary care providers such as internists, pediatricians, family physicians, gynecologists and obstetricians, nurses, and health behavior specialists

5. **Advisory Committee on Immunization Practices (ACIP):** consists of fifteen experts in fields associated with immunization who have been selected by the secretary of the US Department of Health and Human Services to provide advice and guidance to the secretary, the assistant secretary for health, and the CDC on the control of vaccine-preventable diseases

6. **Medicare:** federally funded health care services provided to individuals over the age of sixty-five years

7. **Medicaid:** federally funded health care services provided to individuals living below the poverty line or those who are disabled

8. **Health care service barriers:** any obstacle that prevents individuals from receiving the preventive services recommended for them including time, cost of travel, and lack of available services in their area

REVIEW QUESTIONS

1. What are common conditions or health risks that can be detected early or prevented through recommended clinical preventive services?

2. What are some barriers to individuals getting recommended clinical preventive services?

3. Why are some clinical preventive services recommended for some populations and not for others?

4. What are the entities that recommend evidence-based clinical preventive services identified by the Affordable Care Act?

5. Describe the rating system for preventive care and give examples of A–D ratings.

6. Why does the US government invest in preventive care services?

7. Why, as a health promotion professional, are preventive services important?

STUDENT ACTIVITIES

1. Create a campaign to promote a recommended clinical preventive service for a certain population, keeping in mind the barriers that this population might face.

2. Debate whether families should be allowed to opt out of required vaccinations.

3. Create a chart that details the life stage and the appropriate clinical service needed during that stage.

References

ABIM Foundation. (2013). *Choosing wisely.* Retrieved from www.abimfoundation .org/Initiatives/Choosing-Wisely.aspx

Baker, J. P., & Clements, D. (2013). *Does the MMR vaccine cause autism?* Duke University Health System 2004–2013. Retrieved from http://www.newsforparents .org/expert_mmr_autism.html

Centers for Disease Control and Prevention. (2013). *Heart disease facts.* Retrieved from www.cdc.gov/heartdisease/facts.htm

Centers for Medicare and Medicaid Services. (2010). *Shining a light on health insurance rate increases.* Retrieved from www.healthcare.gov/news/factsheets /2011/02/prevention02092011a.html

Centers for Medicare and Medicaid Services. (2013). *Prevention and getting care.* Retrieved from www.healthcare.gov/prevention/index.html

College of Physicians of Philadelphia. (2013a). *The history of vaccines: Herd immunity.* Retrieved from www.historyofvaccines.org/content/herd-immunity-0

College of Physicians of Philadelphia. (2013b). *The history of vaccines: Measles.* Retrieved from www.historyofvaccines.org/content/articles/measles

Doll R., & Hill, A. B. (1950). Smoking and carcinoma of the lung. *British Medical Journal, 2*(4682), 739–748.

Kolata, G. (2012, August 25). Genes now tell doctors secrets they can't utter. *New York Times.* Retrieved from www.nytimes.com/2012/08/26/health/research/with-rise-of-gene-sequencing-ethical-puzzles.html?pagewanted=all&_r=0

Krist, A., Rothemich, S., Kashiri, P., et al. (2012). *An interactive preventive care record: A handbook for using patient-centered personal health records to promote prevention.* Prepared by the Virginia Commonwealth University, Department of Family Medicine, Virginia Ambulatory Care Outcomes. AHRQ Publication No. 12-0051-EF. Rockville, MD: Agency for Healthcare Research and Quality. Retrieved from http://healthit.ahrq.gov/sites/default/files/docs/page/PreventiveCareHandbook_062912comp.pdf

National Research Council. (2011). *Clinical practice guidelines we can trust.* Washington, DC: National Academies Press. Retrieved from www.iom.edu/Reports/2011/Clinical-Practice-Guidelines-We-Can-Trust.aspx

Office of the US Surgeon General. (2010). *National prevention strategy.* Retrieved from www.surgeongeneral.gov/initiatives/prevention/strategy/preventiveservices.pdf

Text4baby. (2012). Retrieved from www.text4baby.org

Trust for America's Health. (2011, April). *National prevention strategy framework (draft).* Retrieved from http://healthyamericans.org/assets/files/NPS%20Framework.pdf

US Department of Health and Human Services. (2013). *Million hearts.* Retrieved from http://millionhearts.hhs.gov/index.html

US Department of Health and Human Services. (2014, February 12). *What is the history of HHS? When did it get started? What years were the most important in its history?* Retrieved from http://answers.hhs.gov/questions/3049

US National Library of Medicine. (2013). *Genetic testing.* Retrieved from www.nlm.nih.gov/medlineplus/genetictesting.html

US Preventive Services Task Force. (2008). *Grade definitions.* Retrieved from www.uspreventiveservicestaskforce.org/uspstf/grades.htm

US Preventive Services Task Force. (2012a). *Prevention of falls in community-dwelling older adults.* Retrieved from www.uspreventiveservicestaskforce.org/uspstf/uspsfalls.htm

US Preventive Services Task Force. (2012b, November). *Second annual report to Congress on high-priority evidence gaps for clinical preventive services.* Retrieved from www.uspreventiveservicestaskforce.org/annlrpt2/index.html

US Preventive Services Task Force. (2013a). *Understanding how the U.S. Preventive Services Task Force works: USPSTF 101*. Retrieved from www.uspreventiveservices taskforce.org/uspstf101_slides/uspstf101.htm

US Preventive Services Task Force. (2013b). *Procedure manual*. Retrieved from www.uspreventiveservicestaskforce.org/uspstf08/methods/procmanual.htm

US Preventive Services Task Force. (2013c). *Screening for high blood pressure in adults*. Retrieved from www.uspreventiveservicestaskforce.org/uspstf/uspshype .htm

US Preventive Services Task Force. (2013d). *Genetic risk assessment and BRCA mutation testing for breast and ovarian cancer susceptibility*. Retrieved from www.uspreventiveservicestaskforce.org/uspstf/uspsbrgen.htm

US Preventive Services Task Force. (2014). *Our members*. Retrieved from http://www.uspreventiveservicestaskforce.org/members.htm

PART THREE

HEALTH PROMOTION IN ACTION

Chapters 9 through 12 are geared toward introducing you to the broad context of health promotion. Now that you have gained some knowledge on health behavior change theories, models for program development, and have acquired an in-depth view of selected health-promoting behaviors, you will read about government programs consistent with promoting health, certifications and associations in the field, where the jobs are, and then finish with future trends in health promotion as we move through the twenty-first century.

Chapter 9 on national, state, and local activities is rich with examples of how the federal agencies monitor health status, provide broad guidelines, conduct research, and fund programs to promote health. Collectively, there are thousands of federal employees who work across disciplines to study or implement new approaches to improve the health of our society. More initiatives have been started as a result of the Patient Protection and Affordable Care Act. Because the act prioritizes health promotion and disease prevention, more funding has become available to departments of health to implement policies and programs that address healthy lifestyle choices.

Chapter 10 discusses settings where health promotion is taking place, which further exemplifies that health promotion is beginning to be seen everywhere, such as in day care centers, schools, colleges, work sites, food stores, retirement homes, and communities. These health promotion positions can also be categorized by stages in one's life, from starting at a very young age to college students to adults and the elderly. The growth in the field is only just beginning and many professionals believe in the vision of a country in which people are practicing healthy behaviors every day because the healthy choice is the easy choice.

Chapter 11 presents associations, journals, and certifications that can provide you with important information for your life beyond the borders of an academic institution. In time, reading a textbook or listening to a professor's lecture will be in the past. But as a professional, you will need to stay current. This chapter describes many associations and their related journals in areas such as exercise science, nutrition, health education, public health, and health promotion, to name a few. Also, there are numerous certifications for health coaching, personal training, and health education. These certifications are usually earned after you graduate and may require continuing education to maintain the certification. These ongoing educational opportunities will facilitate your continued professional development.

The final chapter is a look into the future, predicting eleven trends that are driving the country to acknowledge and commit to creating a culture of health. These trends will ensure that the Healthy People 2020 goals to "attain high-quality, longer lives free of preventable disease, to improve the health of all groups, to create social and physical environments that promote good health for all, and to promote healthy behaviors across all life stages" will be achieved. The trends are based on the changing demographics of our nation, the rising health care costs, and the shift toward a health care system that prioritizes health promotion and disease prevention strategies.

CHAPTER 9

NATIONAL AND STATE INITIATIVES TO PROMOTE HEALTH AND WELL-BEING

Jennifer Childress and Jill Dombrowski

Throughout the nation, Americans are experiencing declining levels of health. How is this determined? What measurements are used and who measures them? What programs have been developed to address declining health levels? Partnerships and data are key to improving the health of Americans where we live, work, and play.

Healthy People: 1979–2020

Since 1979, the **US Department of Health and Human Services (HHS)** has been setting ten-year national health objectives for Americans, called **Healthy People**. By establishing benchmarks and monitoring progress over time, Healthy People's aims are to do the following:

- Encourage collaboration across communities and sectors.
- Empower individuals toward making informed health decisions.
- Measure the impact of prevention activities.

Since the 1980s, the HHS Healthy People initiatives have built on their predecessors and have addressed new areas of importance related to the health of the nation. Given the comprehensiveness and pervasiveness of health, the development of Healthy People goals involve input from multiple sectors and stakeholders. Most recently, public health; health promotion and prevention experts;

LEARNING OBJECTIVES

After reading this chapter, the student will be able to:

- Discuss the history of the Department of Health and Human Services' Healthy People initiative with an emphasis on Healthy People 2020.

- Describe the work of key federal government agencies to support research, share findings, and develop guidelines for healthy living.

- Identify government programs that promote health.

- Recognize key surveillance surveys and activities that monitor the health of the US population.

- Summarize state-level programs that use national guidelines to promote health.

US Department of Health and Human Services (HHS)
the US government's principal agency tasked with protecting the health of all Americans and providing essential human services

Healthy People
ten-year national health objectives for Americans released by the US Department of Health and Human Services

federal, state, and local government officials; a consortium of more than two thousand organizations; and the general public were invited to provide feedback and input during the drafting of Healthy People 2020 objectives (US Department of Health and Human Services, 2010).

The goals identified in Healthy People 2020 are broad and include objectives for areas that were included in prior Healthy People goals, such as nutrition and physical activity, immunizations, cancer, heart disease, medical insurance coverage, mental health, environmental quality, and substance abuse. In addition, Healthy People 2020 has been expanded to include new areas of focus, such as global health; genomics; adolescent health; older adult health; lesbian, gay, bisexual, and transgender health; and sleep health.

HISTORY OF HEALTHY PEOPLE

- 1979 surgeon general's report, *Healthy People: The Surgeon General's Report on Health Promotion and Disease Prevention*
- Healthy People 1990: Promoting Health/Preventing Disease: Objectives for the Nation
- Healthy People 2000: National Health Promotion and Disease Prevention Objectives
- Healthy People 2010: Objectives for Improving Health

Healthy People 2020

The majority of deaths among Americans are the result of chronic diseases that are preventable through lifestyle behavior modifications. On December 2, 2010, Healthy People 2020 was released with the vision of a society in which all people live long, healthy lives (US Department of Health and Human Services, nd-a).

The mission of Healthy People 2020 is to do the following:

- Identify nationwide health improvement priorities.
- Increase public awareness and understanding of the determinants of health, disease, disability, and the opportunities for progress.
- Provide measurable objectives and goals that are applicable at the national, state, and local levels.

- Engage multiple sectors to take actions to strengthen policies and improve practices that are driven by the best available evidence and knowledge.

- Identify critical research, evaluation, and data collection needs.

Healthy People 2020 has four overarching goals:

- Attain high-quality, longer lives free of preventable disease, disability, injury, and premature death.

- Achieve health equity, eliminate disparities, and improve the health of all groups.

- Create social and physical environments that promote good health for all.

- Promote quality of life, healthy development, and healthy behaviors across all life stages.

Over the next ten years, progress toward these goals will be determined by the following four foundational health measures:

- General health status

- Health-related quality of life and well-being

- Determinants of health

- Health disparities

There are twenty-six leading health indicators within Healthy People 2020 organized under twelve topics. These indicators are being tracked, measured, and reported regularly throughout the decade to better evaluate the nation's progress toward meeting Healthy People 2020 goals. These indicators represent a smaller set of objectives that reflect high-priority issues and associated actions to address them (see table 9.1).

HHS launched the Healthy People website (www.healthypeople.gov) to provide users access to information and resources particular to their needs (e.g., based on sex, age group, setting, population group, intervention agent, health condition, and prevention areas). Although the large number of indicators and associated data and information may seem overwhelming, HHS issued a special challenge for web application developers to create easy-to-use applications to quickly access these data. With easy access to relevant data, health professionals can better assist Americans where they live, work, and learn.

In June 2011, the US surgeon general's office released the National Prevention Strategy, which is aimed at increasing the number of Americans

Table 9.1   Healthy People 2020 Leading Health Indicators

Access to Health Services

* Persons with medical insurance

* Persons with a usual primary care provider

Clinical Preventive Services

* Adults who receive a colorectal cancer screening based on the most recent guidelines

* Adults with hypertension whose blood pressure is under control

* Adult diabetic population with an A1c value greater than 9%

* Children aged nine to thirty-five months who receive the recommended doses of DTaP, polio, MMR, Hib, hepatitis B, varicella, and PCV vaccines

Environmental Quality

* Air quality index exceeding 100

* Children aged three to eleven years exposed to secondhand smoke

Injury and Violence

* Fatal injuries

* Homicides

Maternal, Infant, and Child Health

* Infant deaths

* Preterm births

Mental Health

* Suicides

* Adolescents who experience major depressive episodes

Nutrition, Physical Activity, and Obesity

* Adults who meet current federal physical activity guidelines for aerobic physical activity and muscle-strengthening activity

* Adults who are obese

* Children and adolescents who are considered obese

* Total vegetable intake for persons aged two years and older

Oral Health

* Persons aged two years and older who used the oral health care system in past twelve months

Reproductive and Sexual Health

* Sexually active females aged fifteen to forty-four years who received reproductive health services in the past twelve months

* Persons living with HIV who know their serostatus

Social Determinants

* Students who graduate with a regular diploma four years after starting ninth grade

Substance Abuse
* Adolescents using alcohol or any illicit drugs during the past thirty days
* Adults engaging in binge drinking during the past thirty days

Tobacco
* Adults who are current cigarette smokers
* Adolescents who smoked cigarettes in the past thirty days

who are healthy at every stage of life. It includes comprehensive and evidence-based prevention strategies.

There are four strategic directions:

* Healthy and safe community environments

* Clinical and community preventive services

* Empowered people

* Elimination of health disparities

There are seven targeted priorities:

* Tobacco-free living

* Preventing drug abuse and excessive alcohol use

* Healthy eating

* Active living

* Injury and violence free living

* Reproductive and sexual health

* Mental and emotional well-being (US Department of Health and Human Services, Office of the Surgeon General, National Prevention Council, 2011)

This federal initiative is a component of the Patient Protection and Affordable Care Act (ACA) and is focused on disease prevention. Some of the strategies for disease prevention are the same as those for health promotion, but the outcome measures may be different because the goals are different: preventing disease versus promoting and maintaining good health. Some of these measures may be based on secondary prevention; therefore, the target populations may already have risk factors such as hypertension and obesity. For example, this chapter highlights healthy eating and active living interventions, but the focus of these strategies from the perspective of the National Prevention Strategy would be to avoid diseases or chronic health conditions such as CVD, stroke, and diabetes. The emphasis then would be on behavior change to avoid disease, which may work for some populations but not others, such as adolescents, who are not concerned with development of disease when they are middle-aged.

US Department of Health and Human Services (HHS)

HHS is the United States government's principal agency for protecting the health of all Americans and providing essential human services, especially for those who are least able to help themselves (US Department of Health and Human Services, nd-b). HHS works with state and local governments to provide health and human services through state or county agencies and through private-sector grantees. HHS programs are administered by eleven operating divisions, comprising eight agencies in the US Public Health Service and three human services agencies.

As a department within the federal government, the secretary of HHS sits on the president's cabinet and is a presidential appointee. Every four years the secretary of HHS is responsible for updating a five-year strategic plan that defines the department's missions and goals and the means by which progress will be measured. The most recent strategic plan

HHS STRATEGIC PLAN

- Promote high-value, safe, and effective health care.
- Secure and expand health insurance coverage.
- Eliminate health disparities.
- Promote prevention and wellness.
- Help Americans achieve and maintain healthy weight.
- Prevent and reduce tobacco use.
- Support the national HIV/AIDS strategy.
- Put children and youth on the path for successful futures.
- Promote early childhood health and development.
- Protect Americans' health and safety during emergencies and foster resilience in response to emergencies.
- Implement a twenty-first-century food safety system.
- Accelerate the process of scientific discovery to improve patient care.
- Promote program integrity, accountability, and transparency.

(2010–2015) is available on the HHS website and is designed to be a living, vital document that is updated frequently to reflect progress. The last update to the strategic plan was March 10, 2014 (US Department of Health and Human Services, 2014).

The organizational chart in figure 9.1 identifies the eleven operating divisions and eight agencies under HHS (www.hhs.gov). When visiting the HHS website, you can click on the organizational chart to be directed to the

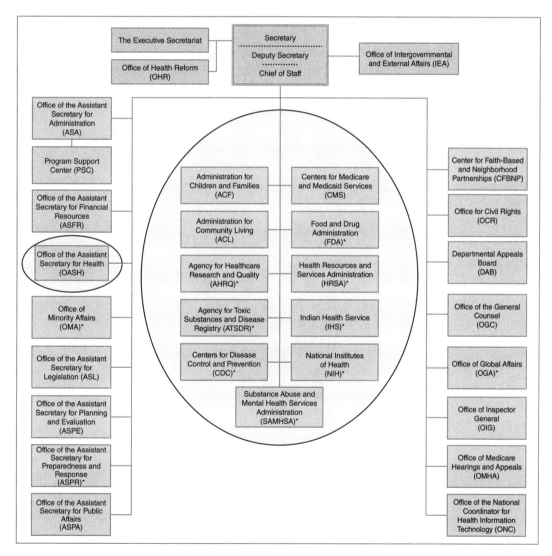

Figure 9.1   HHS Organizational Chart

Note: *Designates that it is a component of the US Public Health Service.

Source: US Department of Health and Human Services (nd-c).

division or agency website and view the sublayers that exist in addition to those pictured in figure 9.1.

HHS-operating divisions and agencies are tasked with carrying out initiatives to support Healthy People 2020 objectives, and the overall mission of HHS is to support and protect the health of Americans through research, public health, food and drug safety, grants, health insurance, and many other actions. Many of the initiatives discussed in this textbook fall under one of the entities of HHS circled in figure 9.1. Following are descriptions of some HHS agencies or divisions that are of particular interest in the field of health promotion.

The Centers for Disease Control and Prevention (CDC)

Centers for Disease Control and Prevention (CDC)
a federal agency under the US Department of Health and Human Services responsible for the public health of the nation; works to protect the public health and safety of people in the United States by tracking, detecting, and responding to threats

The mission of the **Centers for Disease Control and Prevention (CDC)** is to collaborate to create the expertise, information, and tools that people and communities need to protect their health—through health promotion; prevention of disease, injury, and disability; and preparedness for new health threats (Centers for Disease Control and Prevention, 2012a). Working with partners throughout the nation and the world, the CDC seeks to accomplish its mission by doing the following:

- Monitoring health

- Detecting and investigating health problems

- Conducting research to enhance prevention

- Developing and advocating sound public health policies

- Implementing prevention strategies

- Promoting healthy behaviors

- Fostering safe and healthful environments

- Providing leadership and training

The CDC is composed of various centers, an institute, and offices to meet its mission, goals, and objectives, share resources, and effectively address public health concerns. On the CDC website, viewers may examine the plethora of health-related topics addressed. The CDC provides information, publications, multimedia, and tools to support experts, individuals, communities, and organizations as they act to address health concerns. The CDC strives to provide information through various mediums to its audience; for example, in addition to print and online, information is available through podcast. To address a larger audience, many CDC resources are also available in Spanish.

The following examples of CDC information sharing for seasonal influenza and smoking and tobacco use are demonstrative of the types of detailed information typically provided by the CDC.

Seasonal Influenza (Flu) Addressed by CDC

The CDC provides information to the general public regarding flu activity and surveillance. The website provides maps and information through the weekly FluView. Viewers can identify areas of flu outbreaks throughout the United States or customize the information to generate state-specific reports. Information includes the proportion of people visiting health care providers for influenza-like illness (ILI) (see figure 9.2), influenza-related

The CDC Influenza Application for Clinicians and Health Care Professionals (available in the App Store) provides information on the latest recommendations and flu activity updates, videos from subject matter experts, and products to print out and post in the workplace or distribute to patients.

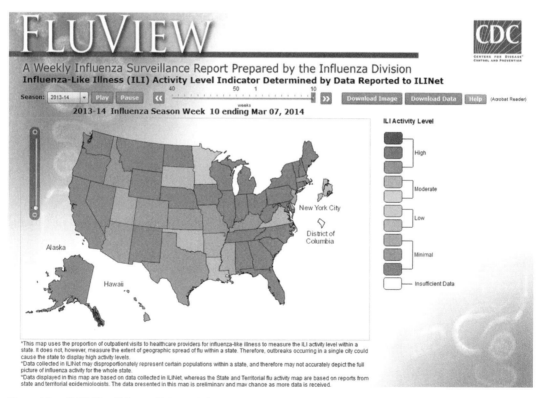

Figure 9.2 CDC FluView Webpage: ILI Activity Indicator Map

Source: Centers for Disease Control and Prevention (2014).

mortality rates, the geographic spread of influenza, and hospitalizations related to influenza.

In addition to tracking influenza patterns, the CDC also provides information and facts regarding prevention and treatment of the flu. Through the "Take 3" campaign, the CDC encourages three actions to prevent and fight the flu. The campaign outlines these three actions, along with steps and research supporting each one:

* Take time to get the flu vaccine.

* Take everyday preventive actions to stop the spread of germs.

* Take flu antiviral drugs if your doctor prescribes them.

Smoking and Tobacco Use Addressed by the CDC

Another area of focus for the CDC is smoking and tobacco use. Similar to addressing influenza, the CDC provides resources to individuals and health professionals, as well as to communities, clinicians, teachers, and workplaces. The State Tobacco Activities Tracking and Evaluation (STATE) system is an interactive application on the CDC website that houses and displays current and historical state-level data on tobacco use prevention and control. It uses data from the Behavioral Risk Factor Surveillance and Youth Risk Behavior Surveillance systems (discussed later in this chapter) to generate graphs and images. Figure 9.3 provides a webshot of the STATE home page.

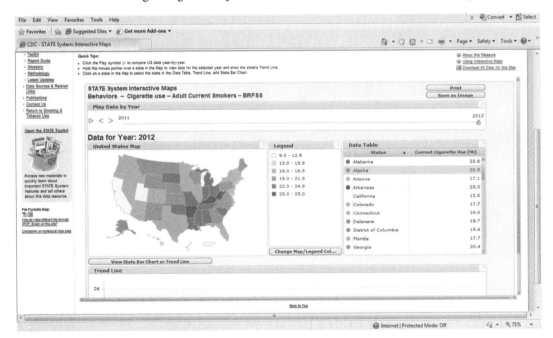

Figure 9.3 STATE System Interactive Map: Behaviors—Cigarette Use—Adult Current Smokers—BRFSS

Source: Centers for Disease Control and Prevention (nd-a).

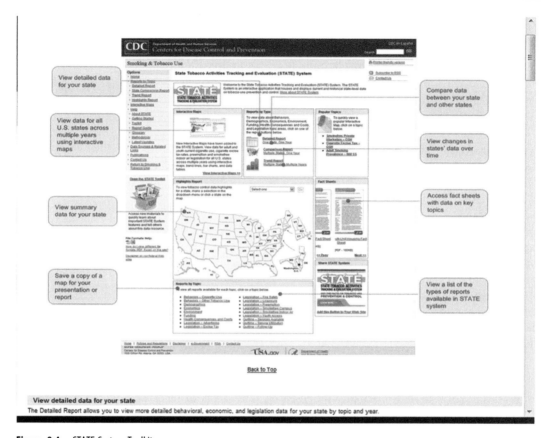

Figure 9.4   STATE System Toolkit

Source: Centers for Disease Control and Prevention (nd-b).

The CDC has developed the STATE system toolkit, which provides users with data for the United States and each state over multiple years, as well as state summaries. The site provides users with the ability to save copies of maps for presentations or reports (see figure 9.4).

For individuals, the CDC provides information on the health consequences of smoking, secondhand smoke, and smokeless tobacco, as well as suggestions to help people quit smoking. The Tobacco-Free Sports Initiative Campaign is designed to help prevent and reduce the number of youth who use tobacco.

The Say It, Share It tobacco-free campaign (www.betobaccofree.gov), targeting teens, uses videos employing storytelling techniques to help prevent teens from smoking and using tobacco products. In addition, it leverages social media (Facebook, Twitter, and a widget) to reach teens.

Through its Healthier Worksite Initiative the CDC (2010b) has developed resources and toolkits to help employers implement tobacco-free campuses and provide employees with information and resources to quit smoking. The information for employers is comprehensive, ranging from making an initial assessment, to planning (e.g., communications, timing, and policies), promoting, implementing, and evaluating their tobacco-cessation programs.

National Institutes of Health (NIH)

National Institutes of Health (NIH)
a federal agency under the US Department of Health and Human Services; the primary medical research agency composed of twenty-seven institutes and centers supporting scientific studies with the theme of turning discovery into health

The **National Institutes of Health (NIH)** is the nation's medical research agency, composed of twenty-seven institutes and centers supporting scientific studies with the theme of turning discovery into health (www.nih.gov). Its mission is to

> seek fundamental knowledge about the nature and behavior of living systems and the application of that knowledge to enhance health, lengthen life, and reduce the burdens of illness and disability. (National Institutes of Health, nd)

The NIH is the leading supporter of biomedical research in the world, with an impact that reaches beyond health to job creation and the US economy. The NIH states that the thirty-year increase in life expectancy of a baby born in the United States today, compared to one born in 1900, is due in large part to NIH research. The areas of research covered by NIH are broad, ranging from the lifelong impact of acute kidney injury, to wonders of the brain, to the landscape of genomics.

Clinical Center

The NIH Clinical Center is the home of NIH clinical research trials and is devoted entirely to clinical research. The Clinical Center facilitates the rapid translation of scientific observations and laboratory discoveries into medical approaches to diagnose, treat, and prevent disease. Findings from clinical trials are also communicated to the public through traditional news channels. Examples of recently successful clinical trial research projects include the HPV anticancer vaccine technology that led to the first FDA-approved vaccine against cancer (Intramural Research Program, nd) and a vaccine to protect against the Ebola virus infection, which was recently proven effective among monkeys and is now being tested in humans.

Chronic Disease Institutes

Health promotion professionals benefit from work conducted by the National Heart, Lung, and Blood Institute (NHLBI) (www.nhlbi.nih.gov) and the National Institute of Diabetes and Digestive and Kidney Diseases

(NIDDK) (www.niddk.nih.gov). The NHLBI's Heart Truth program is widely recognized by the red dress logo during American Heart Month (February). The aim of Heart Truth is to unite women in the fight against their number one killer: heart disease. The campaign increases awareness of risk factors and empowers women and their families to take steps to reduce their risks. NHLBI provides resources and tools for the public on heart disease, cholesterol, heart attacks, high blood pressure, sleep disorders, being overweight, and physical activity.

NIDDK's National Diabetes Program provides resources to individuals, families, and communities on preventing, managing, and treating diabetes. These include questionnaires, publications, and a recommended team approach strategy—which involves businesses, schools, and health care professionals. Through the HealthSense initiative, materials and resources can be personalized based on age, ethnicity, diabetes status, and language (www.ndep.nih.gov). This initiative addresses diabetes from a comprehensive approach, including information on stress and emotions, healthy eating, active living, and weight management.

US Department of Agriculture (USDA)

The **US Department of Agriculture (USDA)** (www.cnpp.usda.gov) is responsible for the development and dissemination of the Dietary Guidelines for Americans, the cornerstone of federal nutrition policy and nutrition education activities. Every five years, USDA and HHS jointly update and issue these guidelines, centered on reducing caloric intake, making informed food choices, and being physically active for individuals aged two years and older. The most recent guidelines were issued in 2010 and will be updated again in 2015 (see table 9.2).

The dietary guidelines recognize that many Americans do not eat foods that are adequately nutritious, even though they are available. The guidelines provide recommendations based on two major concepts:

- Maintain calorie balance over time to achieve and sustain a healthy weight.

- Focus on consuming nutrient-dense foods and beverages (e.g., limiting sodium, solid fats, added sugars, and refined grains while emphasizing fruits, vegetables, whole grains, low-fat or fat-free milk products, seafood, lean meats, poultry, eggs, beans, peas, nuts, and seeds).

Recommendations are provided for the general public and for specific populations (e.g., pregnant or breastfeeding women and individuals over fifty).

US Department of Agriculture (USDA) the US government's primary agricultural agency responsible for supporting America's agriculture and providing safe and nutritious foods to the US public; responsible for the development and dissemination of the dietary guidelines for Americans

Table 9.2   Key Recommendations from the Dietary Guidelines for Americans, 2010

Balancing Calories to Manage Weight; Foods and Food Components to Reduce

* Reduce daily sodium intake to less than 2,300 milligrams (mg) and further reduce intake to 1,500 mg among persons who are fifty-one and older and those of any age who are African American or have hypertension, diabetes, or chronic kidney disease. The 1,500 mg recommendation applies to about half of the US population, including children and the majority of adults.
* Consume less than 10% of calories from saturated fatty acids by replacing them with monounsaturated and polyunsaturated fatty acids.
* Consume less than 300 mg per day of dietary cholesterol.
* Keep trans fatty acid consumption as low as possible by limiting foods that contain synthetic sources of trans fats, such as partially hydrogenated oils, and by limiting other solid fats.
* Reduce the intake of calories from solid fats and added sugars.
* Limit the consumption of foods that contain refined grains, especially refined grain foods that contain solid fats, added sugars, and sodium.
* If alcohol is consumed, it should be consumed in moderation—up to one drink per day for women and two drinks per day for men—and only by adults of legal drinking age.

Foods and Nutrients to Increase
Individuals should meet the following recommendations as part of a healthy eating pattern while staying within their calorie needs:

* Increase vegetable and fruit intake.
* Eat a variety of vegetables, especially dark-green and red and orange vegetables and beans and peas.
* Consume at least half of all grains as whole grains. Increase whole-grain intake by replacing refined grains with whole grains.
* Increase intake of fat-free or low-fat milk and milk products, such as milk, yogurt, cheese, or fortified soy beverages.
* Choose a variety of protein foods, which include seafood, lean meat and poultry, eggs, beans and peas, soy products, and unsalted nuts and seeds.
* Increase the amount and variety of seafood consumed by choosing seafood in place of some meat and poultry.
* Replace protein foods that are higher in solid fats with choices that are lower in solid fats and calories or are sources of oils.
* Use oils to replace solid fats when possible.
* Choose foods that provide more potassium, dietary fiber, calcium, and vitamin D, which are nutrients of concern in American diets. These foods include vegetables, fruits, whole grains, and milk and milk products.

Building Healthy Eating Patterns

* Select an eating pattern that meets nutrient needs over time at an appropriate calorie level.
* Account for all foods and beverages consumed and assess how they fit within a total healthy eating pattern.
* Follow food safety recommendations when preparing and eating foods to reduce the risk of foodborne illnesses.

Monitoring the Nation's Health

The CDC and other HHS divisions use multiple federal datasets to monitor the nation's health. Using these data, federal departments, agencies, and divisions with health-related responsibilities produce reports, publications, and recommendations to address specific areas of focus.

Behavioral Risk Factor Surveillance System (BRFSS)

The **Behavioral Risk Factor Surveillance System (BRFSS)** (www.cdc .gov/brfss) is the world's largest, ongoing telephone health survey system, tracking and reporting on health conditions and risk behaviors in the United States on an annual basis since 1984. Currently, data are collected monthly in all fifty states, the District of Columbia, Puerto Rico, the US Virgin Islands, and Guam. More than 350,000 adults are interviewed annually. Their responses help identify emerging public health problems, track trends, develop objectives, and formulate policies and programs at the national and state levels. These data are made available to researchers and policy makers. As mentioned previously, one of the aims of HHS is to provide relevant data and tools to researchers, practitioners, and the general public to enable them to access and understand available data more readily.

Each month a cross-sectional representation of the US adult population (eighteen years of age and older) is randomly contacted by state health departments. Only one respondent per household is permitted. The questions asked are drawn from a standardized questionnaire related to risk behaviors and health practices. There are core questions that are asked annually, a set of rotating core questions asked every other year, and emerging core questions focused on late-breaking health issues. There are also optional modules that states may choose to administer. State health departments forward data to the CDC, which then compiles a monthly aggregate for each state and publishes the results on the BRFSS website. The BRFSS data and questionnaires are available to view online (see figure 9.5).

Behavioral Risk Factor Surveillance System (BRFSS)
the world's largest, ongoing telephone health survey system, tracking and reporting on health conditions and risk behaviors in the United States on an annual basis

Youth Risk Behavior Surveillance System (YRBSS)

The **Youth Risk Behavior Surveillance System (YRBSS)** (www.cdc.gov /yrbs) is conducted among middle and high school students in the United States to assess health-risk behaviors that typically contribute to the leading causes of death and disability in this age group including the following:

- Behaviors that contribute to unintentional injuries and violence
- Sexual behaviors that contribute to unintended pregnancy and sexually transmitted diseases, including HIV infection
- Alcohol and other drug use
- Tobacco use
- Unhealthy dietary behaviors
- Inadequate physical activity

Youth Risk Behavior Surveillance System (YRBSS)
a survey conducted among middle and high school students in the United States to monitor health-risk behaviors that contribute to the leading causes of death and disability among youth and adults

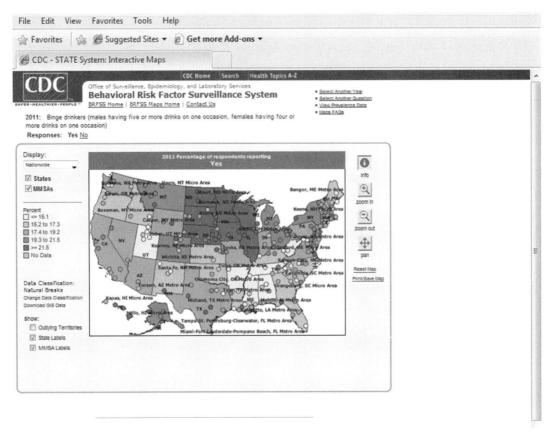

Figure 9.5   BRFSS Map Showing 2010 Data for Alcohol Consumption

Note: Respondents who answered "yes" to binge drinking (males having five or more drinks on one occasion, females having four or more drinks on one occasion)

Source: Centers for Disease Control and Prevention (2010a).

The YRBSS also measures the prevalence of obesity and asthma among youth and young adults and includes a national school-based survey conducted by state, territorial, and local education and health agencies and tribal governments.

Similar to the BRFSS for adults, YRBSS data are used to track progress toward meeting health goals and objectives, identify trends, and develop relevant legislation, policy, and programming. YRBSS data may also be used to seek funding to support new initiatives.

The national YRBSS is conducted every two years during the spring semester. During one class period, a survey administrator distributes survey materials and reads directions to the students. Students complete the questionnaire in approximately thirty-five minutes. Participation is voluntary and anonymous; local parental permission procedures are followed

Trends in the Prevalence of Behaviors that Contribute to Violence
National YRBS: 1991–2011

YRBSS

The national Youth Risk Behavior Survey (YRBS) monitors priority health risk behaviors that contribute to the leading causes of death, disability, and social problems among youth and adults in the United States. The national YRBS is conducted every two years during the spring semester and provides data representative of 9th through 12th grade students in public and private schools throughout the United States.

1991	1993	1995	1997	1999	2001	2003	2005	2007	2009	2011	Changes from 1991–2011[1]	Change from 2009–2011[2]
Carried a weapon on at least 1 day (for example, a gun, knife, or club during the 30 days before the survey)												
26.1 (23.7–28.5)[3]	22.1 (19.8–24.6)	20.0 (18.8–21.4)	18.3 (16.5–20.2)	17.3 (15.4–19.3)	17.4 (15.5–19.5)	17.1 (15.4–19.0)	18.5 (16.9–20.2)	18.0 (16.3–19.8)	17.5 (16.1–19.0)	16.6 (15.4–18.0)	Decreased, 1991–1999 No change, 1999–2011	No change
Carried a gun on at least 1 day (during the 30 days before the survey)												
NA[4]	7.9 (6.7–9.3)	7.6 (6.5–8.7)	5.9 (5.1–6.8)	4.9 (3.8–6.3)	5.7 (4.8–6.8)	6.1 (5.1–7.2)	5.4 (4.6–6.3)	5.2 (4.4–6.0)	5.9 (5.1–6.9)	5.1 (4.6–5.7)	Decreased, 1993–1999 No change, 1999–2011	No change
In a physical fight one or more times (during the 12 months before the survey)												
42.5 (40.0–45.0)	41.8 (39.8–43.8)	38.7 (36.5–40.9)	36.6 (34.7–38.7)	35.7 (33.4–38.1)	33.2 (31.8–34.7)	33.0 (31.1–35.1)	35.9 (34.3–37.4)	35.5 (34.0–37.1)	31.5 (30.1–32.9)	32.8 (31.5–34.1)	Decreased, 1991–2009 No change, 2009–2011	No change
Injured in a physical fight one or more times (injuries had to be treated by a doctor or nurse, during the 12 months before the survey)												
4.4 (3.6–5.3)	4.0 (3.2–5.0)	4.2 (3.6–4.8)	3.5 (3.0–4.1)	4.0 (3.3–4.8)	4.0 (3.6–4.5)	4.2 (3.4–5.3)	3.6 (3.2–4.0)	4.2 (3.7–4.7)	3.8 (3.3–4.3)	3.9 (3.4–4.4)	Decreased, 1991–2011	No change
Carried a weapon on school property on at least 1 day (for example, a gun, knife, or club during the 30 days before the survey)												
NA	11.8 (10.4–13.3)	9.8 (8.9–10.7)	8.5 (7.1–10.2)	6.9 (5.8–8.2)	6.4 (5.5–7.6)	6.1 (5.1–7.4)	6.5 (5.6–7.5)	5.9 (5.2–6.7)	5.6 (5.0–6.3)	5.4 (4.7–6.1)	Decreased, 1993–2003 No change, 2003–2011	No change
In a physical fight on school property one or more times (during the 12 months before the survey)												
NA	16.2 (15.1–17.5)	15.5 (13.9–17.2)	14.8 (13.6–16.2)	14.2 (13.0–15.5)	12.5 (11.5–13.5)	12.8 (11.3–14.4)	13.6 (12.5–14.7)	12.4 (11.5–13.4)	11.1 (10.0–12.2)	12.0 (11.3–12.8)	Decreased, 1993–2009 No change, 2009–2011	No change
Threatened or injured with a weapon on school property one or more times (for example, a gun, knife, or club during the 12 months before the survey)												
NA	7.3 (6.5–8.3)	8.4 (7.3–9.7)	7.4 (6.5–8.3)	7.7 (6.9–8.6)	8.9 (7.9–10.1)	9.2 (7.8–10.8)	7.9 (7.2–8.6)	7.8 (7.0–8.8)	7.7 (6.9–8.5)	7.4 (6.8–8.1)	No change, 1993–2003 Decreased, 2003–2011	No change
Did not go to school because they felt unsafe at school or on their way to or from school on at least 1 day (during the 30 days before the survey)												
NA	4.4 (3.7–5.2)	4.5 (3.8–5.3)	4.0 (3.4–4.7)	5.2 (4.0–6.8)	6.6 (5.7–7.7)	5.4 (4.7–6.3)	6.0 (4.9–7.4)	5.5 (4.7–6.3)	5.0 (4.3–5.7)	5.9 (5.1–6.9)	No change, 1993–2011	No change

Figure 9.6   Sample YRBSS Report

Source: Centers for Disease Control and Prevention (2012b).

prior to the administration of the YRBSS. The data represent all public and private school students in the fifty states and the District of Columbia. An example of the type of data collected by the National YRBS is included in figure 9.6.

National Health and Nutrition Examination Survey (NHANES)

The **National Health and Nutrition Examination Survey (NHANES)** (www.cdc.gov/nchs/nhanes.htm) is a program of studies designed to assess the health and nutritional status of adults and children in the United States. The survey is unique in that it combines interviews and physical examinations. NHANES is administered by the CDC through the National Center for Health Statistics. It was launched in the 1960s, focusing on different populations or health topics. In 1999, it became a continuous program

National Health and Nutrition Examination Survey (NHANES)

a program of studies, including interviews and physical examinations, to assess the health and nutritional status of adults and children in the United States focusing on a variety of changing health and nutrition measurements. Each year, approximately five thousand people from a nationally representative sample are selected across the United States; fifteen counties are visited each year. Each participant receives an exam based on age, gender, and current medical conditions, and the exam results, at no cost. Participants receive compensation for their time. Interviewers determine participants' eligibility, and a one-time health exam at a mobile site is arranged. The tests included in the health exam are listed in table 9.3.

Table 9.3   NHANES Health Exam Tests

Health Measurements by Participant Age and Gender
- Physician's exam—all ages
- Blood pressure—ages 8 years and older
- Bone density—ages 8 years and older
- Condition of teeth—ages 5 years and older
- Vision test—ages 12 years and older
- Hearing test—ages 12–19 years and 70 years and older
- Height, weight, and other body measures—all ages
- Ophthalmology exam for eye diseases—ages 40 and older
- Breathing tests—ages 6–79 years

Lab Tests on Urine: (6 Years and Older)
- Kidney function tests—ages 6 years and older
- Sexually transmitted disease (STD)
- Chlamydia and gonorrhea—ages 14–39
- Exposure to environmental chemicals—selected persons ages 6 and older
- Pregnancy test—females 12 years and older and girls 8–11 years who have periods

Lab Tests on Blood: (1 Year and Older)
- Anemia—all ages
- Total cholesterol and HDL—ages 6 years and older
- Glucose measures—ages 12 years and older
- Infectious diseases—ages 2 years and older
- Kidney function tests—ages 12 years and older
- Lead—ages 1 year and older
- Cadmium—ages 1 year and older
- Mercury—ages 1 year and older
- Liver function tests—ages 12 years and older
- Nutrition status—ages 1 year and older

- Thyroid function test—ages 12 years and older
- Prostate specific antigen (PSA)—males ages 40 years and older
- Sexually transmitted diseases (STD)
- Genital herpes—ages 14–49 years
- Human immunodeficiency virus (HIV)—ages 18–49 years
- Human papillomavirus (HPV) antibody—ages 14–59 years
- Exposure to environmental chemicals—selected persons ages 6 years and older

Lab Tests on Water
- Environmental chemicals—ages 12 years and older in half of households

Other Lab Tests
- Vaginal swabs (self-administered)—females ages 14–59 years
- Human papillomavirus (HPV)—ages 14–59 years

Private Health Interviews
- Health status—ages 12 years and older
- Questions about drug and alcohol use—ages 12 years and older (No drug testing will be done.)
- Nutrition—all ages
- Reproductive health—females ages 12 years and older
- Questions about sexual experience—ages 14–69 years
- Tobacco use—ages 12 years and older

After the Visit to the NHANES Examination Center
- Persons asked about the foods they eat will receive a phone call 3–10 days after their exam for a similar interview, all ages.
- Then participants, or an adult for participants 1–15 years old, will be asked about food shopping habits.
- Persons who test positive for hepatitis C will be asked to participate in a brief telephone interview 6 months after the exam. Parents will respond for children.

Source: Centers for Disease Control and Prevention (2010c).

All information for the home interview and exam are confidential. Data collected are used to identify information and track trends in areas such as birth weight and height charts, diabetes, obesity, and high blood pressure.

State Initiatives

In addition to federal health initiatives, states have their own initiatives aimed at improving the health of their citizens. State health departments primarily provide data-based information and resources to their citizens. Examples of specific state initiatives and activities are provided in the following sections.

Arizona

The Arizona Department of Health Services' Division of Behavioral Health Services has introduced quarterly health initiatives to integrate physical health with behavioral health to improve the general health of individuals (www.azdhs.gov/bhs/qhi). Monthly partnerships are formed between a physical health content expert and the tribal and regional behavioral health authorities to introduce health topics that affect consumers receiving behavioral health services. The first quarter of 2013 focused on mental health and weight; the Division of Behavioral Health Services developed a handout for citizens, along with resources and questions for patients to ask their doctors.

Maine

The Maine Department of Health and Human Services (nd) provides seasonal information to citizens. For example, "Stay Healthy This Winter" provides information and resources regarding burning wood smart and healthy, preventing carbon monoxide intake, and preventing hypothermia.

Florida

Combining data with information for public health partners and stake-holders, Florida has developed a State Health Improvement Plan 2012–2015. Action items include health protection, chronic disease prevention, community relationships and partnerships, access to care, and health finance and infrastructure. Their aims align with the Healthy People 2020 goals, the CDC Community Guide, the CDC Winnable Battles, and the US Preventive Services Task Force guidelines. The Florida plan effec-tively identifies data, coordinating agencies, partners, and stakeholders to provide information that can help make a difference in the health of their state.

EXCERPT FROM THE FLORIDA STATE HEALTH IMPROVEMENT PLAN 2012–2015

Health begins with healthy communities with safe streets, freedom from violence, and parks where kids can play. Health begins with a good education, where children learn not only how to read, write, and prepare for fulfilling, prosperous lives, but how to treat each other with dignity and respect. And health begins with safe jobs and fair wage, where people derive a sense of personal satisfaction from their work and connection to their co-workers . . .

Association of State and Territorial Health Officials (ASTHO)

From an association perspective, the **Association of State and Territorial Health Officials (ASTHO)** (www.astho.org) is the national nonprofit organization representing state-level public health agencies in the United States, the US Territories, and the District of Columbia, and the more than one hundred thousand public health professionals these agencies employ. ASTHO members, the chief health officials of these jurisdictions, formulate and influence sound public health policy and ensure excellence in state-based public health practices. ASTHO's primary function is to track, evaluate, and advise members on the impact and formation of public or private health policy that may affect them and to provide them with guidance and technical assistance on improving the nation's health (Association of State and Territory Health Officials, nd-c). Recent topics include medical marijuana (figure 9.7) and newborn screening for congenital heart defects (figure 9.8).

Association of State and Territorial Health Officials (ASTHO) a national nonprofit organization representing state-level public health agencies in the United States, the US territories, and the more than one hundred thousand public health professionals these agencies employ

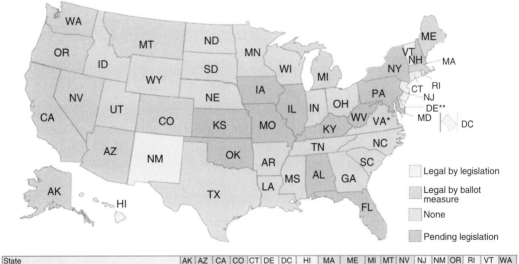

State	AK	AZ	CA	CO	CT	DE	DC	HI	MA	ME	MI	MT	NV	NJ	NM	OR	RI	VT	WA
Year of enactment	98	10	96	00	12	11	11	00	12	99	08	04	00	10	07	98	06	04	98
Affirmative defenses or decriminalization	•	•	•	•	•	•	•	•	•	•	•	•	•	•	•	•	•	•	•
Health Agency Responsibilities — Dispensary permitting		•			•	•		•	•						•	•	•		
Health Agency Responsibilities — Patient registry	•	•	•	•	•	•		•		•	•	•	•	•	•	•			
Health Agency Responsibilities — Caregiver registry	•	•	•	•	•	•			•	•	•	•	•	•	•				
Health Agency Responsibilities — Addition of medical conditions	•	•		•		•	•		•	•	•	•			•	•	•	•	•

Figure 9.7   Legalization of "Medical" Marijuana Map

Notes: *Virginia was the first state to pass a medical marijuana law in 1979. It exempts physicians and pharmacists from state prosecution for prescribing marijuana during the course of treatment for glaucoma or cancer. While on the books, this law has little practical effect.

**The governor of Delaware has suspended implementation due to the possibility of criminal charges against state employees.

Source: Association of State and Territory Health Officials (nd-a).

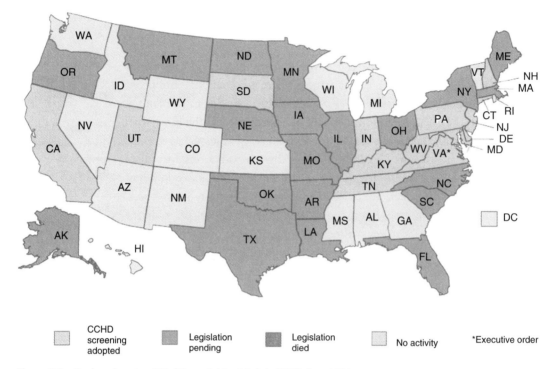

Figure 9.8   Newborn Screening: Critical Congenital Heart Defects (CCHD), Current Status

Source: Association of State and Territory Health Officials (nd-b).

ASTHO also develops annual state legislative and regulatory prospectuses that review available prefiled legislation and survey state health agency legislative liaisons to identify legislative priorities and issues. ASTHO provides an annual summary of findings to facilitate information sharing among states (Association of State and Territory Health Officials, 2013). In the 2013 state legislative and regulatory prospectus, emerging issues such as violence prevention and mental health, drug shortages, and regulation of compounding pharmacies were identified. Health reform implementation, promoting healthy behaviors, food safety, newborn screening, prescription painkiller abuse, misuse and overdose, and synthetic drugs were identified as ongoing issues.

The National Conference of State Legislatures (NCSL)

National Conference of State Legislatures (NCSL)
a bipartisan organization that serves the legislators and staff of the nation's states and territories

The **National Conference of State Legislatures (NCSL)** (www.ncsl.org) is a bipartisan organization that serves the legislators and staff of the nation's states and territories. NCSL provides research, technical assistance, and opportunities for policy makers to exchange ideas on the most pressing state issues. The health topics covered by the NCSL are broad in scope.

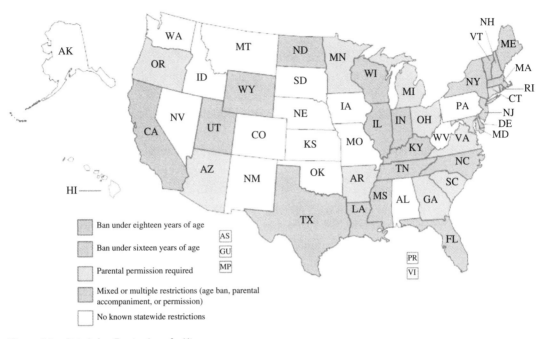

Figure 9.9   State Indoor Tanning Laws for Minors

Source: National Conference of State Legislatures (2012).

Information and data provided to policy makers include bill summaries, articles, news releases, briefs, meetings, and reports. Health conditions covered by NCSL include AIDS/HIV; cancer; chronic disease; diabetes; disability; disease management; heart, stroke, and cardiovascular disease; infectious disease; influenza; obesity; osteoporosis; respiratory diseases; and sexually transmitted diseases.

NCSL provides an overview of information on data and bills. Figure 9.9 shows a US map with information related to state indoor tanning laws for minors.

Local Programs

Programs established in communities through organizations such as YMCAs or Jewish community centers support healthier individuals and communities by providing resources, which may include space, information, and activities for community members. Chapter 10 provides detailed information regarding community-level physical activity initiatives sponsored by the YMCA. Other local programs supporting the health of communities include local farmers' markets and food cooperatives, as well as local health advocacy nonprofits. One example of such an organization is

DC Greens (www.dcgreens.org), an organization based in Washington, DC, that is working to bridge the gaps in the local food system to ensure that all residents of the district have a deeper connection to the sources of their food and can afford fresh, local fruit and vegetables through farmers' markets, school gardens, and farm-to-school programs.

In conjunction with state health departments, cities and districts often implement programs directed to specifically address health issues within a defined area. For example, in Richmond, Virginia, the Richmond City Health Department offers programs that address adolescent health and teen pregnancy prevention (Virginia Department of Health, 2013). The Richmond Environmental Health Division regulates and inspects all city food establishments and vendors to ensure quality service and sanitation. Through the Richmond Emergency Preparedness and Response program, activities are planned to help prepare rapid and effective response to public health emergencies, such as disease outbreaks or natural disasters.

On another level, local Chambers of Commerce often assist business members in providing health insurance to their employees. This is particularly helpful for small business owners who otherwise cannot afford health insurance. With the ACA, the landscape of health care coverage is changing. However, up until 2013, provision of employee health insurance coverage had been an important health support at the local level.

Summary

Using data collected by federal organizations such as the CDC can help health promoters and policy makers identify leading health threats. Health issues facing communities affect the nation as a whole. HHS has developed the Healthy People 2020 goals as a guidepost for the nation to meet certain levels of health. Using these goals, health promotion professionals can develop plans, policies, and programs to help improve the health of individuals, businesses, churches, schools, communities, states, and, ultimately, the health of all Americans.

KEY TERMS

1.   **US Department of Health and Human Services (HHS):** the US government's principal agency tasked with protecting the health of all Americans and providing essential human services

2. **Healthy People:** ten-year national health objectives for Americans released by the US Department of Health and Human Services

3. **Centers for Disease Control and Prevention (CDC):** a federal agency under the US Department of Health and Human Services responsible for the public health of the nation; works to protect the public health and safety of people in the United States by tracking, detecting, and responding to threats

4. **National Institutes of Health (NIH):** a federal agency under the US Department of Health and Human Services; the primary medical research agency composed of twenty-seven institutes and centers supporting scientific studies with the theme of turning discovery into health

5. **US Department of Agriculture (USDA):** the US government's primary agricultural agency responsible for supporting America's agriculture and providing safe and nutritious foods to the US public; responsible for the development and dissemination of the dietary guidelines for Americans

6. **Behavioral Risk Factor Surveillance Survey (BRFSS):** the world's largest, ongoing telephone health survey system, tracking and reporting on health conditions and risk behaviors in the United States on an annual basis

7. **Youth Risk Behavior Surveillance Survey (YRBSS):** a survey conducted among middle and high school students in the United States to monitor health-risk behaviors that contribute to the leading causes of death and disability among youth and adults

8. **National Health and Nutrition Examination Survey (NHANES):** a program of studies, including interviews and physical examinations, to assess the health and nutritional status of adults and children in the United States

9. **Association of State and Territorial Health Officials (ASTHO):** a national nonprofit organization representing state-level public health agencies in the United States, the US territories, and the more than one hundred thousand public health professionals these agencies employ

10. **National Conference of State Legislatures (NCSL):** a bipartisan organization that serves the legislators and staff of the nation's states and territories

REVIEW QUESTIONS

1. How would you describe the history of the Healthy People initiative?

2. What are the leading health indicators for Healthy People 2020?

3. What is the importance of monitoring health practices of people in the United States?

4. How is this information connected to program planning discussed in chapter 3?

5. What is the mission of the National Institutes of Health?

6. What are the Dietary Guidelines for Americans?

7. How do the Dietary Guidelines for Americans connect with the nutrition-related chronic diseases discussed in chapter 5?

8. What is the contribution of social marketing campaigns to health behavior change?

9. What are the state-level activities that drive health promotion?

10. What does the acronym NHANES stand for and what is it?

11. How important is it to visually represent health behaviors using a US map?

STUDENT ACTIVITIES

1. The initiative of Healthy People has a long history. How important is it that the Department of Health and Human Services establish goals each decade? Who is the target audience? How does the target audience engage in the process?

2. Review the Department of Health and Human Services' organizational chart and identify each person by name.

3. For the state you are from, identify three facts using the BRFSS and three using the YRBFSS.

References

Association of State and Territory Health Officials. (2013). *2013 state legislative and regulatory prospectus.* Retrieved from www.astho.org/Advocacy/2013-Prospectus

Association of State and Territory Health Officials. (nd-a). *Legalization of "medical" marijuana map.* Retrieved from www.astho.org/Public-Policy/State-Health -Policy/Medical-Marijuana-State-Map

Association of State and Territory Health Officials. (nd-b). *Newborn screening— Congenital heart disease, current status.* Retrieved from www.astho.org/Public -Policy/State-Health-Policy/Newborn-Screening-Heart-Defects-Map

Association of State and Territory Health Officials. (nd-c). *State health policy.* Retrieved from www.astho.org/Public-Policy/State-Health-Policy

Centers for Disease Control and Prevention. (2010a). *Behavioral risk factor surveillance system.* Retrieved from http://apps.nccd.cdc.gov/gisbrfss/select_question .aspx

Centers for Disease Control and Prevention. (2010b). *Healthier worksite initiative.* Retrieved from www.cdc.gov/nccdphp/dnpao/hwi

Centers for Disease Control and Prevention. (2010c). *National health and nutrition examination survey, health exam tests.* Retrieved from www.cdc.gov/nchs /nhanes/testcomp.htm

Centers for Disease Control and Prevention. (2012a, December 14). *CDC organization.* Retrieved from www.cdc.gov/about/organization/cio.htm

Centers for Disease Control and Prevention. (2012b). *Trends in the prevalence of behaviors that contribute to violence national YRBS: 1991–2011.* Retrieved from www.cdc.gov/healthyyouth/yrbs/pdf/us_violence_trend_yrbs.pdf

Centers for Disease Control and Prevention. (2014). *FluView.* Retrieved from http:// gis.cdc.gov/grasp/fluview/main.html

Centers for Disease Control and Prevention. (nd-a). *State tobacco activities tracking and evaluation (STATE) system.* Retrieved from http://apps.nccd.cdc.gov/state system/InteractiveReport/InteractiveReports.aspx?MeasureID=4

Centers for Disease Control and Prevention. (nd-b). *Getting started.* Retrieved from http://apps.nccd.cdc.gov/statesystem/help/help_gettingstarted.aspx

Florida Department of Health. (2012). *Florida state health improvement plan 2012– 2015.* Retrieved from www.doh.state.fl.us/Planning_eval/Strategic_Planning /SHIP/FloridaSHIP2012-2015.pdf

Intramural Research Program. (nd). *Clinical trials.* Retrieved from http://irp.nih .gov/nih-clinical-center/clinical-trials

Maine Department of Health and Human Services. (nd). *Stay healthy this winter.* Retrieved from www.maine.gov/dhhs/mecdc/environmental-health/heat-2008 .shtml

National Conference of State Legislatures. (2012). *State indoor tanning laws for minors.* Retrieved from www.ncsl.org/issues-research/health/indoor-tanning -restrictions.aspx

National Institutes of Health. (nd). *About NIH.* Retrieved from www.nih.gov/about /mission.htm

US Department of Health and Human Services. (2010, December 2). *HHS announces the nation's new health promotion and disease prevention agenda.* Retrieved from www.hhs.gov/news/press/2010pres/12/20101202a.html

US Department of Health and Human Services, Office of the Surgeon General, National Prevention Council. (2011). *National prevention strategy.* Retrieved from www.healthcare.gov/prevention/nphpphc/strategy/report.pdf

US Department of Health and Human Services. (2014, March 10). *HHS strategic plan and secretary's strategic initiatives.* Retrieved from www.hhs.gov/strategic -plan/priorities.html

US Department of Health and Human Services. (nd-a). *Healthy people 2020*. Retrieved from www.healthypeople.gov/2020/about/default.aspx

US Department of Health and Human Services. (nd-b). *About HHS*. Retrieved from www.hhs.gov/about

US Department of Health and Human Services. (nd-c). *HHS organizational chart*. Retrieved from www.hhs.gov/about/orgchart

Virginia Department of Health. (2013). *Programs*. Retrieved from www.vdh.state.va .us/LHD/richmondcity/programs.htm

CHAPTER 10

SETTINGS FOR HEALTH PROMOTION

David Stevenson

Inspirational and effective health promotion programs and services may be offered in many different settings where healthy lifestyle habits can be developed, nurtured, and sustained. The unique characteristics and strengths of environments where people live, learn, work, relax, recover, and worship can be used in teaching, modeling, and supporting positive health behaviors. Although settings may be very different, characteristics common to all effective health promotion programs include competent and enthusiastic leadership, a feeling of being welcome and safe, camaraderie among participants and with staff, involvement and adherence to proven programs and services, and measures of success leading to a sense of achievement. Health promotion programs and settings also offer excellent opportunities for professional and volunteer leaders to make a positive effect on the health and well-being of others. Let's explore diverse settings where healthy lifestyles can be developed, promoted, and supported (Breckon, Harvey, & Lancaster, 1998; Floyd & Allen, 2004).

The Home

An individual's place of residence is likely to be the most important setting for the development of positive health behaviors. Including time for sleep, most individuals spend twelve to fifteen hours at home each day (U.S. Department of Labor, 2011). The development of new technology including improved access to information

LEARNING OBJECTIVES

After reading this chapter, the student will be able to:

- Identify the major settings where health promotion occurs.

- Describe each setting and the opportunities where health promotion professionals can promote health.

- Discuss how the major settings reach people in different places.

- Explain how the settings complement each other.

- Describe how the targeted behaviors are uniquely incorporated into the settings.

- Summarize opportunities for employment and volunteerism in various health promotion settings.

In 2010, the US Department of Health and Human Services launched Healthy People 2020 (www.HealthyPeople.gov) presenting new objectives for improving the health of all Americans. Many of the health promotion settings and concepts presented in this chapter, such as early childhood centers, schools, work sites, physical activity, policies, and structural environments, are included in the new national objectives for improving health and well-being.

(the Internet), expanded opportunities for entertainment (cable television), and new opportunities to interact with others using social media have led to more time being spent in the home. Also contributing to this trend is an expanded use of business technology and home-based offices, enabling individuals to work from home while reducing costs for employees and employers (Matthews et al., 2008). It is also known that more individuals are using their home as a place to exercise. In fact, the Sport and Industry Fitness Association (www.SGMA.com) reports that the purchase of home exercise equipment far outpaces the purchase of exercise equipment by commercial health clubs and other institutions.

Family

Relationships with those held most closely in a person's life can have a profound effect on one's health and wellness. It is understood, therefore, that an individual's family or those whom they live with will play a vital role in their well-being (Umberson, 1987). To explore this concept, we must recognize that society's understanding of the word *family* has changed dramatically since the 1950s. In addition to the traditional family of parents and children, today's home often supports a new definition of family. Multigenerational families, foster homes, same-sex families, group homes, and homes supporting individuals with disabilities are a few examples of the diversity in the composition of today's modern family.

In families led by adults, the modeling and leadership offered by a parent, guardian, or caregiver is critical to the healthy development of the child (Golan & Crow, 2004). Children who live in a household where healthy foods are served, where fun physical activity is modeled and encouraged, where access to screen time (television, computers, hand-held devices) is limited, and where the day begins after a good night's sleep will have a great foundation for lifelong well-being. Inversely, living in a home with easy access to unhealthy foods, where little physical activity takes place, where family members are glued to screens in a motionless state for many hours each day, and where family members start the day without proper rest can have a devastating effect on the health and well-being of all in the home.

Physical Space

The **physical space** of the home may also support or detract from an individual's pursuit of a healthy lifestyle. Modern inventions designed to minimize physical exertion have achieved their goal. Conveniences such as the power garage door opener, washing machine, TV remote, and self-propelled lawn mower facilitate the completion of life's daily chores, often with just the lift of a finger. The physical requirements of daily chores for many in modern American society have been reduced to such an extent that exercise must be intentionally pursued to maintain health and wellness. Many leading health experts have pointed to this physical inactivity crisis as a major contributor to the epidemic of overweight and obesity taking place in developed countries (van Sluijs, McMinn, & Griffin, 2007).

physical space
the physical makeup of the home, office, or other environment; changes to one's personal space can make daily activities easier to complete, but require less physical movement, making exercise a task to be intentionally pursued

personal trainer
a fitness professional involved in exercise prescription and instruction; motivates clients by setting goals and providing feedback and accountability

According to the National Association of the Remodeling Industry (www.NARI.com), adding or renovating a home exercise space offers the owner a major advantage—convenience. As the number of home exercisers continues to grow, the dedication of space for fitness activities in the American home is becoming more common.

Personal Training

Services provided by a **personal trainer** in the home or other venues can offer the encouragement, support, and guidance necessary for improvement of an individual's health and wellness. Excellent personal trainers possess sound **interpersonal communication skills**, knowledge in exercise science, and understand how to inspire individuals to adopt and maintain healthy living habits. Personal trainers should be certified in emergency response including cardiopulmonary resuscitation and often possess certification through the American College of Sports Medicine (www.ACSM.org), National Strength and Conditioning Association (www.NSCA.com), YMCA (www.YMCA.net), National Academy of Sports Medicine (www .NASM.org), or other certifying organizations. Chapter 11 provides more detail on personal training certifications and other health promotion related certifications.

interpersonal communication skills
the process by which people exchange information, feelings, and meaning through verbal and nonverbal messages; message content can be seen as equally important as how it is said, including the tone of voice, facial expressions, gestures, and body language

Physical Safety

Serious accidents can take place in the home, particularly involving young children and older adults. Special precautions can be employed to minimize safety risks in the home by installing adequate lighting and skid protection, limiting access to stairways, securing hazardous chemicals, and ensuring safe access and use of ladders, appliances, and swimming pools. Safety measures in homes where older adults live may include walking surfaces free of obstructions such as extension cords, grab bars in bathrooms enabling safe use, access to handrails and other support around stairways, and communications systems that can be easily accessed in case of an emergency. Excellent home safety tips are offered by organizations such as the American Association of Retired Persons (AARP) and the National Association of Home Builders (NAHB).

Communities

communities

defined as families and individuals living or working in close proximity and who share common services

Defined as families and individuals living or working in close proximity and who share common services, **communities** serve as an excellent setting for the promotion of health. Grassroots community health initiatives have proven to be very effective in reducing health risks and promoting healthy lifestyles (Kaiser Permanente, 2008). Strategies and programs developed by not-for-profit organizations, schools, health care providers, and local government agencies have led to community-wide health promotion opportunities including the following:

- Health education through community health fairs and seminars

- New opportunities for physical activity through community walks and fun runs, expanded green spaces, bike lanes, and better sidewalks

- Easier access to healthy foods grown in community gardens or sold at local farmers' markets

We have also learned that comprehensive community wellness initiatives developed and offered by organizations working in partnership will expand and strengthen the impact desired in improved community health (Perkins, 2002). Not-for-profits, schools, health care providers, and government agencies each bring unique and complementary strengths to providing a comprehensive and collaborative approach to address community health and wellness. When working together, these organizations can have a powerful impact on the lives of many. Funding for community health programming can be particularly challenging because few health and wellness initiatives generate revenue from the users. Local health departments wishing to develop and implement health promotion strategies and programs are often able to secure necessary funding through government grants and support from generous foundations wishing to improve community health. One such organization is the Robert Wood Johnson Foundation (www.RWJF.org), which has funded many community health promotion initiatives throughout the United States.

Health Fairs

A community **health fair** offers an excellent example of organizations coming together to assess the health of local residents and to offer educational services to improve health and well-being.

health fair
an educational and interactive event designed for outreach to provide basic preventive medicine and medical screening to people in the community or employees at a work site

Local hospitals often play a leadership role in organizing health fairs, which can be held in community gathering places such as senior centers, shopping malls, recreation centers, libraries, employee cafeterias, and schools, to name a few. In addition to local hospitals, partners in community health fairs often include physician groups, physical therapy and chiropractic groups, public health departments, weight management groups, and educational and research organizations including the American Heart Association and American Cancer Society among others. Working in an open-space setting where individuals can move from booth to booth, health fair participants can visit with providers in a relaxed and more comfortable environment that contributes to a sense of community.

Targeted Community Initiatives

The Young Men's Christian Association (the Y) offers an excellent model aimed at improving community health through the Diabetes Prevention Program (www.ymca.net/diabetes-prevention) supported by local Y staff leadership and in partnership with a national health insurer. The goal of the program is to identify and coach those at risk for type 2 diabetes through education and coaching programs over the course of one year. The program is multifaceted because local Ys work with health care providers and other local organizations to encourage participation and program adherence.

Another example of an excellent community health initiative can be found in urban biking programs through which physical activity is increased and the use of automobiles is decreased, thereby reducing traffic congestion and carbon emissions. Effective collaborations among biking enthusiasts, local government, bicycle manufacturers, and local bike shops have led to improved biker safety including new bike lanes, the availability of bikes for rent at convenient locations, and improved awareness and acceptance of bicycles in cities and towns.

Farmers' Markets and Community Gardens

Farmers' markets and community gardens are great examples of settings for health promotion. This is especially true in urban areas that may be struggling to provide residents with easy access to healthy foods. Growers who bring their harvest and other goods to a local community serve many purposes in addition to providing a variety of healthy food at reasonable prices. The opportunities to learn about the health benefits of different foods, for socialization (also a component of good health!), and to stimulate the local economy are all positive benefits of farmers' markets. Community gardens also expand a community's healthy food choices, promote socialization, and increase physical activity.

Volunteer Opportunities

Programs and services designed to strengthen community health and wellness offer exciting opportunities for volunteerism. Offering one's time to work at health fairs, lead a community wellness initiative, or support a farmers' market or community garden can lead to great personal satisfaction and program success, and can positively affect the program's financial picture. National health organizations, including the American Heart Association (www.Heart.org), American Lung Association (www.Lung.org), American Cancer Society (www.Cancer.org), and many others, offer excellent volunteer development opportunities.

Early Childhood Centers

It is well accepted that a significant portion of an individual's development takes place in the early years of life. Bonding with loved ones, learning how to socialize with other children, and developing learning skills are all characteristics of healthy development at a young age. The early childhood setting, which can include full- and part-day child care as well as nursery or prekindergarten programs, also offers an excellent opportunity to teach, model, and provide opportunities for healthy activities that can lead to positive lifetime habits. Characteristics of early childhood programs that offer excellent health promotion components include the following:

- Validation of a child's current health status before entering a program including a health history, preenrollment physician clearance, and proper immunizations

- Leadership from staff members who teach and model positive health behaviors including proper hygiene and safety

- Opportunities for physical play that are embedded in the early childhood program experience
- Offerings of healthy and flavorful foods
- Opportunities for health examinations including vision and hearing assessments

Hygiene and Safety Habits

Quality-based not-for-profit and for-profit early childhood centers, including nationwide providers such as the Y and KinderCare, incorporate intellectual, physical, social, and emotional development into their curriculum for preschool children. In most states, child care teachers and support staff are required to meet stringent certification requirements in all areas of child development and administration including components of healthy development through physical activity, nutrition, and proper safety practices. Excellent child care organizations encourage modeling by their staff in proper hygiene, such as hand washing, proper handling of food, and how to protect others when sneezing or coughing. Staff members are required to follow safety practices thereby demonstrating to children how to avoid accidents. Special attention is given to the safe use of sharp objects such as scissors, toys, arts and crafts supplies, and the proper use of equipment including playgrounds, sports gear, bicycles, and tricycles.

Physical Activity

Quality-based child care programs will include scheduled times for structured physical activity and free-play time for children throughout the day. Organized programs are led by trained professionals and may include activities ranging from group games to swimming lessons. Fair play, sportsmanship, safety, and the joy of physical activity are modeled and rewarded by staff leaders. Equally important to a child's well-being and development is time spent in free play (Ginsburg, 2007). Also referred to as free-range play or recess, unstructured playtime enables children to have fun and enjoy physical activity while expressing themselves, building new relationships, exploring new environments, and developing new skills and abilities.

Nutrition and Healthy Eating Habits

Proper nutrition and healthy eating are vital components of the early childhood experience. Many children enrolled in a full-day child care program will eat two to three meals and one or more snacks during their time at the center. To ensure a healthy diet, special care should be given to developing a menu that is well balanced, flavorful, and age appropriate. Serving food to young children that tastes good including fruits and vegetables will begin good eating habits that can last for a lifetime. For those children who bring food to the center, staff members are encouraged to educate parents or guardians about proper nutrition for a developing child. Serving an occasional meal to the entire family at the early childhood center will enable families to spend time together while enjoying a healthy meal and reinforcing good health habits. It will also give staff time to interact with parents or guardians on a more relaxed basis (other than drop off or pickup). Serving food also presents opportunities to teach children about safe ways in which to handle and store food and the postmeal procedures for cleanup and dishwashing.

Health Assessments

health assessments
a plan of care that identifies the specific needs of the client and how these needs will be addressed by the health care system or skilled nursing facility; in an early childhood setting may include annual on-site examinations for general health, vision, hearing, dental, and speech

Early childhood programs serving low-income families, such as Head Start (www.acf.hhs.gov/programs/ohs), offer important opportunities to assess the health and wellness of the preschooler. Often required by the organization's curriculum or licensing agency, **health assessments** may include annual on-site examinations for general health, vision, hearing, dental, and speech. These services offer a valuable benefit to the child and the family who may be uninsured, underinsured, or may not have the funds to pay for or the ability to schedule regular health assessments.

Schools

The use of the elementary, middle, and high school settings to positively affect health habits and future success holds tremendous potential for students, as well as faculty, staff, and members of the community. It is well established that early development of positive health behaviors will likely lead to better health and well-being as an adult and that good health and physical fitness benefit children in many ways including their ability to learn and perform academically (Chomitz, Slining, McGowan, Mitchell, Dawson, & Hacker, 2009).

Quality-based health promotion in a school setting involves far more than what traditional physical education classes typically address. Characteristics of an effective school-based health promotion program include the following:

+ Support from the school principal and governing board who are committed to each child's health, education, and development through health and wellness policy development, curriculum structure, and program funding

- Guidance and support from faculty members and staff to teach and reinforce positive health habits throughout the school day

- Opportunities throughout the day for children to get up and move their bodies; special emphasis is based on progressive physical education programs that teach lifetime fitness skills and daily recess when children can physically play in an unstructured environment

- Offerings of healthy and flavorful foods in the school cafeteria

- Active involvement by the school nurse or health care team to ensure that children have received appropriate exams and screenings and have been identified for follow-up based on their health history or physical exams

- Celebration of improvements in individual and group health, wellness, and fitness with a special emphasis on participation

- Use of school buildings and grounds after traditional school hours (evenings and weekends) to support public recreation, exercise, and other wellness programs

Academics and Health

Elementary and secondary schools are experiencing significant challenges because many of the demands of modern society are placed at their doorsteps. Funding support, increased costs, curriculum demands, political pressures, student performance, the education achievement gap, graduation rates, and aging facilities are but a few of the problems facing today's school boards and administrators. Although improved health and wellness are known to strengthen academic performance, many school systems have reduced or eliminated time dedicated to physical education, health, wellness, and other time for physical activity including recess (National Association for Sport and Physical Education, 2009). Part of this challenge relates to the fact that teachers and administrators are accountable for student *academic* performance and not necessarily for the health and well-being of the student. Time, therefore, is spent on curriculum, classes, and programs that will improve academic test scores. There are exceptions to this trend, and many school districts fully recognize the great value of health promotion in the school setting. These schools offer daily physical education, excellent health education curriculum and programs, and free time for physical activity (recess). Sadly, many school districts have reduced time devoted to these important components of elementary and secondary education.

School Policy Supporting Health

Schools that offer well-developed health, physical education, and health promotion curricula and programs to their students typically enjoy professional and elected leadership who understand the relationship between investment in student health and well-being and the resulting positive effect on academic performance. These school superintendents and boards have developed and adopted **school wellness policies** designed to strengthen student health and wellness, and have worked hard to maintain adequate funding for these important programs. In fact, federal law enacted in 2006 requires all public school districts to adopt and implement a wellness policy including goals for nutrition education, nutrition guidelines, physical activity, parental and community involvement in policy development and review, and a plan to measure the implementation of the wellness policies. Although modest progress has been made, only 46% of students attended schools in 2010–2011 with a wellness policy that included all of the required elements (Robert Wood Johnson Foundation, 2013). Excellent school administrators understand that student health and wellness mean more than athletics and sports teams. Curriculum addresses current-day health challenges facing youth including overweight and obesity, physical inactivity, poor eating habits, and substance abuse, to name a few. Great school-based health promotion programs also offer physical activity programs designed for *all* students, not just the select few on the competitive sports teams.

school wellness policies

an important tool for parents, local educational agencies, and school districts in promoting student wellness, preventing and reducing childhood obesity, and providing assurance that school meal nutrition guidelines meet the minimum federal school meal standards

Teachers' Roles

Schools offering excellent student health promotion programs have also gained the enthusiastic support of faculty members and staff who model, teach, and encourage healthy behaviors and activities within their student populations. Often times, these teachers do more than simply talk about health and well-being; they are personally committed to living a healthy lifestyle and use the greatest teaching tool known—personal example. In fact, many progressive school districts have implemented comprehensive health promotion programs for faculty members and staff based on the philosophy that an investment in an individual's health and well-being will lead to improved performance in the workplace—in this case, the classroom.

Healthy Food Choices

Offering healthy and flavorful foods that students want to eat is a vital component of an effective school-based health promotion program. The often-maligned school lunch has endured many negative stereotypes in which children have shunned the bland and tasteless food offered by the school in favor of sweet or salty items such as snack foods and dessert items available in the cafeteria. Sadly, some administrators view their cafeteria or food service as a profit center to generate revenue through the sale of popular yet often unhealthy foods. Doughnuts in the morning, vending machines selling high-sugar drinks, and ice cream bars may add to a school's bottom line, but they do not contribute to students' health and wellness. In response to growing concerns from parents and others about healthy food choices, and youth overweight and obesity, the Healthy Hunger-Free Kids Act was passed in 2010 to improve school nutrition standards. Many school districts have reinvented the school meal offerings to include foods lower in fat and calories, higher in complex carbohydrates, and use locally grown produce (often coming from the school garden!), colorful food choices, and foods that are prepared using healthy cooking techniques. Enlightened school administrators, nutritionists, and cafeteria managers are creating a healthy school meal experience that kids enjoy and that contributes to student well-being.

School Health Care Services

The role played by the school nurse and health care team has become more than simply making sure that students have gotten their shots and that the medical forms are filled out properly. Efficient administration is still required, but many school districts have expanded the role of the school nurse to include identification of students who may exhibit serious health concerns and developing programs targeted toward students based on health challenges. Working as a team, the school nurse, principal, health and physical education teacher, and classroom teacher can develop individualized health plans for students aimed at addressing specific concerns. Many schools have adopted plans to identify students with high **body mass index (BMI)** and have developed programs in partnership with hospitals, Ys, and others in an effort to help students gain and maintain ideal body weight. A popular program used by many school districts is the **Let's Go! 5210 program** in which on a daily basis students strive to eat five servings of fruits and vegetables, limit screen time to two hours, be physically active for one hour, and consume zero sugared drinks (www.letsgo.org). Programs such as the 5210 Club are strengthened when families are invited to participate.

Health Promotion Initiatives

Recognition and celebration inspire students to continue in the pursuit of healthy living and can come in many forms. Simple recognition for student

body mass index (BMI) a weight-to-height ratio, calculated by dividing one's weight in kilograms by the square of one's height in meters; it is used as an indicator of overweight, obesity, ideal weight, and underweight status

Let's Go! 5210 program program in which on a daily basis students strive to eat five servings of fruits and vegetables, limit screen time to two hours, be physically active for one hour, and consume zero sugared drinks

or class success can include a mention of goal achievement in the morning announcements, and more formal celebration can include certificates or other awards or prizes during formal ceremonies such as graduation. Schools with great health promotion programs are always finding new and exciting ways to regularly celebrate success and inspire adherence to healthy living practices.

School After-Hours

School districts committed to health promotion often recognize the opportunity to contribute to community health and wellness by making school buildings and grounds available to the public and not-for-profit organizations who offer recreation, exercise, and wellness programming. Communities that have access to low or no-cost evening and weekend activities and programs held in the school gym, all-purpose room, or on the athletic field enjoy great opportunities to strengthen individual and family health and wellness.

Coordinated School Health

The Centers for Disease Control and Prevention (www.cdc.gov) offers an excellent resource for the development of comprehensive health promotion programs in the school setting. The CDC's (2010) *Components of Coordinated School Health* addresses school-based health education and physical education, health and nutrition services, psychological and social services, a safe school environment, health promotion for staff, and family and community involvement (Marx & Wooley, 1998).

Professional Opportunities

Elementary, middle, and high school settings offer many opportunities for the professional wishing to make a positive impact on the health and wellness of young people. Most school-based teaching positions will require a four-year bachelor's degree in disciplines such as health education or physical education, and a school nurse position will often require a bachelor's degree as well as certification as a school nurse (National Association of Registered School Nurses, nd).

Colleges and Universities

Many public and private institutions of higher education, including two-year community colleges and four-year colleges and universities, now offer formal health promotion programs, services, and facilities to their students, faculty, and staff. Students entering colleges or universities face many new opportunities including decisions about their personal health and wellness, and college administrators recognize their responsibility and the opportunity to guide students toward positive lifestyle choices. Characteristics of quality-based comprehensive health promotion programs in the college and university setting include the following:

- Commitment from administrators to develop, fund, implement, and evaluate health promotion programs and services

- Recognition of all aspects of campus life including the student health center, dining hall, clubs and activities, and sports and recreation in developing a collaborative approach to improving and supporting healthy habits within the college or university community

- Development of the college campus to encourage physical activity through new or renovated recreation, fitness and sports facilities, safe sidewalks, bike lanes, and so on

Safe and Healthy Environment

Students entering college often enjoy many new freedoms that they had not experienced during their high school years. The ability to use time as one wants, to move about freely regardless of the time of day, to make decisions without parental oversight, and to have access to foods, alcohol, drugs, and other substances that may range from unhealthy to dangerous create many crossroads for the college student. Administrators understand that although these new freedoms are part of a student's individual development, an environment must be developed and maintained that will lead students toward safe and healthy choices. Excellent college presidents will lead a regular dialogue (speeches, social media, student newspapers, small groups, etc.) about student health and safety including responsibilities held by students and the college. Campus communication systems, interpersonal relationships and dating, student counseling and support groups, policies regarding alcohol and drugs are but a few of the topics that are continually addressed by astute college administrators. Funding necessary to develop and support these efforts will be included in the yearly budget and regular evaluation will be completed to ensure that initiatives and programs are effective and are meeting the safety, health, and wellness needs of the college student.

Coordinated Health Promotion

Great **coordinated health promotion programs** offered in the college and university setting use all of the resources of the institution through a

coordinated health promotion programs programs that use all of the resources of the institution through a well-coordinated offering of programs and services

well-coordinated offering of programs and services. Campus leaders meet to share how their departments are contributing to student health and well-being and discuss ways in which they may be able to work together to strengthen the college-wide health promotion experience. In addition to caring for students who are ill, the student health center should offer proactive educational programs, including ways to avoid diseases and disorders, and can serve as a resource for preventive services such as flu shots. Dining halls will offer healthy and delicious foods when students want to eat. Clubs and college event planners should consider student safety, health, and well-being as criteria when developing new activities. Student intramurals, club sports, and other physical activities will be viewed as fun and safe and should be developed to encourage participation by all students.

Physical Environment

College and university campuses have experienced explosive growth in athletic and recreation facilities over the past few decades (Bogar, 2008). Major universities have built huge stadiums and arenas to support their teams, especially for football and basketball. As colleges and universities strive to attract the best students, campus facilities such as classrooms, labs, libraries, dormitories, dining halls, and health centers have been built or updated. This trend in campus redevelopment has created opportunities to enhance the wellness experience by improving and encouraging pedestrian and biker safety, as well as constructing new fitness, wellness, and intra-mural sports centers for all students.

Professional Opportunities

The diversity of college life creates many opportunities to positively affect the health and wellness of students, faculty, and staff. Health care profes-sionals, including physicians, physician assistants, and nurses, work in the campus health center offering prevention and care of illnesses and injuries. Many campus-based wellness and fitness centers and intramural programs are led by degreed and certified professionals and are often staffed by college students earning degrees in health, physical education, recreation, or related fields.

The Work Site

A large portion of adult life is devoted to professional pursuits; thus, the work site offers a special opportunity to positively affect health and wellness.

An employer's commitment to investing in programs and activities that strengthen wellness and minimize job-related health hazards can produce excellent results for the employee and the employer. From a human relations' perspective, employers who offer health promotion programs are often perceived as caring leaders who are interested in the well-being of their workers. Additionally, organizations that invest in employee health through proven programs will strengthen their company's bottom line. In fact, a review of the research shows that for every $1 invested in quality-based health promotion leadership, programs, and facilities, $3 to $5 will be saved through reduced employee health care costs (Linnan, 2010). Beyond the return on investment, many professionals are connecting health and human capital and encouraging work site health promotion professionals to expand the benefits to quality of life (Chenoweth, 2007).

The continued evolution of the work site, including varied full-time and part-time work schedules, telecommuting, and remotely based staff, pose new challenges for the effective delivery of health promotion programs and services. Quality-based work site health promotion has adapted rapidly to the constantly changing nature of the workplace with solid health promotion strategy and flexible delivery of services that are meaningful to employees at their place of work.

Work site health promotion has evolved dramatically since the 1940s. At that time, business leaders recognized the benefit of staying fit and began to develop gymnasiums and fitness facilities primarily for executives. With the explosion of the fitness industry in the 1970s, work site wellness grew through many businesses as well as deeper into employee populations. Recognizing the benefit to the employee *and* the organization, companies began to develop comprehensive wellness and recreation programs for all in their workforce.

Characteristics of an effective work site health promotion include the following:

- Ongoing support from the organization's leadership, including the clear identification of employee health and wellness as a priority and allocation of leadership, funds, space, and other resources to operate an effective health promotion program

- The creation of a culture of health that promotes health and one that minimizes health risks in the workplace (industrial accident prevention, protection against exposure to unhealthy work environments and materials, opportunities for periodic activity breaks for those in sedentary jobs, etc.)

- Opportunities to participate in effective programs and activities such as exercise, nutrition counseling, smoking cessation, stress management, and low back injury prevention

- An assessment system including guidance by a health coach to ensure targeted programming that will lead to regular participation and measurable results

- The use of technology, electronic media, and the Internet to educate, inspire, and provide continuous feedback on success, thereby improving program adherence

- An incentive system through which participation is rewarded by meaningful recognition or other more tangible means such as reduced health care insurance premiums

Leadership

Regardless of mission or profit motives, excellent employers understand the benefit of a healthy workforce. For-profit companies, not-for-profit organizations, government agencies, schools, and other strong organizations demonstrating solid employee productivity share a commitment to employee health and wellness, including leadership and support from the chief executive officer. For a new business, product, or company initiative to be successful, leadership from the top of the organization is vital, and comprehensive and effective employee health promotion programs are no exception. Often leading by example, chief executives will dedicate the time, personnel, funds, space, equipment, and other resources necessary to promote, develop, and maintain good health and well-being within the employee population.

Effective work site health promotion programs can range from offering basic health screenings and wellness education programs to highly developed strategies including sophisticated health assessments and comprehensive wellness facilities. Excellent work site health promotion programs often provide fitness facilities and equipment to their employees, and many organizations have integrated employee wellness incentives and improvement into their strategic plans and measures of overall organizational success.

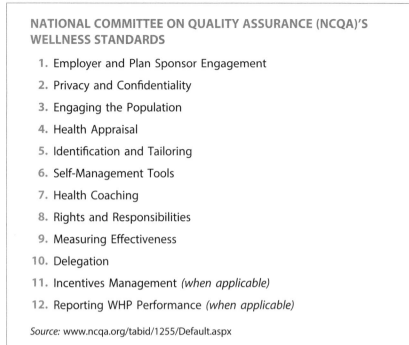

NATIONAL COMMITTEE ON QUALITY ASSURANCE (NCQA)'S WELLNESS STANDARDS

1. Employer and Plan Sponsor Engagement
2. Privacy and Confidentiality
3. Engaging the Population
4. Health Appraisal
5. Identification and Tailoring
6. Self-Management Tools
7. Health Coaching
8. Rights and Responsibilities
9. Measuring Effectiveness
10. Delegation
11. Incentives Management *(when applicable)*
12. Reporting WHP Performance *(when applicable)*

Source: www.ncqa.org/tabid/1255/Default.aspx

Work Site Safety

An important component of an employee health promotion program can be found in the commitment of many health care providers to their patients, "First, do no harm." Great employers create a culture of safety and protect their employees from potentially hazardous or unhealthy environments. This is especially true for manufacturing and construction organizations, where employees may work with and be exposed to heavy equipment and tools, chemicals, building materials, and harsh weather. To prevent workers from being killed or seriously harmed at work, the Occupational Safety and Health Act was passed in 1970. The law created the Occupational Safety and Health Administration (OSHA), which established and enforces protective safety and health standards in the workplace. OSHA also provides employers and their workers with information, training, and assistance to improve workplace safety.

An employer's first responsibility to the health and well-being of its workforce is to ensure that risks are identified and that reasonable safeguards are in place to protect workers. After identification, the next step is to educate all employees about the potential hazards they may face in the workplace. Ensuring that employees fully understand the potential dangers of the tools or machines they work with, the chemicals and materials that they are exposed to, and the history and type of accidents that can happen on the job will serve as a solid foundation in protecting employee safety, health, and well-being. Basic cautionary measures, such as wearing protective gear (safety glasses, proper clothing, protective footwear, etc.) and periodic breaks to ensure that employees are rested and alert, are well accepted in most workplaces. More advanced safeguards may include regular safety reviews and inspections, drug and alcohol screening, fall protection, and driving training and tests. To prevent accidents and other chronic injuries or disorders in the workplace, employers will strive to develop the physical conditioning and strength of their employees as well as educating their employees about the importance of performing certain physical tasks properly (e.g., lifting). By developing a culture of safety, employers can minimize health risks, reduce and eliminate accidents, contribute to employee morale and productivity, and increase profits.

Health Promotion

Employers fully committed to comprehensive health promotion will offer a wide range of programs and services designed to target specific health concerns and strengthen employee health and well-being. Program offerings may address topics such as healthy eating and weight loss, smoking cessation, stress management, type 2 diabetes prevention, as well as programs targeting injury prevention. A program can be as simple as a brown-bag lunch talk when a fifteen- to thirty-minute program is offered during the lunch break or it can be a more in-depth exploration over the course of weeks or months learning about the causes of an unhealthy behavior and specific steps that can be adopted for improvement.

Excellent employee health promotion programs will also use a variety of opportunities to encourage, monitor, and celebrate employee participation in physical activities and fitness programs. Many well-resourced companies offer a full range of fitness facilities, including gymnasiums, swimming pools, group exercise centers, athletic fields, and locker rooms, and wellness centers often include a variety of cardiovascular exercise and strength-training equipment. Organizations that are not able to offer these kinds of facilities and equipment must be creative in identifying and developing other opportunities for physical activity and exercise. Organizing groups within the workforce that share common interests such as walking, biking, hiking, and so on is a great way to promote physical activity either on company time or on personal time. Many organizations including the Y, Jewish community centers (JCCs), public recreation centers, and for-profit fitness centers offer employee wellness programs and group rates.

Health Coaches

Facilities and equipment can be terrific resources for the employee health promotion program. More important, however, is the guidance and counsel provided by a health promotion professional. Often referred to as **health coaches**, the health promotion professional provides programs and services at the work site and offers advice and support that will inspire employees to improve and maintain a good level of health, physical conditioning, and well-being. Effective coaches develop a personal relationship with employees through an understanding of the individual's background, work requirements, and motivations, which can be used in building adherence to healthy lifestyle practices. Through this relationship, the coach and the employee can focus on particular areas for improvement and can track and celebrate milestones and achievements together. The coach builds a solid level of trust with employees and can be counted on to protect confidential information. Excellent coaches have received education in the health sciences and psychology and always demonstrate a caring, enthusiastic, and outgoing personality and attitude.

Employee Assistance Programs

Employee assistance programs (EAPs) are offered by many employers to help workers and their families manage issues in their personal lives. Originally established in the 1950s to support workers struggling with alcohol dependency, EAPs have evolved to help employees address issues such as substance abuse, emotional distress, major life events, health care concerns, personal financial problems, and family and personal relationships to name a few. EAPs typically use counselors to provide assessment, support, and referrals to employees and family members facing serious challenges. In many cases, employers work through a third party to provide EAP services. Confidentiality must be maintained during the process of seeking and gaining guidance and support, and EAPs can serve as an excellent benefit to workers and their employers.

Technology and Social Media

The use of technology and social media offers a great tool supporting the improvement and maintenance of good employee health and wellness (see "The Internet"). Special company websites for employees can be used to promote new health promotion programs and services and can serve as a platform to track group progress and to announce and celebrate achievements. Tools such as e-mail, text messaging, Twitter, and Facebook can be

health coaches provide programs and services at the work site and offer advice and support that will inspire employees to improve and maintain a good level of health, physical conditioning, and well-being; effective coaches develop a personal relationship with employees through an understanding of the individual's background, work requirements, and motivations, which can be used in building adherence to healthy lifestyle practices

Employee assistance programs (EAPs) offered by many employers to help workers and their families manage issues in their personal lives; originally established in the 1950s to support workers struggling with alcohol dependency, EAPs have evolved to help employees address issues such as substance abuse, emotional distress, major life events, health care concerns, personal financial problems, and family or personal relationships, to name a few

used by coaches and employees to communicate with each other on a regular basis. Technology providers such as FitLinxx (www.FitLinxx.com) and MobileFit (www.MobileFit.com) offer excellent applications that will enable participants to record, track, and celebrate fitness milestones including the use of cardiovascular exercise and strength-training equipment.

Measuring and Celebrating Success

Tracking, evaluating, and celebrating success are hallmarks of a comprehensive quality-based work site health promotion program. During times when organizations are challenged to show a return on investment, employee health promotion programs must continually demonstrate a positive benefit to the workforce and to the organization's bottom line. Employee feedback should be collected using in-house surveys or evaluations administered by third-party professionals and analyzed to measure the qualitative and quantitative benefits of the work site health promotion program. Through use of this data, organizations can focus resources on areas in which the greatest impact can be made. Historically, these areas have included increased employee productivity and morale and decreased health care use, sick leave, and accidents. Recognition and reward systems can also be developed using data. Some employers will recognize participation and improvement of individual health and wellness through financial rewards such as bonuses or decreased health insurance costs for employees. Others may use the powerful tools of praise or public recognition to celebrate success and encourage continued participation and growth.

Professional Opportunities

Health promotion professionals working in a work site–based wellness program will often possess a hybrid of skills, abilities, and certifications. In addition to possessing skills and certification in the field of health promotion, including wellness assessment, exercise programming, and nutrition counseling, work site wellness professionals must possess business acumen and excellent communication skills. By fully understanding the mission and culture of the organization where they are working, professionals can relate to, communicate with, and support the employees they are serving.

Health Care Providers

The opportunities for health care providers, such as physicians in offices and hospitals, therapists in physical therapy and rehabilitation centers, and those who work in long-term care centers, to positively affect health and wellness are boundless. This is especially true for those health care organizations that have adopted preventive health care as a primary focus. Unique opportunities for health promotion exist in health care settings because most clients and patients are searching for care or treatment because of disease, disorder, or discomfort. In other words, individuals are seeking help and are motivated to improve their health.

A major obstacle to improving an individual's health and well-being is the requirement of change. Changing one's lifestyle can be daunting and is often looked on negatively. The advantage held by health care organizations or professionals is that they are usually viewed favorably and are held in high regard because of their reputation, training, expertise, and sincere interest in the patient's health and well-being. This perception positions professional health care organizations or providers very well in leading and supporting positive change in a patient's health.

Physicians

The physician may have the greatest opportunity to inspire improvement in an individual's health and well-being. People usually like and respect their doctor and will take action based on the advice he or she offers. The challenge for the physician is to move beyond treating a specific disease or disorder by educating patients about the benefits of healthy lifestyle habits and then helping their patients through the process of making positive changes. Simply *telling* a patient to lose weight (most patients already know this!) will rarely lead to successful weight loss. Successful weight loss is more likely to occur if the physician and support staff show the patient *how* to lose weight through education, guidance, support, and regular follow-up.

Other Health Care Providers

Other health care and long-term care providers, including hospitals, rehabilitation centers, chiropractic centers, assisted-living homes, and nursing homes, can make significant contributions to an individual's health and well-being through the unique strengths possessed by each organization. Hospitals enjoy a wide range of complementary programs and services that can be offered on-site. In fact, hospitals that have rebranded as health care organizations or systems often offer preventive services and facilities, including fitness centers, rehabilitation centers, and health promotion programs such as nutrition education and smoking cessation. Long-term care centers, such as assisted-living and nursing homes, can lead and support residents on their journeys toward healthier living by serving nutritious foods, encouraging physical activity, and building social relationships centered on positive health habits.

Faith-Based Centers

Health promotion programs and services offered in a faith-based setting can provide meaningful benefits to participants, particularly those seeking spiritual growth or the improvement of the whole person in spirit, mind, and body. Research suggests there can be a benefit to the inclusion of faith or spiritual growth as a contributing component to improvement of whole-person wellness initiatives (Powell, Shahabi, & Thoreson, 2003). Faith-based settings such as religious institutions hold characteristics that have contributed to strong success in improving wellness:

+ A belief that strengthening the spirit, mind, and body is part of the religion that one practices

+ Offering a setting where people feel comfortable and may gather with others who share common beliefs

+ The development of wellness facilities, including gymnasiums and fitness centers, as part of a religious institution's physical facilities

Many religions recognize the relationship among healthy spirit, mind, and body and take proactive steps to strengthen these three core components of total health and wellness. Churches, synagogues, mosques, and other centers of worship often provide educational, wellness, physical fitness, and other health promotion programs to their followers in comfortable and nonthreatening environments. Other faith-based organizations, including the Y and the JCC, were founded to promote spiritual beliefs and have grown to offer many educational and wellness programs, services, and facilities. A study of the Y's history shows the evolution of the organization from one that simply proclaimed the teachings of Jesus Christ to an organization that developed and promotes the concept of fulfillment of the whole person through growth in spirit, mind, and body and is exemplified in the Y triangle. Today, with a mission "to put Christian principles into practice through programs that build a healthy spirit, mind, and body for all" (Young Men's Christian Association, 2014), the Y is the largest nonprofit organization in the United States.

The Internet

Recognition of the Internet (websites, search engines, social media, blogosphere, e-mail, texting, etc.) as a setting for health promotion invites interesting discussion. Although the Internet is not characterized as a physical space, it does serve as a tool through which we can be inspired and entertained, gather information, communicate with others, store data, and track progress. In fact, the Internet, now available to most US citizens, has, arguably, changed the way Americans lead their lives. How, then, is the Internet used as a setting to positively affect health and well-being?

Access to Information and Data

An important characteristic of any quality-based setting for health promotion is the opportunity to gather information and learn. The Internet provides limitless opportunities for access to information regarding wellness topics such as physical activity, healthy eating, stress management, substance abuse prevention, spiritual wellness, and safety. A key strength of the Internet is instantaneous access to information through hand-held devices such as cellular telephones and laptop computers. Using search engines such as Google and Bing, we simply enter key words or phrases such as *fitness, nutrition, preventive screening,* or *stress management* and can begin to learn about all of the components of healthy living. The use of an incredible variety of websites can also be helpful in educating ourselves about health and well-being. Most health and wellness organizations in America have well-developed websites that offer information about their mission, programs, and services and may include interactive tools to help educate the visitor. These tools can be as simple as entering a few numbers to receive a basic health measure such as body mass index (BMI) or more sophisticated, such as entering comprehensive biometric information that may produce a complete profile identifying health risks and areas for improvement.

Although the Internet offers incredible tools for the promotion of health, the health seeker and professional must emphasize the importance of confidentiality and the quality of information being gathered. One must exercise caution in storing and sharing data as well as viewing information gathered and maintain a critical eye. Using multiple sources to validate information is prudent, particularly when an individual's health is being addressed.

Tracking Personal Health Data

Many health and wellness websites also offer opportunities to store and track personal health data. Wellness centers will use technology to enable the participant to enter physical activity information including type of exercise, intensity, and minutes and will provide feedback on ways to improve the participant's program to achieve desired results more effectively. Sophisticated programs offer websites that include personal coaching from trained professionals who maintain regular contact with the participant through messaging tailored to the individual's goals and objectives. Weight loss programs such as Jenny Craig (www.JennyCraig.com), Nutrisystem (www.Nutrisystem.com), and Weight Watchers (www.WeightWatchers.com) make excellent use of their websites and other communication technologies to educate their clients about effective weight loss, track progress, and celebrate success.

Social Media

The use of social media can be very powerful in the pursuit of a healthy lifestyle and holds special opportunities for health promotion leaders and organizations. Progressive health promotion organizations have recognized the value in maintaining a presence on Facebook, LinkedIn, Twitter, and other social media because an increasing number of individuals use social media as a primary form of communication. Organizations use these media to attract new clients, disseminate information in a timely manner, and inspire clients and the public with messages of encouragement, praise, and recognition. Social media is also used as an excellent tool to connect individuals with each other based on common characteristics such as shared health challenges, activity preferences, geographic locations, and so on. The use of tools that help to connect people holds special value because we understand the benefit of positive personal relationships and the feeling of belonging to like-minded groups of people striving to develop and maintain healthy lifestyles.

Summary

Settings where we live, learn, work, relax, recover, and worship each present unique and powerful opportunities to positively affect the health and wellness of individuals and groups. Although varied in location, structure, and offerings, environments supporting and contributing to healthy lifestyles are most effective when they become part of our daily life. Those individuals who enjoy a healthy home, school, workplace, and other positive settings are likely to experience the compounding effect of continued wellness education, inspiration, and support throughout the day. The health promotion setting also offers exciting opportunities for employment and volunteerism through which committed leaders can positively affect the health and wellness of others by providing ongoing encouragement, education, coaching, and evaluation. Outstanding health promotion settings enable individuals to learn, build healthy and positive relationships, inspire us to move our bodies and eat healthy foods, and foster a sense of achievement and growth.

KEY TERMS

1. **Physical space:** the physical makeup of the home, office, or other environment; changes to one's personal space can make daily activities easier to complete, but require less physical movement, making exercise a task to be intentionally pursued

2. **Personal trainer:** a fitness professional involved in exercise prescription and instruction; motivates clients by setting goals and providing feedback and accountability

3. **Interpersonal communication skills:** the process by which people exchange information, feelings, and meaning through verbal and nonverbal messages; message content can be seen as equally important as how it is said, including the tone of voice, facial expressions, gestures, and body language

4. **Communities:** defined as families and individuals living or working in close proximity and who share common services

5. **Health fair:** an educational and interactive event designed for outreach to provide basic preventive medicine and medical screening to people in the community or employees at a work site

6. **Health assessments:** a plan of care that identifies the specific needs of the client and how these needs will be addressed by the health care system or skilled nursing facility; in an early childhood setting may include annual on-site examinations for general health, vision, hearing, dental, and speech

7. **School wellness policies:** important tools for parents, local educational agencies, and school districts in promoting student wellness, preventing and reducing childhood obesity, and providing assurance that school meal nutrition guidelines meet the minimum federal school meal standards

8. **Body mass index (BMI):** a weight-to-height ratio, calculated by dividing one's weight in kilograms by the square of one's height in meters; it is used as an indicator of overweight, obesity, ideal weight, and underweight status

9. **Let's Go! 5210 Program:** program in which on a daily basis students strive to eat five servings of fruits and vegetables, limit screen time to two hours, be physically active for one hour, and consume zero sugared drinks

10. **Coordinated health promotion programs:** programs that use all of the resources of the institution through a well-coordinated offering of programs and services

11. **Health coach:** provides programs and services at the work site and offers advice and support that will inspire employees to improve and maintain a good level of health, physical conditioning, and well-being; effective coaches develop a personal relationship with employees through an understanding of the individual's background, work

requirements, and motivations, which can be used in building adherence to healthy lifestyle practices

12. **Employee assistance programs (EAPs):** offered by many employers to help workers and their families manage issues in their personal lives; originally established in the 1950s to support workers struggling with alcohol dependency, EAPs have evolved to help employees address issues such as substance abuse, emotional distress, major life events, health care concerns, personal financial problems, and family or personal relationships, to name a few

REVIEW QUESTIONS

1. How can elementary, middle, and high schools promote health?

2. What health issues are of concern on college and university campuses?

3. What are the guidelines for health promotion at the work site?

4. How does a work site evaluate its health promotion programs?

5. What guidelines would you provide to someone when searching for health information on the Internet?

STUDENT ACTIVITIES

1. Describe what a health-promoting community would offer its residents.

2. Health issues are many times age specific. Identify the health issues a health promotion program would target for the following settings:

   a. Work site

   b. College campus

   c. Day care setting

3. Identify one setting you believe is important for individuals and then find one example of this setting in the literature that can be used as a model program for a similar setting.

4. Track the life span of a person and describe health promotion opportunities as the person ages.

References

Bogar, C. T. (2008). Trends in college recreation facilities. *The Sport Journal, 11*(4).

Breckon, J., Harvey, J. R., & Lancaster, R. B. (1998). *Community health education: Settings, roles, and skills for the 21st century.* Gaithersburg, MD: Aspen Publishers.

Centers for Disease Control and Prevention (CDC). (2010). *Components of coordinated school health.* Retrieved from www.cdc.gov?HealthyYouth/CSHIP

Chenoweth, D. H. (2007). *Worksite health promotion* (2nd ed.). Champaign, IL: Human Kinetics.

Chomitz, V. R., Slining, M. M., McGowan, R. J., Mitchell, S. E., Dawson, G. F., & Hacker, K. A. (2009). Is there a relationship between physical fitness and academic achievement? Positive results from public school children in the northeast United States. *Journal of School Health, 79,* 30–37.

Floyd, P. A., & Allen, B. J. (2004). *Careers in health, physical education and sport.* Belmont, CA: Wadsworth-Thompson Learning.

Ginsburg, K. R. (2007). The importance of play in promoting healthy child development and maintaining strong parent-child bonds. *Pediatrics, 119*(1), 182–191.

Golan, M., & Crow, S. (2004). Parents are key players in the prevention and treatment of weight-related problems. *Nutrition Reviews, 62*(1), 39–50.

Kaiser Permanente. (2008, December). *Kaiser Permanente community health initiative: Interim report.* Retrieved from http://share.kaiserpermanente.org /media_assets/pdf/communitybenefit/assets/pdf/our_work/global/chi/CHI%20 Interim%20Report%20FINAL%203–6–09.pdf

Linnan, L. A. (2010). The business case for employee health: What we know and what we need to do. *North Carolina Medical Journal, 71*(1), 69–74.

Marx, E., & Wooley, S. F. (Eds.). (1998). *Health is academic: A guide to coordinated school health programs.* New York: Teachers College Press.

Matthews, C. E., Chen, K. Y., Freedson, P. S., Buchowski, M. S., Beech, B. M., Pate, R. R., & Troiano, R. P. (2008). Amount of time spent in sedentary behaviors in the United States, 2003–2004. *American Journal of Epidemiology, 167*(7), 875–881.

National Association of Registered School Nurses. (nd). *School nurse certification.* Retrieved from www.nasn.org/RoleCareer/SchoolNurseCertification

National Association for Sport and Physical Education. (2009). *Reducing school physical education programs is counter-productive to student health and learning and to our nation's economic health.* Retrieved from www.blindbrook.org/cms /lib07/NY01913277/Centricity/Domain/61/REDUCING-SCHOOL-PHYSICAL -EDUCATION-PROGRAMS-IS-COUNTER-11-25–09-FINAL-2-3.pdf

Perkins, T. (2002). *Comprehensive community initiatives (CCI): A comparison of community implementation plans.* University of Nebraska Public Policy Center, Paper 71. Retrieved from http://digitalcommons.unl.edu/publicpolicypublica tions/71

Powell, L. H., Shahabi, L., & Thoreson, C. E. (2003), Religion and spirituality: Linkage to physical health. *American Psychologist, 58*(1), 36–52.

Robert Wood Johnson Foundation. (2013, February). *School district wellness policies: Evaluating progress and potential for improving children's health five years after the federal mandate.* Chicago: Bridging the Gap. Retrieved from www .bridgingthegapresearch.org/_asset/13s2jm

Umberson, D. (1987). Family status and health behaviors: Social control as a dimension of social integration. *Journal of Health and Social Behavior, 28,* 306–319.

US Department of Labor. (2011). *American time use survey.* Retrieved from www .bls.gov/tus/datafiles_2011.htm

van Sluijs, E.M.F., McMinn, A. M., & Griffin, S. J. (2007). Effectiveness of interventions to promote physical activity in children and adolescents: Systematic review of controlled trials. *BMJ, 335,* 703.

Young Men's Christian Association. (2014). *About the Y.* Retrieved from www.ymca .net/about-us

CHAPTER 11

HEALTH PROMOTION–RELATED ORGANIZATIONS, ASSOCIATIONS, AND CERTIFICATIONS

Anastasia Snelling and Michelle Kalicki

This chapter introduces a number of different associations and organizations that broadly support health promotion. Most commonly, nonprofit health-related associations or organizations target the general public or a subset of the general public to advocate for a specific health condition or topic through fund-raising, sponsoring research, lobbying to advance legislation, and raising awareness about a health condition. Professional health associations specifically target professionals who work directly in the field of health promotion, public health, and health education. Professionals in the field may become members of these associations, which offer continuing education through local, regional, and national conferences, newsletters, journals, and e-mail lists. Some associations or organizations focus exclusively on the publication of scholarly journals, providing critical information and research to health promotion practitioners and policy makers in the field. In addition, other organizations offer health-related certifications in the areas of exercise science, health coaching, nutrition education, or to become wellness specialists. These organizations may be national or international in scope. This chapter explores how these organizations and associations contribute to the field of health promotion.

One of the most frequently asked questions by any prospective health promotion student is, "Where do health

LEARNING OBJECTIVES

After reading this chapter, the student will be able to:

• Describe how associations and organizations contribute to health promotion activities.

• Define the purpose of different associations and how they relate to health promotion.

• Identify the variety and role of certifications related to the field of health promotion.

• Discuss why and how an individual becomes a member of a certain organization or association.

• Summarize the benefits of joining a professional association.

promotion professionals work?" The truth is, health promotion is more visible than most people think. As described in chapter 10, health promotion activities are taking place in many different settings. Health promotion is an immensely prevalent field, focusing on many different behaviors and occurring in almost all communities across the country. Promoting healthy lifestyles is a field that has a long, interesting, and encouraging history. Many active organizations and associations have been contributing in different ways to the health of our nation for many decades. These entities respond to our ever-changing health culture and play a critical role in moving our nation toward a healthier society.

Nonprofit Health Associations

nonprofit health organizations associations that target the general public or a subset of the general public to advocate for a specific health condition or topic through fund-raising, sponsoring research, lobbying to advance legislation, and raising awareness about a health condition

There are hundreds of **nonprofit health organizations** and associations aimed at promoting different aspects of health. Many are well known because of the popular events they regularly hold or the marketing they do to promote a specific health concern. Organizations such as the American Heart Association and the American Cancer Society are good examples of organizations that receive significant public attention because of their important role of raising money through various charitable events and funding critical medical research. As of this writing, heart disease and cancer are the top two leading causes of death in the United States, respectively. Fortunately, many, though not all, of the risk factors associated with the development of these diseases are preventable or their prevalence can be reduced through living healthy lifestyles. The American Heart Association and American Cancer Society address these issues in terms that are more readily understood by the majority of Americans. These associations operate local chapters that serve communities around the nation. They are active, well-managed organizations that operate and support numerous programs and efforts to achieve their missions.

American Heart Association (AHA)

The mission of the American Heart Association (AHA) is to "build healthier lives, free of cardiovascular diseases and stroke." Recognizing the need for a national organization to share research findings and promote further study, six cardiologists representing several smaller groups founded the American Heart Association in 1924. To broaden its scope, the AHA reorganized in 1948 and brought in nonmedical volunteers with skills in business management, communication, public education, community organization, and fund-raising.

The AHA focuses on addressing the many conditions that fall under the "heart disease" umbrella through numerous campaigns and continuous education. One AHA goal is to provide credible heart disease and stroke information for effective prevention and treatment. The National Wear Red Day initiative, started in 2002, is an official campaign to raise awareness and inform women about the risk factors of heart disease. The Start! campaign promotes walking and being active to support heart health. Life's Simple 7 Check—a program designed to help Americans get and stay healthy—promotes the use of a simple tool that quickly assesses a person's current health status and provides suggestions as to how to improve his or her score. The Simple 7 behaviors comprise getting active, controlling cholesterol, managing blood pressure, eating better, losing weight, reducing blood sugar, and quitting smoking. All of these behaviors are described in this textbook and are related not only to heart disease but also to other chronic diseases, including cancer and diabetes.

These are just a few examples of American Heart Association activities. Volunteers are paramount to the AHA's success, but there are also a variety of career positions available, from fund-raising to health services to marketing.

Other Nonprofit Health Organizations

There are many other nonprofit organizations that address a variety of chronic diseases at the national, state, and local levels. Organizations such as the AHA and the others listed in table 11.1 are valuable institutions in the realm of health promotion; they act as advocates for the public at large. These organizations strive to bridge that critical knowledge gap between the professional health community and the general public.

Professional Health Associations

Although the specific mission of each **professional health association** varies, they all share the common goal of advocating and educating professionals by holding national conferences, regional and local meetings, and educational summits; publishing journals or periodicals; hosting webinars and facilitating discussions; and taking positions on public policy to promote health. For an extensive list of professional associations, see table 11.2.

This section identifies important professional health associations by aspects of health behaviors associated with chronic disease, such as nutrition, physical activity, and health education. At this time, the field of health

professional health association
an association that specifically targets and represents professionals who work directly in the field of health promotion, public health, and health education

Table 11.1   Nonprofit Health Associations

Association	Website
American Heart Association	www.heart.org
American Diabetes Association	www.diabetes.org
American Lung Association	www.lung.org
National Osteoporosis Foundation	www.nof.org
Susan G. Komen Foundation	www.komen.org
American Cancer Society	www.cancer.org
Mental Health America	www.nmha.org
American Health Care Association	www.ahcancal.org
American Association of Retired Persons	www.aarp.org
Leukemia and Lymphoma Society	www.lls.org
The American Institute of Stress	www.stress.org
American Institute for Cancer Research	www.aicr.org
Stroke Foundation	www.stroke.org

promotion does not have an association specific for the field; however, many organizations integrate the field of health promotion into their specific content area.

Nutrition

The overall imbalance of nutrition in the country correlates with our nation's rising chronic health problems. Food desert issues, the rise in type 2 diabetes, and the obesity epidemic are all aspects that can, at least in part, be attributed to nutrition. As discussed in chapter 5, trends in our nation's diet have changed dramatically since the 1950s. The role of nutrition-related associations is to organize and clearly disseminate timely information that is constantly being discovered and published regarding the role of nutrition in health.

Academy of Nutrition and Dietetics (AND)

The Academy of Nutrition and Dietetics, the world's largest organization of food and nutrition professionals (Academy of Nutrition and Dietetics,

Table 11.2   Select Health Professional Associations

Agency	Website
Nutrition	
Academy of Nutrition and Dietetics	www.eatright.org
American College of Nutrition	www.americancollegeofnutrition.org
Society for Nutrition Education and Behavior	www.sneb.org
Global Alliance for Improved Nutrition	www.gainhealth.org
National Association of Nutrition Professionals	www.nanp.org
School Nutrition Association	www.schoolnutrition.org
American Society for Nutrition	www.americannutritionassociation.org
Physical Activity	
SHAPE America	www.shapeamerica.org
American College of Sports Medicine	www.acsm.org
National Association for Health and Fitness	www.physicalfitness.org
National Coalition for Promoting Physical Activity	www.ncppa.orge-newsletters
National Health and Exercise Science Association	www.nhesa.org
Health, Education, and Wellness	
Wellness Council of America	www.welcoa.org
International Association for Worksite Health Promotion	www.iawhp.org
American Public Health Association	www.apha.org
Institute of Health and Productivity Management	www.ihpm.org
American College Health Association	www.acha.org
American School Health Association	www.ashaweb.org
National Wellness Institute	www.nationalwellness.org
Society for Public Health Education	www.sophe.org
International Union for Health Promotion and Education	www.iuhpe.org
Partnership for Prevention	www.prevent.org
American Health Care Association	www.ahcancal.org

2014). was founded in 1917 with a goal to improve the nation's health by empowering its members to become the leading figures in the field. The academy's primary activities in support of their mission are as follows:

- Providing reliable and evidence-based nutrition information for the public

- Accrediting undergraduate and graduate programs

- Credentialing dietetic professionals

- Advocating for public policy

- Publishing a peer-reviewed periodical

In order to become a member of the Academy of Nutrition and Dietetics, individuals must comply with very specific guidelines. This strict process ensures that only the most qualified individuals are awarded membership and become actively contributing members. The academy and its members work to provide the most accurate and up-to-date information about food and nutrition, disease management and prevention, food safety, and related topics to the general public.

American College of Nutrition (ACN)

Another prominent association in the world of nutrition education is the American College of Nutrition (ACN). The ACN works to "stimulate nutrition research and publication, elevate nutrition knowledge among researchers and clinicians, and provide practical guidance on clinical nutrition" (American College of Nutrition, 2014). The ACN provides a platform for professionals to come together and exchange knowledge, views, experiences in the field, and research findings to broaden their scope of understanding. A unique feature of the ACN is that they recognize the importance of nutrition education and research to the medical community. The ACN accepts no funding from for-profit corporations in an effort to provide the most accurate information without compromise.

Society for Nutrition Education and Behavior (SNEB)

The Society for Nutrition Education and Behavior (SNEB) is an international organization of nutrition professionals who work in a variety of different settings, including schools, government agencies, volunteer organizations, and the food industry. Founded in 1968, SNEB works toward bridging research findings and practitioner work in the field to promote nutrition behavior change. This is significant because changing behavior is also part of the underlying principle of health promotion. SNEB publishes the *Journal of Nutrition Education and Behavior* as a way to disseminate scientific research findings to interested parties worldwide.

Physical Activity

Nearly two-thirds of people in the United States are either overweight or obese due to poor nutrition and a lack of exercise. As technology and innovation have expanded, lives have become increasingly sedentary as discussed in chapter 6. Organizations focused on promoting physical activity and encouraging active lifestyles among adults and children have become more prevalent. The role of these organizations is to educate people on the importance of regular physical activity and to encourage everyone to lead active lifestyles. By offering continuing **professional development** and fostering the work of health promoters in the field, these associations are playing a huge role in the ongoing efforts to reverse the current health trends in the country.

professional development
the combination of experiences, memberships, and connections one makes to advance his or her career

SHAPE America

One of the most recognized and far-reaching associations in this area is the Society of Health and Physical Educators or SHAPE America, formerly known as the American Alliance for Health, Physical Education, Recreation, and Dance (AAHPERD). SHAPE America understands the importance of addressing health and physical activity from many different points, working "to advance professional practice and promote research related to health and physical education, physical activity, dance, and sport" (SHAPE America, 2014). The association hosts annual conventions, publishes a number of different journals, tenders accreditations, and offers a variety of educational opportunities.

SHAPE America was founded in 1885 as the Association for the Advancement of Physical Education (AAPE). At the time of its inception, AAPE consisted of forty-nine members, all physical educators. After going through multiple restructurings and name changes, SHAPE America is now twenty thousand members strong of professionals involved in a multitude of areas related to achieving an active, healthy lifestyle including physical education, physical activity, dance, sport, and more.

Historically, the organization's main roles have been to provide numerous professional development opportunities, maintain a strong **advocacy** presence, disseminate research in physical activity and health through its research council, and work to advance national standards and guidelines in the areas of health and physical education. However, as the landscape of health and physical activity continues to change so does SHAPE America.

advocacy
a technique used by many health organizations to influence policy making decisions

SHAPE AMERICA'S AREAS OF FOCUS

- Physical education
- Physical activity
- Health education
- Research
- Early childhood education
- Sport coaching
- Dance

On reorganizing in 2014, SHAPE America has added early childhood education to its repertoire. SHAPE America strives to maintain its leadership position in the area of physical activity and will continue to provide the latest tools for its members and their beneficiaries.

American College of Sports Medicine (ACSM)

Another prominent physical activity organization is the American College of Sports Medicine (ACSM). According to their mission, ACSM "advances and integrates scientific research to provide educational and practical applications of exercise science and sports medicine" (American College of Sports Medicine, 2014). ACSM members are professionals and students working and studying in scientific and clinical settings, academia, and the health and fitness industry. ACSM is considered the gold standard by many in the industry because their guidelines and positions on relevant policy issues are widely used and cited by professionals around the world, in addition to the quality of their certifications. ACSM initiatives focus on a range of issues, from antidoping in sports to childhood obesity. Although ACSM primarily focuses on sports medicine and exercise science, improving quality of life for all is a goal ACSM shares with all of the associations discussed in this chapter. ACSM holds conferences and summits, supports regional chapters, and has created interest groups to initiate discussion forums on topics such as aging, minority health research, and work site health promotion, among many others. These interest groups are essentially subcommittees of ACSM that have a particular focus area and meet annually at the ACSM conference. ACSM is also widely recognized for its professional certifications, discussed later in this chapter.

Health, Wellness, and Education

The large number of professional health associations underscores the dynamic and all-encompassing field of health promotion. The organizations described in this section address broader health, wellness, and education efforts in a variety of settings.

American Public Health Association (APHA)

An emerging aspect of health promotion is its relationship with public health. Although the fields have distinct characteristics and goals, they do intersect and it is important to recognize this fact. Historically, public health officials' emphasis was on the prevention of infectious disease and for access to health care, as discussed in chapter 1. However, since the 1990s, this focus has expanded to include chronic conditions; currently, there is more overlap between health promotion and public health. With the growing obesity epidemic and its associated health complications, it is essential for all health professionals to collaborate to formulate solutions. The American Public Health Association (APHA) is the oldest public health association in the United States; APHA members have a rich history of striving to achieve the vision of "a healthy global society" (http://apha.org). Founded in 1872 with a goal to advance science to reveal the causes of communicable diseases, the APHA laid the foundation for the public health profession and for the infrastructure to support its work. From its inception, the APHA has been dedicated to improving the health of all US residents.

The APHA is composed of a diverse group of health professionals that includes educators, environmentalists, and policy makers whose aims are not only to prevent serious health threats but also to advocate for families and communities to receive proper health care, find adequate funding for health services, and eliminate health disparities. The association holds an annual meeting and exposition to provide its members the opportunity to connect face-to-face and enhance their knowledge of all aspects of public health. APHA achieves its goals with the help of state **affiliates**.

As discussed in chapter 10 two major settings for health promotion are education settings and work sites. Programs in these settings focus on all aspects of health and wellness to encourage and facilitate lifestyle and behavior changes in students and staff and work site employees. Work in these settings is often associated with public health activities.

affiliates
state- or local-level subgroups of a national organization

Society for Public Health Education (SOPHE)

For more than sixty years, the Society for Public Health Education (SOPHE) has served a diverse membership of health education professionals and students in the United States and other countries. The organization promotes healthy behaviors, healthy communities, and healthy environments through its membership, its network of local chapters, and its numerous partnerships with other organizations. Members work in a number of settings such as elementary and secondary schools, universities, voluntary organizations, health care settings, work sites, and local, state, and federal government agencies.

Wellness Councils of America (WELCOA)

The Wellness Councils of America (WELCOA) is a leading association for work site health promotion in the United States. In the 1980s, WELCOA's founders were among the first to make the connection between health and well-being and its impact within the workplace. WELCOA bases its mission on the belief that a healthy workforce is essential to America's growth and that by investing in employee health and well-being our nation will be more productive and health care costs will be better controlled. Healthy employees benefit a company or organization; WELCOA's 3,200 members work to promote healthy work sites and work site health promotion programs. WELCOA is a dominant source of information for work site wellness programs in the United States.

American College Health Association (ACHA)

The American College Health Association (ACHA) may be of particular importance to health promotion students enrolled in this course. The mission of the ACHA is to provide advocacy, education, communications, products, and services, as well as promote research and culturally competent practices to enhance its members' ability to advance the health of all students and the campus community (American College Health Association, 2014). Members include two- and four-year institutions, individual health professionals and students, and corporations and nonprofits dedicated to college health.

American School Health Association (ASHA)

The American School Health Association (ASHA) and its members have never been more vital. ASHA's goals are to promote interdisciplinary collaboration between health and academic professionals, advocate for coordinated school health programs, offer professional development opportunities for its more than two thousand members around the world, support and disseminate research initiatives, and provide crucial resources to

BENEFITS OF ASSOCIATION MEMBERSHIP

- Network with other professionals in similar positions or areas
- Stay current on research and best practices of the profession
- Network for job opportunities
- Attend local, regional, and national conferences for continuing education credits
- Learn more about the profession and the variety of jobs and opportunities
- Discounts on conference fees
- Opportunities to present information to colleagues in order to promote best practices

Most associations require an annual membership fee so it is important to select the association most beneficial to you and your career.

support its members and their mission. Members come from a wide range of backgrounds, including school administrators, counselors, health and physical educators, psychologists, nurses, and physicians, among others.

Table 11.2 identifies health professional associations and lists their websites for additional information.

Scholarly and Professional Health Journals

In addition to nonprofit health organizations and health professional associations, there is a diverse array of **scholarly and professional health journals** to disseminate health promotion research and information. These journals include publications covering a range of broad topics, such as the *American Journal of Health Promotion,* to more specific topics such as the *American Journal of Clinical Nutrition.* Access to many of these journals is free of charge to students at academic institutions through university library databases. Peer-reviewed journals are considered the most accurate and desirable resources for papers, projects, and presentations because of the rigorous review process each article must undergo prior to publication. Upon submission, articles are critiqued for research content by multiple peer reviewers as well as the editors for accuracy, clarity, and relevance. Thus, although many mainstream media outlets offer valid information, most have not been reviewed as thoroughly as articles published in peer-reviewed journals. Table 11.3 lists a selection of journals.

scholarly and professional health journals
typically peer-reviewed publications that publish research articles and commentaries

Table 11.3   Select Scholarly Journals

Journal	Association	Website
Nutrition		
Journal of the Academy of Nutrition and Dietetics	Academy of Nutrition and Dietetics	www.adajournal.org
Journal of the American College of Nutrition	American College of Nutrition	www.jacn.org
Journal of Nutrition Education and Behavior	Society of Nutrition Education and Behavior	www.jneb.org
Journal of Child Nutrition & Management (SNA)	School Nutrition Association	www.schoolnutrition.org
American Journal of Clinical Nutrition (ASN)	American Society for Nutrition	www.acjn.nutrition.org
Physical Activity		
American Journal of Health Education *Journal of Physical Education, Recreation, and Dance* *Women in Sport and Physical Activity Journal*	SHAPE America	www.shapeamerica.org/publications /journals/
Medicine & Science in Sport & Exercise	American College of Sports Medicine	www.acsm.org/access-public-information /acsm-journals
General Health Promotion and Education		
Health, Education and Wellness		
American Journal of Public Health	American Public Health Association	http://ajph.aphapublications.org
Journal of Health and Productivity	Institute of Health and Productivity Management	www.ihpm.org/jhp/index.php
Journal of American College Health	American College Health Association	www.acha.org/Publications/JACH.cfm
Journal of School Health	American School Health Association	www.ashaweb.org/i4a/pages/index.cfm ?pageid=3341
Health Education and Behavior	Independent	http://heb.sagepub.com
Health Promotion International and *Global Health Promotion*	International Union For Health Promotion and Education	http://heapro.oxfordjournals.org http://ped .sagepub.com
Childhood Obesity	Independent	www.liebertpub.com/overview/childhood obesity/384/???
Health Affairs	Project HOPE	www.healthaffairs.org
Health Communication	Independent	www.tandfonline.com/toc/hhth20/current

American Journal of Health Promotion	Independent	www.healthpromotionjournal.com
American Journal of Health Behavior	Independent	www.ajhb.org
Journal of Community Health	Independent	www.springer.com/public+health/journal /10900
International Journal of Occupational and Environmental Health	Center of Occupational and Environmental Health	www.ijoeh.com

Becoming familiar with these publications as a student, especially those of particular interest to you and your career, will assist you upon graduation; journals are a source of continuing education for professionals in the field.

Certifications

Obtaining a degree in health promotion is the first step to beginning a career in this exciting field. However, in a society that requires specific educational standards from its graduates, attaining a certification in the preferred field of interest may be a recommended next step. As the health industry expands, professional certifications are one of its fastest growing aspects. **certification** come in all shapes and sizes for individuals, organizations and institutions and are offered through many of the associations identified in this chapter. If an individual's career aspirations are to work in an academic setting or a public health department, becoming a Certified Health Education Specialist (CHES) may be a perfect fit. If an individual chooses to work in the field of personal training or fitness instruction, a fitness-based certification is usually a prerequisite for employment.

certification
an endorsement of qualifications obtained by an individual or organization showing a degree of expertise in a particular field

The following sections explore a few of the health promotion certifications available for various paths.

Health Promotion Certifications

The National Wellness Institute (NWI), founded in 1977, provides resources and services to support and foster health promotion and wellness professionals in their fields. The NWI offers a certified work site wellness specialist (CWWS) certification to acquire the skills needed to run a successful work site health promotion program and a certified work site wellness program manager (CWWPM) certification for those pursuing a work site wellness management role. Additionally, the NWI offers a general wellness practitioner certification for professionals dedicated to continuing their wellness education and leadership experience. For more information, check out the NWI website at www.nationalwellness.org.

Certified Worksite Wellness Specialist (CWWS)

The CWWS is the first step in NWI's work site wellness certification programming and delivers the tools required to carry out a successful work site wellness program. Program participants include work site wellness coordinators and managers, human resource professionals, occupational health nurses, employee assistance professionals, insurance and benefit providers and brokers, and other individuals seeking training and certification in work site wellness.

Certified Work site Wellness Program Manager (CWWPM)

The CWWPM is geared toward professionals who are currently in a work site wellness manager-supervisor role or who are working toward a manager-supervisor role. It is the next step in work site wellness certification following completion of the CWWS program. The program covers critical competencies in managing the planning, design, implementation, and measurement of a comprehensive work site wellness–health management program.

Certified Wellness Practitioner (CWP)

The CWP is not specific to work site wellness programs but is rather a designation for those who have strong academic and professional credentials and have shown a commitment to continuing their overall development. With the CWP designation, a professional in the field is certified to create and evaluate programs using sound health promotion models and theories and help to create "health-enhancing environments" (www.nationalwellness.org). To become a certified wellness practitioner, an individual has to either (1) apply and be selected by the review committee or (2) be a graduate of an NWI-accredited academic program.

Health Education Certifications

The objective of the National Commission for Health Education Credentialing (NCHEC) (2010) is to facilitate the enhancement of an upstanding health education system.

Certified Health Education Specialist (CHES)

The CHES designation is obtained by demonstrating competency with the standards issued by the NCHEC and passing the exam. To take the exam an

Health education specialists are professionals who design, conduct and evaluate activities that help improve the health of all people. These activities can take place in a variety of settings that include schools, communities, health care facilities, businesses, universities, and government agencies. Health education specialists are employed under a range of job titles such as patient educators, health education teachers, health coaches, community organizers, public health educators, and health program managers. (www.nchec.org)

SEVEN AREAS OF RESPONSIBILITY FOR HEALTH EDUCATION

Area 1: Assess needs, assets, and capacity for health education.

Area 2: Plan health education.

Area 3: Implement health education.

Area 4: Conduct evaluation and research related to health education.

Area 5: Administer and manage health education.

Area 6: Serve as a health education resource person.

Area 7: Communicate and advocate for health and health education.

Continuing education is required for certain certifications or degrees. Continuing education is usually completed through attending local or national conferences or reading articles published in journals.

individual must have a bachelor's, master's, or doctorate's degree from an accredited institution and have an official transcript clearly showing a major in health education or an official transcript showing at least twenty-five semester hours of course work in the seven areas of responsibility for health education (see the sidebar). The certification is valid for five years, with the caveat that seventy-five hours of **continuing education** must be completed during that time. For more information, see the National Commission for Health Education Credentialing at www.nchec.org.

continuing education
a requirement for maintaining certifications; can be obtained through attending conferences, taking various classes, and so on

Master CHES (MCHES)

Beyond the entry-level CHES certification is the Master CHES certification. Candidates for this exam are either current CHES recipients or non-CHES recipients. As a CHES recipient, candidates need to have five continuous years of health education employment. For a non-CHES recipient, candidates must have a master's degree or higher. Additionally, candidates must have five years of documented experience as a health education specialist. Similar to maintaining the CHES certification, continuing education credits are necessary for the MCHES.

Fitness-Based Certifications

There are a number of fitness-based certifications available through a variety of associations. The focus, expertise, and prestige of each certifying organization are varied so it is important to identify one's interests and specific professional requirements prior to committing to a certain certification. In general, a high level of comprehension of human anatomy and exercise physiology is necessary to pass the exam, as well as a strong knowledge of the specific guidelines for that organization's theory of best practice. For those individuals planning to work at a fitness facility or start an independent personal training company, the credibility provided through a formal certification process is essential. Additionally, many certifying organizations offer more than one certification option for personal training. Group fitness instructors, strength and conditioning specialists, and professionals focusing on certain age groups, such as seniors or youth, may also benefit from a certification or specific credential.

Some of the most recognizable and respected fitness-based certification organizations are listed in table 11.4.

Table 11.4   Fitness-Based Certification Organizations

Organization	Website
American College of Sports Medicine	www.acsm.org
National Strength and Conditioning Association	www.nsca.com
National Association of Sports Medicine	www.nasm.org
American Council on Exercise	www.acefitness.org
Aerobics and Fitness Association of America	www.afaa.com
American Fitness Professionals and Associates	www.afpafitness.com
National Exercise and Sports Trainers Association	www.nestacertified.com

Nutrition Certifications

Certified Nutrition Specialists (CNS) use medical nutrition therapy to combat obesity and the chronic diseases widely associated with poor nutrition habits. The Certification Board of Nutrition Specialists administers exams twice each year to interested and qualified candidates. A graduate degree in nutrition or a clinical health care–related field with specific course work in nutrition, biochemistry, physiology, and clinical, life, or physical sciences, and supervised nutrition experience are required to obtain the CNS credential.

As the health industry continues to grow, different organizations are offering nutrition specialist certifications as well. As a professional working more generally to help people improve eating habits or lose weight, certain certifications may be beneficial. As it becomes clearer that a combination of physical activity and better eating habits is the only proven formula for healthy living, many of the fitness-based organizations listed in table 11.4 have begun to offer nutrition or weight management certifications. A few of these certifications are described in the following:

- The American Fitness Professionals & Associates (AFPA) has multiple certifications that enhance one's knowledge and credibility in the field. AFPA offers a weight management consultant certification, nutrition and wellness consultant certification, and a sports nutrition consultant certification.
- The National Association of Sports Medicine (NASM) offers a fitness nutrition specialist and weight loss specialist credential.
- The American Council on Exercise (ACE) offers a weight management specialist certification.

Again, as with any certification, these do not guarantee employment. Continuing education, broadening one's knowledge base, and professional experience will most benefit your career.

Health Coaching

Health coaching is another growing area in the field. Health coaching combines evidence-based practice interventions with the science of motivational interviewing in an effort to reduce costs, change behaviors, and improve health outcomes. The occupation initially appeared in the late 1990s and continues to evolve. Work site health promotion programs are the primary employers of health coaches, along with health care organizations and human resources departments.

Table 11.5   Health Coaching Certification Organizations

Organization	Description	Website
International Coach Federation (ICF)	• Gold standard for coaching certifications • Evaluate other programs according to a specific criterion	www.coachfederation.org/ICF
Coach Training Alliance (CTA)	• Certified coach program • Teleconferencing, online media, and interactive software • Six months • ICF approved the course to be worth thirty-six hours	www.coachtrainingalliance.com
The Coaches Training Institute (CTI)	• ICF accredited • Two components: core curriculum and certification program • Telephonic, six months	www.thecoaches.com
Wellcoaches	• Telephonic course • Ten weeks • CHES accepts certification as continuing education hours	www.wellcoaches.com
National Society of Health Coaches (NSHC)	• Online program based on motivational interviewing • Created for health professionals who must have specific degrees to qualify	www.nshcoa.com

Table 11.5 shows some of the certifying agencies for health coaching and the specific requirements for each.

Academic Institute Certifications

academic institution
an educational body dedicated to teaching and research and also grants degrees

In addition to the aforementioned individual certifications, **academic institution** are also eligible to become accredited. The National Wellness Institute Council on Wellness Accreditation and Education (CWAE) provides recognition to health promotion programs within a college or university. For schools, accreditation demonstrates that they have met or exceeded the standards issued by the CWAE, contributing to recognition in the academic community. For students, on graduation they are eligible to be an NWI-certified wellness practitioner as a result of the program's accreditation, and employers can hire these graduates with assurance that they are competent for entry-level positions in the field. More information on the National Wellness Institute's accreditations and certifications can be found at www.nationalwellness.org.

As mentioned previously, public health is increasingly involved in health promotion. The academic accreditation from the Council on Education for Public Health (CEPH) is recognized by the US Department of Education to accredit schools and programs of public health at the undergraduate and graduate levels. As with the CWAE accreditation, it is a great benefit for the school to attain a CEPH accreditation. Students graduating from CEPH-accredited universities or colleges can be expected to have a high level of public health knowledge based on the standards that must be met for accreditation, found at www.ceph.org.

Summary

This chapter identified a variety of different associations that support the field of health promotion. Understanding that the field is diverse and overlaps with other fields, students might consider learning more about and joining a number of different associations. These associations provide many educational and networking opportunities that keep professionals current in the field. The chapter also introduced several different personal certifications that students might consider as they progress through their careers. The diverse certifications are for general work site health promotion, health education, personal training, health coaching, and nutrition, among others. Each certification requires a different set of prerequisites, variable costs, and continuing education credits. The importance of associations, journals, conferences, and certifications will become more apparent as health promotion students and professionals develop their careers. Now is the time to explore these opportunities.

KEY TERMS

1. **Nonprofit health organizations:** associations that target the general public or a subset of the general public to advocate for a specific health condition or topic through fundraising, sponsoring research, lobbying to advance legislation, and raising awareness about a health condition

2. **Professional health association:** an association that specifically targets and represents professionals who work directly in the field of health promotion, public health, and health education

3. **Professional development:** the combination of experiences, memberships, and connections one makes to advance his or her career

4. **Advocacy:** a technique used by many health organizations to influence policy decision making

5. **Affiliates:** state- or local-level subgroups of a national organization

6. **Scholarly and professional health journals:** typically peer-reviewed publications that publish research articles and commentaries

7. **Certification:** an endorsement of qualifications obtained by an individual or organization showing a degree of expertise in a particular field

8. **Continuing education:** a requirement for maintaining certifications; can be obtained through attending conferences, taking various classes, and so on

9. **Academic institution:** an educational body dedicated to teaching and research and also grants degrees

REVIEW QUESTIONS

1. Why would someone join the Society of Nutrition Education and Behavior or the American Public Health Association?

2. If you wanted to attend a conference sponsored by the Society for Public Health Education, what would the registration cost be for members? Is there a special rate for students? Do they accept interns?

3. There are a number of personal training certifications available to consumers. What criteria would you use to select a personal training certification?

4. What is the role of nonprofit health associations in health promotion?

5. What is the overall importance of associations in the field of health promotion?

STUDENT ACTIVITIES

1. List the five leading causes of disease and identify two nonprofit organizations dedicated to reducing death and disability related to that condition.

2. Discuss the reasons why you might consider a certification in addition to receiving your bachelor's degree.

3. Find a job listing that includes the phrase "CHES preferred." Describe the position.

4. Select two personal certifications and compare and contrast the eligibility requirements for these two certifications.

5. Select two journals, and find two articles of interest and write an abstract for each journal article.

References

Academy of Nutrition and Dietetics. (2014). *Who we are and what we do*. Retrieved from www.eatright.org/About/Content.aspx?id=7530

American College Health Association. (2014). *Who we are*. Retrieved from www .acha.org/About_ACHA/Who_We_Are.cfm

American College of Nutrition. (2014). *About the college*. Retrieved from http:// americancollegeofnutrition.org/content/about-college

American College of Sports Medicine. (2014). *Who we are*. Retrieved from www .acsm.org/about-acsm/who-we-are

American Heart Association. (nd-a). *My life check*. Retrieved from http://mylife check.heart.org/Multitab.aspx?NavID=3

American Heart Association. (nd-b). *Start!* Retrieved from www.startwalkingnow .org

National Commission for Health Education Credentialing. (2010). *Health education profession*. Retrieved from http://nchec.org/credentialling/profession

SHAPE America. (2014). *About us*. Retrieved from www.shapeamerica.org

CHAPTER 12

TRENDS IN HEALTH PROMOTION

David Hunnicutt

Although health promotion is a relatively new concept and largely considered by many to still be an emerging discipline, according to many experts there is little question that this area will continue to grow in need and popularity over the next several decades. In fact, several significant trends will drive the expansion of the field of health promotion. Specifically, there are eleven trends that have the potential to contribute to the growth of health promotion and prevention:

Trend 1: The population will get much older in the next three decades.

Trend 2: The health status of aging adults will decline steadily if we don't do things differently.

Trend 3: Adults won't be the only ones who are losing their health status.

Trend 4: Health care costs will remain an issue of significant concern far into the future.

Trend 5: Prevention will become a national priority.

Trend 6: Medical self-care will gain rapid popularity.

Trend 7: Physical activity will become the most commonly prescribed medicine.

Trend 8: Financial incentives and disincentives will go mainstream.

LEARNING OBJECTIVES

After reading this chapter, the student will be able to:

- Identify how shifts in the population will affect health promotion.

- Describe how health promotion will affect the changing health status of children and adolescents.

- Explain how the focus on disease prevention and health promotion will address rising health care costs.

- Identify different strategies to engage people in health promotion efforts.

- Describe key statistics and trends that will influence the health promotion field.

Trend 9: Physical environments will be altered radically.

Trend 10: Efforts to curb obesity will intensify greatly.

Trend 11: The need for talented health promotion professionals will skyrocket.

The following paragraphs document each one of these emerging trends, which will reveal numerous personal, professional, and societal implications. After reading this chapter, you should have a much better grasp of what the future holds for health promotion, prevention, and wellness in the United States.

Trend 1: The Population Will Get Much Older in the Next Three Decades

Over the course of the next three decades, the mean age of the United States' and world's population will increase. To provide the context for this phenomenon, it is important to understand the present makeup of the current US population. At the time of this writing, there are presently some 313 million citizens in this country—and perhaps the most significant segment of the population that will drive the aging phenomenon is that of the baby boomers. In fact, the **baby boomers**—those born between 1946 and 1964—are made up of about eighty million people and, again, will be the fastest-growing segment of the aging population (Haaga, 2002).

baby boomers
Americans born between 1946 and 1964; about eighty million people and the fastest growing segment of the aging population

According to the US Census Bureau, there are roughly forty-three million Americans who are presently sixty-five years and older residing in the United States (US Census Bureau, 2013). By 2020, that number will grow to approximately fifty-six million; by 2025, sixty-five million; and by 2030, seventy-three million (US Census Bureau, 2012). Indeed, at the time of this writing, one US citizen is turning sixty every eight seconds and that trend will continue for years into the future. Moreover, some ten thousand people are retiring *each day* in the United States.

Without question, this rapidly aging wave of Americans will have a transformational impact across many institutions and segments of society—not least of which will be the discipline of health promotion. Indeed, the unprecedented aging of the US population will bring with it health and medical care issues that have never needed to be addressed in this country—until now.

In simpler terms, without good health, the aging of the American population could bring dire consequences for individuals and our society at large. In fact, consider this quote from one of the nation's leading economists, Dr. Laurence Kotlikoff, in his book, *The Coming Generational Storm:*

> It's 2030 . . . you see a country where the collective population is older than that of Florida today. You see a country where people in wheelchairs will outnumber kids in strollers. You see a country with twice as many retirees but only 18% more workers to support them. You see a country with large numbers of impoverished elderly citizens languishing in understaffed, overcrowded, substandard nursing homes. . . .
>
> (Kotlikoff & Burns, 2005)

By coming to grips with the reality that we are aging rapidly as a society, it is easy to see how the need for better health promotion and collective preventive practices will grow over the next three decades. For starters, we will need an army of health promotion and allied health professionals who are well trained and motivated to keep an aging population healthy, happy, and productive. Moreover, we'll need our nation's citizens to step up and embrace the responsibility for managing their own health and well-being. The key question is whether or not we can start the engines fast enough to produce an adequate supply of talented and capable health promotion professionals. Similarly, there is a very real concern as to whether our nation's citizens are willing to accept responsibility for better health practices.

Trend 2: The Health Status of Aging Adults Will Decline Steadily If We Don't Do Things Differently

The second trend to watch for is the very real possibility that the **health status** of more than eighty million aging adults will decline unless we do some things very differently. This notion of the danger of declining health status is substantiated by the fact that there are a number of high-profile, well-respected experts who are in general agreement that this will indeed be the case.

For example, one of the nation's preeminent health promotion researchers—Dr. Dee Edington, former director of the University of Michigan's Health Management Research Center—highlights the stark reality that, as people get older, they generally move from relatively good health to compromised health to poor health. In other words, as individuals age in this country, they systematically and predictably migrate from low-risk to moderate-risk to high-risk status. And although this idea of health status migration is interesting in and of itself, consider for a moment the

health status
the measurement of the health of an individual or population as subjectively assessed by the individual or by more objective measures, including life expectancy and presence of disease conditions

implications of having eighty million baby boomers all getting old at the same time and the vast majority of them being in poor health (Edington, 2013).

Believe it or not, as the boomers age, the Centers for Disease Control and Prevention (2013b) estimate the following will happen:

- One-quarter of all Americans will have heart disease.

- One in twelve Americans will have asthma.

- One in fourteen Americans will have diabetes.

- One in seven Americans will develop Alzheimer's.

- Approximately one in five Americans will have arthritis, already the country's leading cause of disability.

Almost implausibly, Kotlikoff's bold prediction of an elderly population languishing in understaffed, substandard nursing homes begins to make sense.

But could this really happen? Could eighty million people—all of whom are getting old at the same time—potentially put such a strain on our society (and specifically our health care system) to bring us to our knees? Truth be told, this is already occurring. Consider for a moment just a few of the statistics that indicate our population is indeed migrating from low-risk to moderate-risk to high-risk health status.

For example, at the time of this writing, there are over eighteen million people in the United States who have been medically diagnosed with type 2 diabetes. Add to that another seven million US citizens who are presently undiagnosed and that brings the total to twenty-five million people with type 2 diabetes in the United States. The real concern, however, is the fact that some eighty million Americans are considered to be prediabetic and, if left unaddressed, these people will most assuredly progress to type 2 diabetes. This means that of our nation's approximately 313 million citizens, more than 100 million are wrestling with type 2 diabetes. If left unchecked, type 2 diabetes will manifest itself in terms of heart disease, vascular problems, blindness, and amputations (Hoffman, Salerno, & Moss, 2012).

As can be plainly seen, the potential catastrophic human, economic, and social consequences of an aging population only further solidifies the need for placing a greater emphasis on health promotion and better preventive practices in this country. With a greater emphasis being placed on developing and delivering comprehensive health promotion interventions will also come a renewed interest in better understanding and mastering the various well-documented theoretically-based behavior change models such as Prochaska's transtheoretical model as well as Bandura's social cognitive theory, which were described in chapter 2.

Trend 3: Adults Won't Be the Only Ones Who Are Losing Their Health Status

Although it's one thing to witness the US adult population losing their health status, it's quite another to imagine the health status of children being severely compromised. Unfortunately, this is indeed the case at the time of this writing.

For example, consider observations from former US Surgeon General Richard Carmona (2004):

> Over the past 20 years, the rates of overweight doubled in children and tripled in adolescents. Today nearly two out of every three American adults and 15 percent of American kids are overweight or obese. That's more than 9 million children—one in every seven kids—who are at increased risk of weight-related chronic diseases. These facts are astounding, but they are just the beginning of a chain reaction of dangerous health problems—many of which were once associated only with adults.

> Today pediatricians are diagnosing an increasing number of children with Type 2 diabetes—which used to be known as adult-onset diabetes. Research indicates that one-third of all children born in 2000 will develop Type 2 diabetes during their lifetime. Tragically, people with Type 2 diabetes are at increased risk of developing heart disease, stroke, kidney disease, and blindness. These complications are likely to appear much earlier in life for those who develop Type 2 diabetes in childhood or adolescence. Because of the increasing rates of obesity, unhealthy eating habits, and physical inactivity, we may see the first generation that will be less healthy and have a shorter life expectancy than their parents.

Fortunately, there is still time to address these serious and rapidly multiplying adolescent health issues—and the answers in large part revolve around promoting better preventive practices. Consider the findings of the Department of Health and Human Services' Diabetes Prevention Program in which clinical trials showed that people with prediabetes can delay and even prevent type 2 diabetes by losing just 5% to 7% of their body weight through moderate changes in diet and exercise. These lifestyle changes worked for people of every ethnic or racial group who participated in the study. The changes—such as walking for thirty minutes a day five days a week—are simple and prove that small steps can indeed bring big rewards (National Institute of Diabetes and Digestive and Kidney Diseases, 2008).

Although children in this country comprise a smaller percentage of the population, they are 100% of our future. Better health promotion practices will ensure that today's children reach their full potential—and to be successful as a country we will need our children to learn and carry good health into their adult years. This will become a significant priority as we move into the future. Chapter 10 gave several examples of where health promotion is happening to affect the health of children of all ages.

Trend 4: Health Care Costs Will Remain an Issue of Significant Concern Far into the Future

There's an old adage that states, "It doesn't take a sharp ear to hear thunder." Certainly, this is the case when it comes to forecasting the societal implications of a rapidly aging population that is losing its health status at the same time. And, as a result of the three aforementioned trends, a fourth significant trend will no doubt emerge—that **health care costs** will continue to remain an issue of significant concern far into the future.

Presently, the United States spends almost $3 trillion annually on health care. This is more than three times the $714 billion spent in 1990, and over eight times the $253 billion spent in 1980. To put this into perspective, the nearly $3 trillion of health care expenditures in the United States represents more than 17% of our economy's annual spending (gross domestic product) and is more than four times what we spend on national defense. Almost incomprehensibly, in 2010, US health care spending was about $8,233 for every man, woman, and child—or more than $30,000 for a family of four (Kaiser Family Foundation and Health Research and Educational Trust, 2012).

With respect to the future, experts predict that those expenditures will increase to $4.2 trillion by 2016. Certainly these projected expenditures are not only mind-numbing but alarming as well, because most Americans will be hard-pressed to afford access to quality health care if this trend remains unabated. However, one of the goals of the Patient Protection and Affordable Care Act (ACA) is to make health care more affordable to American citizens. More time is needed to understand if the ACA is able to offer affordable care to consumers (Centers for Medicare and Medicaid Services, 2012; Kaiser Family Foundation and Health Research and Educational Trust, 2012).

health care costs
the actual costs of providing services related to the delivery of health care, including the costs of procedures, therapies, and medications; differentiated from health expenditures, which refers to the amount of money paid for the services, and from fees, which refers to the amount charged, regardless of cost

To address the expenditures, health promotion will become integral to how America conducts its daily affairs because chronic diseases—preventable illnesses such as heart disease, cancer, stroke, and so on—are now responsible for approximately 70% of the deaths in America and consume three-fourths of health care spending. To further build the case for better health-promoting practices, we know definitively that lifestyle-related chronic diseases—heart disease, cancer, and diabetes—are also the leading causes of disability in the United States. Last but certainly not least, approximately 40% of all deaths in the United States are premature and, again, largely preventable—at least nine hundred thousand deaths annually are related to tobacco use, poor diet, sedentary lifestyle, misuse of alcohol and drugs, and accidents (Centers for Disease Control and Prevention, 2013b).

Nearly 70% of health care expenditures is estimated to be largely preventable; thus, health promotion brings with it significant opportunity to contain at least a portion of these escalating costs. Moreover, because lifestyle behaviors—such as smoking, exercise, and dietary choices—contribute to 50% of an individual's overall health status, it is reasonable to think that the rapid adoption of better health practices in the United States can bring with it numerous benefits—not least of which is the containment of health care costs. Indeed, by widely promoting better health practices, many believe it is possible to have a profound impact not only on the two leading causes of death in the United States—heart disease and cancer—but on numerous other conditions as well.

Furthermore, what is certain to emerge as a result of escalating health care costs is an increasing interest in approaches and methodologies that will demonstrate concrete **return on investment** for those who invest heavily in health promotion interventions. This represents a significant opportunity for those who are preparing to enter the field of health and wellness, because many employers, health care administrators, and public health leaders will be searching for talented individuals who can orchestrate such outcomes.

return on investment
a performance measure used to evaluate the efficiency of an investment or to compare the efficiency of a number of different investments

Trend 5: Prevention Will Become a National Priority

There is little question that, when it comes to the health and well-being of our nation's citizens, we are standing at a crossroads. Without significant change and a much greater emphasis on health promotion and more intensive preventive practices, it is likely that many of our nation's citizens will suffer the devastating effects of ill health—much of which is, ironically, largely preventable. Although the individual consequences of poor health are tragic by themselves, it is far from the true impact that an aging population and increasing health care costs could have on the country's economic future.

Consider this: the eighty million baby boomers who are now in their fifties and sixties are largely unprepared to meet the financial demands of retirement. In fact, at the time of this writing, the typical baby boomer has less than $35,000 saved for retirement. To add fuel to the fire, health care costs in retirement are estimated to cost boomers more than $250,000. These financial realities mean that a large percentage of the baby boomer population will be required to work much longer than they had originally anticipated in order to make ends meet.

To meet this demand, tens of millions of boomers will rely greatly on their health status in order to keep working. To be sure, if one's health is failing, it is unlikely that they will be able to productively contribute at work—and even less likely that they will be able to hold down a job at all.

The ramifications of this scenario are profound and immediate. If an aging America is unable to work, who will provide for them? Will there be enough workers to keep our nation's economy moving forward? How will the already overburdened health care system absorb this additional demand?

With this in mind, unless we change how we address health and well-being in this country, the forecast is not a rosy one. However, and to the contrary, if we as a nation are able to make sweeping changes in the very near term, there is a chance we can avert disaster. In light of these realities, much of the population will immediately see the need for better health practices and embrace the value of good health. As a result, many employers, policy makers, and working Americans will begin to advocate for better health practices not just as a good idea but also as a necessity to ensure that America will continue to be able to remain productive and a global economic power.

Trend 6: Medical Self-Care Will Gain Rapid Popularity

To date, Americans have relied far too heavily on the US health care system to address minor, self-treatable health concerns—ailments such as colds, upset stomachs, and minor aches and pains. In fact, recent research reveals that there were 123 million emergency room (ER) visits in 2008 (the most recent year for which data are available). These ER visits resulted in eighty-three million diagnostic tests including forty-three million x-rays and eighteen million CT scans. The typical cost per visit was $1,265 (in 2008 dollars). The most shocking part of this analysis revealed that about 30% of all ER visits were unnecessary (Centers for Disease Control and Prevention, 2012).

Comparably, there were 1.2 billion physician visits in 2007. The average cost per visit was approximately $120. Similar to ER visits, it is estimated by experts that approximately 30% of all physician visits were unnecessary. Moreover, seven in ten visits resulted in at least one prescription or 2.7 billion prescriptions overall. As of 2010, it is estimated that approximately seventy million Americans take at least one prescription daily (Centers for Disease Control and Prevention, 2013a).

As a consequence of Americans' overreliance on the US health care system, emergency rooms and hospitals are bursting at the seams. In fact, 91% of hospitals reported overcrowding and some 70% of ambulance drivers had to be diverted because of overcrowding. What's more, at the time of this writing, it takes on average about fifty-five days to schedule an appointment to see a **primary care physician**. Similarly, due to over-crowding, it takes more than 3.5 hours to be seen in an ER (Hammergren & Harkins, 2008).

Although not usually included in the vernacular of traditional health promotion programs and approaches, with the present state of overuse of our health care system, **medical self-care** programs will gain in popularity as Americans will have fewer disposable dollars available to offer up to unnecessary treatments—and insurance companies will become increasingly stingy with reimbursing unnecessary treatments. As a result, treating minor medical issues will become standard practice among the vast majority of Americans.

primary care physician
a physician, such as a family practitioner or internist, who is chosen by an individual to provide continuous medical care, trained to treat a wide variety of health-related problems, and responsible for referrals to specialists as needed

medical self-care
the care of oneself without medical, professional, or other assistance or oversight

Trend 7: Physical Activity Will Become the Most Commonly Prescribed Medicine

According to one of the nation's leading health promotion experts and founder of the Cooper Institute, Dr. Ken Cooper explains, "Physical activity is one of the greatest bargains the world has ever known. When people are fit and physically active the world is a different place—you can do the things you want and lead the kind of life that has purpose and meaning. There's no question that physical activity really is one of the central components necessary for living a productive life" (Wellness Councils of America, 2010b).

As to the power and efficacy of physical activity as a legitimate medical prescription, Dr. Steve Aldana, work site wellness expert and founder of WellSteps, states, "If you could take this component of exercise and sell it as a pill, it would be the single most effective medication ever devised in the history of mankind. Exercise affects so many conditions, and it affects them so much that the dose would be considered the most powerful medication and the most beneficial medication ever devised. Is it a magic bullet? It's as close to a magic bullet as anything we have" (Wellness Councils of America, 2010a).

Despite the overwhelming evidence as to the power of physical activity to improve human health and delay the onset of disease and disability, the message has been slow to catch on with the American public. In fact, recent statistics from the CDC indicate that only three in ten adults get the recommended amount of physical activity during the course of any given day. To make matters worse, Dr. Wayne Westcott—a noted US exercise scholar—revealed in a recent interview that our already dismal participation in physical activity might be significantly lower than current US estimates indicate.

accelerometers
instruments for measuring acceleration used to assess the daily level of activity of an individual

Westcott and colleagues put **accelerometers** on two groups of five thousand Americans of all ages and found that only 3.5% were getting thirty minutes of modest-level activity. States Westcott, "This is very disconcerting, as it's not a lot of activity. For those over 60, it was less than 2.5 percent . . ." (Wellness Councils of America, 2010c). In an age of poor health and increasing costs, this is certainly discouraging—especially given the fact that walking thirty to forty-five minutes on most, preferably all, days of the week will delay the onset of disability by ten to twelve years.

In the years ahead, there's no question that physical activity will be the most commonly prescribed medicine that is available—and for good reason. In fact, according to Dr. Steven Blair, one of the most celebrated exercise physiologists in the world, "Physical inactivity and low fitness is perhaps the most important predictor of morbidity and mortality that we know of. Low fitness levels account for more sickness and deaths in the population than anything else that we've studied . . . The best insurance you can get to stay out of a nursing home where you will become frail, feeble and incontinent is to be physically active. Physical activity improves brain health, reduces the risk of senile dementia and preserves your function so that you can continue on with life's activities" (Wellness Councils of America, 2010d).

As can be easily seen, given its benefits and high accessibility, physical activity will become the most commonly prescribed medicine in America.

Trend 8: Financial Incentives and Disincentives Will Go Mainstream

For decades, incentives of all kinds were frowned upon by health practitioners. Often it was argued that people should participate in health promoting behaviors because of the potential positive benefits alone—to offer up incentives would dilute the real meaning of health promotion programs. Although that may have been the reigning sentiment for decades, the thinking on incentives is rapidly evolving.

For example, the use of **financial incentives** such as water bottles, t-shirts, merchandise, and cash has been shown to significantly increase participation—at least in the short term—in a number of recent wellness programs. Indeed, there is now a small cadre of organizations that boast more than 90% participation in wellness programs—largely due to incentive-based designs (O'Donnell & Mitts, 2013).

With these successful outcomes in mind, and given the fact that we are struggling as a country to engage our citizens in taking part in meaningful health-promoting activities, it would be prudent to assume that a greater emphasis will be placed on incentives. Indeed, at the time of this writing, insurance companies are already waiving the costs of preventive exams for individuals in an attempt to encourage individuals to see their physicians early to identify potential problems before they progress to catastrophic health issues. Moreover, substantial incentives have been written into the Patient Protection and Affordable Care Act and more time will reveal the impact of these incentives on changing health status.

And if incentives aren't enough, it is reasonable to anticipate that much more severe measures will be taken—including penalizing those who do not take part in health promotion programs. In fact, in a recent national corporate benefits survey, a significant number of employers indicated that they would take stronger measures of imposing penalties on people who do not take part in health-promoting programs. This shows that incentives and disincentives will become commonplace in the years ahead.

financial incentives the use of monetary compensation or goods as incentive for participation in a health promotion program; examples include water bottles, t-shirts, merchandise, and cash

Trend 9: Physical Environments Will Be Altered Radically

Although not emphasized strongly enough in recent years, altering physical environments will play an increasingly larger role in the decades to come—and for good reason. Changing physical environments to promote wellness and facilitate healthier lifestyles works extremely well in bringing about long-term and lasting change.

Several examples immediately come to mind. Take for instance the CDC's successful approach in motivating their employees to use the stairs throughout the workday rather than taking the elevators and/or escalators. By modifying the physical environment—and leveraging comprehensive communications campaigns—health researchers at the CDC were able to significantly increase the number of people who used stairwells throughout

**environmental
modification**

changes made to the
physical environment to
promote wellness and
facilitate healthier
lifestyles, such as
motivating employees to
use stairs instead of the
elevator, adding bike
lanes and walking trails
to a city's urban
environment, and passing
legislation prohibiting
unhealthy behaviors such
as eliminating trans fats
or taxing soda

the day. Although a seemingly small—but without question successful—**environmental modification**, this modest example executed by the CDC has inspired many others to attempt even larger scale environmental changes (Kerr, Yore, Ham, & Dietz, 2004).

Cities such as Omaha, Nebraska, with its "Activate Omaha" movement (www.activateomaha.com), have begun to create and physically engineer healthier communities by adding bike and walking trails to the city's urban environment. Further, the Association of American State Highway and Transportation Officials are working with the Adventure Cycling Association to connect thirty states and more segments are being added to extend the bicycle routes (American Association of State Highway and Transportation Officials, 2013).

As part of engineering healthier environments, there are even more aggressive measures being taken—including passing legislation prohibiting once commonly accepted practices. For example, consider New York City's aggressive measures to eliminate trans fats from all of the city's restaurant offerings as well as increasing taxes on soda and requiring menu labeling in fast food eateries (Wood, 2012).

As a result of the serious health challenges that our society is facing, it comes as no surprise that modifying physical environments will take on a very high priority in our nation's efforts to increase health-promoting behaviors. More examples of changes of the physical environment are described in part 2 on health behaviors.

Trend 10: Efforts to Curb Obesity Will Intensify Greatly

More than one-third of adults and almost 17% of youth were obese in 2009–2010. Sadly, this translates into over 78 million US adults and about 12.5 million adolescents who are carrying too much weight. Obesity increases the risk of a number of health conditions, including hypertension, adverse lipid concentrations, and type 2 diabetes. Of most concern is the fact that the prevalence of obesity in the United States has increased dramatically during the last decades of the twentieth century (Kotlikoff & Burns, 2005; US Census Bureau, 2012). Although, more recently, there appears to have been a slowing in the rate of the increase—or even a leveling off—there is still significant work to be done (Ogden, Caroll, Kit & Flegal, 2012).

Hence, given the health risks of obesity and its high prevalence, it is important for health promotion professionals, policy makers, educators, and business leaders to continue to develop and implement aggressive strategies to combat this major public health concern. To date, much of the effort to reduce the incidence and prevalence of obesity in the United States has centered on personal change efforts designed to modify individual behaviors. For example, diet-based interventions such as Weight Watchers, Atkins, and a variety of others diets have attracted tens of millions of individuals seeking to shed pounds. Despite the popularity and appetite for these types of interventions, the long-term outcomes have been disappointing at best.

Over the course of the next two decades, strategies to reduce obesity among the US population will change significantly. Specifically, it is realistic to think that—given the potential seriousness of the problem—the obesity dialogue will begin to meaningfully engage restaurateurs, soda manufactures, grocers, and the fast food industry. Indeed, with the advent of compelling treatises, such as Eric Schlosser's *Fast Food Nation* and David Kessler's *The End of Overeating,* greater attention has been given to engaging these important players in the fight against obesity.

To date, small but important victories have been won on this battlefield. For instance, the voluntary elimination of trans fats from certain food products by food companies as well as packaging and product modifications that contribute to smaller portions being consumed are but a few of the examples of the type of progress that are possible in the years ahead. However, given the fact that obesity has now become the second leading cause of preventable death in the United States, it stands to reason that we will see a substantial intensification of efforts to stop the spread of obesity in this country.

Trend 11: The Need for Talented Health Promotion Professionals Will Skyrocket

As we look to the future, one final thing becomes strikingly apparent—doing what we have done in the past will not get us to our desired destination. Treating disease after it has already taken hold has driven health care costs in the United States to unprecedented levels—not to mention the fact that the untold millions of individual health consequences have been heartbreaking.

Moving forward, health promotion and prevention will become a standard way of doing business in this country. In fact, the dominos have already been kicked over and momentum is being gained on a variety of fronts. Hospitals and physicians are now making concerted efforts to address primary prevention in a system that has traditionally focused solely on treating disease. Health insurance companies are now beginning to reimburse for primary prevention interventions. National legislation, as witnessed by the passage of the Affordable Care Act, now incorporates significant incentives for prevention and healthier lifestyles. Millions of businesses in the United States are hard at work designing results-oriented wellness initiatives in an attempt to contain costs, improve health, and create healthier cultures.

There's no question that a big part of the future of the United States centers on the notion of health promotion because it has become glaringly obvious to everyone that we need healthy citizens in order to compete on a global level. Indeed, health promotion is no longer just an interesting idea— it has become a national imperative. To sustain the momentum that has been achieved by the pioneers of this movement, it is essential that training programs be put into place to ensure that talented and effective professionals are available to step into the opportunities that are now emerging. To meet the demand, institutions of higher education, medical schools, community colleges, and a variety of other professional preparation programs will need to dedicate substantial resources toward developing capable men and women who will possess the knowledge, skills, acumen, and desire to step into these programs and lead the way to better health (Hunnicutt & Chenoweth, 2013).

Summary

In this chapter, eleven trends for the future of health promotion have been presented. When taken together, it is evident that there is still much work to be done if we are to keep our nation's citizens healthy and our country globally competitive. At the same time, it is also important to see that there are substantial opportunities for individuals to play meaningful and necessary roles that will not only help others remain healthy but also provide long and satisfying careers for those who choose to accept the call.

KEY TERMS

1. **Baby boomers:** Americans born between 1946 and 1964; about eighty million people and the fastest growing segment of the aging population

2. **Health status:** the measurement of the health of an individual or population as subjectively assessed by the individual or by more objective measures, including life expectancy and presence of disease conditions

3. **Health care costs:** the actual costs of providing services related to the delivery of health care, including the costs of procedures, therapies, and medications; differentiated from health expenditures, which refers to the amount of money paid for the services, and from fees, which refers to the amount charged, regardless of cost

4. **Return on investment:** a performance measure used to evaluate the efficiency of an investment or to compare the efficiency of a number of different investments

5. **Primary care physician:** a physician, such as a family practitioner or internist, who is chosen by an individual to provide continuous medical care, trained to treat a wide variety of health-related problems, and responsible for referrals to specialists as needed

6. **Medical self-care:** the care of oneself without medical, professional, or other assistance or oversight

7. **Accelerometers:** instruments for measuring acceleration used to assess the daily level of activity of an individual

8. **Financial incentives:** the use of monetary compensation or goods as incentive for participation in a health promotion program; examples include water bottles, t-shirts, merchandise, and cash

9. **Environmental modification:** a change made to the physical environment to promote wellness and facilitate healthier lifestyles, such as motivating employees to use stairs instead of the elevator, adding bike lanes and walking trails to a city's urban environment, and passing legislation prohibiting unhealthy behaviors such as eliminating trans fats or taxing soda

REVIEW QUESTIONS

1. How will the demographics of our society change in the next thirty to fifty years?

2. What do the terms *low-risk status* and *high-risk status* mean?

3. What did former surgeon general Carmona state about the status of childhood health?

4. What percentage of the gross domestic product is spent on health care?

5. What percent of health care expenditures is associated with health behaviors?

6. How does the Affordable Care Act work to address health behaviors associated with chronic disease?

7. Should we provide incentives for people to engage in healthy behaviors?

8. What are some individual- and industry-level obesity efforts?

9. What trend is the most surprising to you, and why?

STUDENT ACTIVITIES

1. If physical activity becomes recognized as a "common medical intervention," should health insurance companies subsidize exercise programs? Why or why not?

2. Identify what government programs are already in place to reverse chronic disease trends.

3. Describe three additional environmental modifications that you would recommend to increase physical activity for Americans.

4. Based on the trends outlined in this chapter, write a 250-word call to action on what Americans should know about societal health.

References

American Association of State Highway and Transportation Officials. (2013). *AASHTO committee approves new U.S. bicycle route system segments.* Retrieved from www.aashtojournal.org/Pages/110813USBikeRoutes.aspx

Carmona, R. H. (2004). *The growing epidemic of childhood obesity.* Hearing before the Subcommittee on Competition, Infrastructure, and Foreign Commerce of the Committee on Commerce, Science, and Transportation, United States Senate, 108th Cong. 2. Retrieved from www.surgeongeneral.gov/news/testimony/childobesity03022004.html

Centers for Disease Control and Prevention. (2012). *FastStats: Emergency department visits.* Retrieved from www.cdc.gov/nchs/fastats/ervisits.htm

Centers for Disease Control and Prevention. (2013a). *Ambulatory care use and physician visits.* Retrieved from www.cdc.gov/nchs/fastats/docvisit.htm

Centers for Disease Control and Prevention. (2013b, February 8). *Data & statistics.* Retrieved from www.cdc.gov/DataStatistics

Centers for Medicare and Medicaid Services. (2012). *National health expenditures data.* Retrieved from www.cms.gov/Research-Statistics-Data-and-Systems/Statistics-Trends-andReports/NationalHealthExpendData/downloads/tables.pdf

Edington, D. (2013). *Zero trends: Health as a serious economic strategy.* Ann Arbor, MI: Health Management Research Center.

Haaga, J. (2002). *Just how many baby boomers are there?* Population Reference Bureau. Retrieved from www.prb.org/Publications/Articles/2002/JustHowManyBabyBoomersAreThere.aspx

Hammergren, J., & Harkins, P. (2008). *Skin in the game: How putting yourself first today will revolutionize health care tomorrow.* Hoboken, NJ: John Wiley & Sons.

Hoffman, J., Salerno, J. A., & Moss, A. (2012). *The weight of the nation: Surprising lessons about diets, food, and fat from the extraordinary series from HBO.* New York: St. Martin's Press.

Hunnicutt, D., & Chenoweth, D. (2013). *What wellness professionals earn.* White paper. Omaha, NE: Wellness Council of America.

Kaiser Family Foundation and Health Research and Educational Trust. (2012, September 11). *2012 employer health benefits survey.* Retrieved from http://kff.org/private-insurance/report/employer-health-benefits-2012-annual-survey

Kerr, N. A., Yore, M. M., Ham, S. A., & Dietz, W. H. (2004). Increasing stair use in a worksite through environmental changes. *American Journal of Health Promotion, 18*(4), 312–315.

Kotlikoff, L. J., & Burns, S. (2005). *The coming generational storm: What you need to know about America's economic future.* Cambridge, MA: MIT Press.

National Institute of Diabetes and Digestive and Kidney Diseases. (2008, October). *Diabetes prevention program.* Retrieved from http://diabetes.niddk.nih.gov/dm/pubs/preventionprogram

O'Donnell, M., & Mitts, L. (2013, February 18). Should employees get insurance discounts for completing wellness programs? *Wall Street Journal.* Retrieved from http://online.wsj.com/news/articles/SB10001424127887324610504578273673319849976

Ogden, C. L., Caroll, M. D., Kit, B. K., & Flegal, K. M. (2012, January). *Prevalence of obesity in the United States, 2009–2010.* National Center for Health Statistics. Data Brief no. 82. Retrieved from www.cdc.gov/nchs/data/databriefs/db82.pdf

US Census Bureau. (2012). *Table 2: Projections of the population by selected age groups and sex for the United States: 2015 to 2060.* 2012 National Population Projections: Summary Tables. Retrieved from www.census.gov/population/projections/data/national/2012/summarytables.html

US Census Bureau. (2013). *Annual estimates of the resident population for selected age groups by sex for the United States, states, counties, and Puerto Rico Commonwealth and Municipios: April 1, 2010 to July 1, 2012.* Retrieved from http://factfinder2.census.gov/faces/tableservices/jsf/pages/productview.xhtml?src=bkmk

Wellness Councils of America. (2010a). Culture clash: How we win the battle for better health; An expert interview with Dr. Steve Aldana. *WELCOA's News & Views.* Retrieved from welcoa.org/freeresources/pdf/steve_aldanapart2.pdf

Wellness Councils of America. (2010b). Dr. Ken Cooper speaks out on getting (and keeping) Americans healthy: An expert interview with Dr. Ken Cooper. *WELCOA's News & Views.* Retrieved from www.absoluteadvantage.org/uploads/files/newsviews_kcooper.pdf

Wellness Councils of America. (2010c). The good, the bad, and the just plain scary: An expert interview with Dr. Wayne Westcott. *WELCOA's News & Views.* Retrieved from www.absoluteadvantage.org/uploads/files/newsviews_westcott.pdf

Wellness Councils of America. (2010d). Taking a stand on sitting down: An expert interview with Dr. Steven Blair. *WELCOA's News & Views*. Retrieved from www .absoluteadvantage.org/uploads/files/interview_blair_hazards_of_sitting.pdf

Wood, R. W. (2012, September 15). If soda tax can make it in NY it can make it anywhere. *Forbes*. Retrieved from www.forbes.com/sites/robertwood/2012/09 /15/if-soda-tax-can-make-it-in-ny-it-can-make-it-anywhere

Chapter 1: Health Promotion

American Public Health Association

www.apha.org

Centers for Disease Control and Prevention

www.cdc.gov/about/history/tengpha.htm

www.cdc.gov/nchs/fastats/lifexpec.htm

www.cdc.gov/chronicdisease

www.cdc.gov/socialdeterminants

Infectious Disease Society of America

www.idsociety.org/Index.aspx

National Association of Chronic Disease Directors

www.chronicdisease.org

Office of Disease Prevention and Health Promotion

http://odphp.osophs.dhhs.gov

Society of Public Health Education

www.sophe.org

US Department of Health and Human Services

www.hhs.gov/healthcare/rights

World Health Organization

www.who.org

www.who.int/topics/infectious_diseases/en

www.who.int/topics/chronic_diseases/en

www.who.int/topics/health_promotion/en

Chapter 2: Health Behavior Change Theories and Models

Education

   www.education.com/reference/article/social-cognitive-theory

Euromed Info

   www.euromedinfo.eu/the-health-belief-model.html

Instructional Design

   www.instructionaldesign.org/theories/social-learning.html

National Cancer Institute: Theory at a Glance

   www.cancer.gov/cancertopics/cancerlibrary/theory.pdf

Pro-Change Behavior Systems

   www.prochange.com/transtheoretical-model-of-behavior-change

Substance Abuse and Mental Health Services Administration

   www.samhsa.gov/co-occurring/topics/training/change.aspx

Chapter 3: Program Planning Models

American College Health Association

   www.acha.org/healthycampus/ecological_model.cfm

Centers for Disease Control and Prevention

   www.cdc.gov/hrqol/featured-items/match.htm

   www.cdc.gov/violenceprevention/overview/social-ecologicalmodel.html

   www.cdc.gov/healthcommunication/healthbasics/whatishc.html

Making Health Communications Programs Work

   www.cancer.gov/cancerstopics/cancerlibrary/pinkbook

PRECEDE-PROCEED Model

   www.lgreen.net/precede.htm

Weinreich Communications

   www.social-marketing.com/Whatis.html

Chapter 4: Tobacco Use

American Cancer Society

   www.cancer.org

American Legacy Foundation

   www.legacyforhealth.org

American Lung Association

    www.lung.org

American Nonsmokers' Rights Foundation

    www.anrf.org

National Cancer Institute

    www.cancer.gov

SmokeFree.gov

    www.smokefree.gov

Smoking Cessation Leadership Center

    http://smokingcessationleadership.ucsf.edu

Tobacco Free Kids

    www.tobaccofreekids.org

Chapter 5: Eating Behaviors

Center for Science in the Public Interest

    www.cspinet.org

Cornell University Food and Brand Lab

    http://foodpsychology.cornell.edu

Food Politics Blog by Marion Nestle of New York University

    www.foodpolitics.com

Leanwashing

    www.leanwashingindex.com

MyPlate

    www.choosemyplate.gov

National Heart, Lung, and Blood Institute (NHLBI) Portion Distortion

    http://hp2010.nhlbihin.net/portion

Nutrition Source—Harvard School of Public Health

    www.hsph.harvard.edu/nutritionsource

The Nutrition Transition Program at The University of North Carolina at Chapel Hill

    www.cpc.unc.edu/projects/nutrans

2010 Dietary Guidelines for Americans

    http://health.gov/dietaryguidelines/2010.asp

Yale Rudd Center for Food Policy and Obesity

www.yaleruddcenter.org/what_we_do.aspx?id=7

Chapter 6: Physical Activity Behaviors

Active Living Research

http://activelivingresearch.org/policies-and-standards-promoting
-physical-activity-after-school-programs

Alliance for a Healthier Generation

www.healthiergeneration.org

American Alliance for Health, Physical Education, Recreation, and Dance

www.aahperd.org

Healthy Children

www.healthychildren.org/English/ages-stages/gradeschool/fitness
/Pages/Promoting-Physical-Activity-as-a-Way-of-Life.aspx

Let's Move!

www.letsmove.org

National Coalition for Promotion Physical Activity

www.ncppa.org

National Physical Activity Plan

www.physicalactivityplan.com

President's Council on Fitness, Sport, & Nutrition

www.fitness.gov

Robert Wood Johnson Foundation

www.rwjf.org

2008 Physical Activity Guidelines for Americans

www.health.gov/paguidelines

Chapter 7: Stress, Emotional Well-Being, and Mental Health

American Institute of Stress

www.stress.org

American Psychiatric Association

www.psychiatry.org

American Psychological Association

www.apa.org

The Center for Mind-Body Medicine

www.cmbm.org

MentalHealth.gov

www.mentalhealth.gov

National Alliance on Mental Illness

www.nami.org

National Institute on Mental Health

www.nimh.nih.gov

The Substance Abuse and Mental Health Services Administration

www.samhsa.gov

Chapter 8: Clinical Preventive Services

American Health Insurance Plans

www.ahip.org

Centers for Disease Control and Prevention

www.cdc.gov

The Community Guide

www.thecommunityguide.org

National Institutes of Health—Office of Disease Prevention

http://prevention.nih.gov

National Prevention Strategy

www.surgeongeneral.gov/initiatives/prevention/strategy

Partnership for Prevention

www.prevent.org

US Preventive Services Task Force

www.uspreventiveservicestaskforce.org

Chapter 9: National and State Initiatives to Promote Health and Well-Being

Association of State and Territorial Health Officials

www.astho.org

Centers for Disease Control and Prevention

www.cdc.gov

Healthy People 2020

www.healthypeople.gov

National Association of City and County Health Officials

www.naccho.org

National Conference of State Legislatures

www.ncsl.org

National Institutes of Health

www.nih.gov

US Department of Agriculture

www.usda.gov

US Department of Health and Human Services

www.hhs.gov

Chapter 10: Settings for Health Promotion

American College Health Association

www.acha.org

American Community Garden Association

www.communitygarden.org

American School Health Association

www.ashaweb.org/i4a/pages/index.cfm?pageid=1

Center on Developing Children, Harvard University

http://developingchild.harvard.edu/resources/reports_and
_working_papers/foundations-of-lifelong-health

Centers for Disease Control and Prevention

www.cdc.gov/family

www.cdc.gov/nationalhealthyworksite/index.html

Coordinated School Health (CDC)

    www.cdc.gov/HealthyYouth/cshp

Food and Nutrition Service, USDA

    www.fns.usda.gov/cnd/governance/legislation/cnr_2010.htm

International Association for Worksite Health Promotion

    www.acsm-iawhp.org/i4a/pages/index.cfm?pageid=1

International Health, Racquet and Sport Association

    www.ihrsa.org

National Association for Community Health

    www.nachc.com

National Wellness Institute

    www.nationalwellness.org

Wellness Councils of America

    www.welcoa.org

YMCA

    www.ymca.net

Chapter 11: Health Promotion–Related Organizations, Associations, and Certifications

The Academy of Nutrition and Dietetics

    www.eatright.org

American Alliance for Health, Physical Education, Recreation, and Dance

    www.aahperd.org

American Association of School Health

    www.ashaweb.org

American College of Nutrition

    www.americancollegeofnutrition.org

American College of Sports Medicine

    www.acsm.org

American Heart Association

    www.heart.org

American Public Health Association

    www.apha.org

Institute of Health and Productivity Management

www.ihpm.org

Society for Public Health Education

www.sophe.org

Chapter 12: Trends in Health Promotion

Administration on Aging

www.aoa.gov/AoARoot/%28S%282ch3qw55k1qylo45dbihar2u
%29%29/Aging_Statistics/index.aspx

American Health Insurance Plans

www.ahip.org

American Medical Association

www.ama-assn.org

The Center for Public Education

www.centerforpubliceducation.org/You-May-Also-Be-Interested
-In-landing-page-level/Organizing-a-School-YMABI/The-United
-States-of-education-The-changing-demographics-of-the-United
-States-and-their-schools.html

Centers for Disease Control and Prevention

www.cdc.gov/workplacehealthpromotion/businesscase/reasons
/changing.html

Health Care Cost Institute

www.healthcostinstitute.org

Institute of Health and Productivity Management

www.ihpm.org

Kaiser Family Foundation

http://kff.org

National Business Group on Health

www.businessgrouphealth.org/toolkits/et_financialincentives.cfm

National Center for Health Statistics

www.cdc.gov/nchs

US Department of Labor

www.dol.gov/oasam/programs/history/herman/reports
/futurework/conference/trends/trendsi.htm

World Population on Aging

www.un.org/esa/population/publications/worldageing19502050

INDEX